FOURTH EDITION

Comprehensive Lactation Consultant
EXAM REVIEW

Linda J. Smith, MPH, IBCLC, FACCE, FILCA

Owner and Director
Bright Future Lactation Resource Centre Ltd.

Director of Perinatal Policy
American Breastfeeding Institute

Adjunct Instructor
Boonshoft School of Medicine
Wright State University
Dayton, Ohio

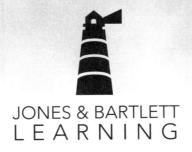

JONES & BARTLETT
LEARNING

World Headquarters
Jones & Bartlett Learning
5 Wall Street
Burlington, MA 01803
978-443-5000
info@jblearning.com
www.jblearning.com

Jones & Bartlett Learning books and products are available through most bookstores and online booksellers. To contact Jones & Bartlett Learning directly, call 800-832-0034, fax 978-443-8000, or visit our website, www.jblearning.com.

Substantial discounts on bulk quantities of Jones & Bartlett Learning publications are available to corporations, professional associations, and other qualified organizations. For details and specific discount information, contact the special sales department at Jones & Bartlett Learning via the above contact information or send an email to specialsales@jblearning.com.

Production Credits
VP, Executive Publisher: David D. Cella
Executive Editor: Amanda Martin
Acquisitions Editor: Teresa Reilly
Editorial Assistant: Lauren Vaughn
Senior Production Editor: Amanda Clerkin
Production Assistant: Rebecca Humphrey
Marketing Communications Manager: Katie Hennessy

Production Services Manager: Carolyn Downer
Product Fulfillment Manager: Wendy Kilborn
Composition: S4Carlisle Publishing Services
Cover Design: Scott Moden
Rights & Media Specialist: Wes DeShano
Cover Image: © romrf/Shutterstock
Printing and Binding: McNaughton & Gunn
Cover Printing: McNaughton & Gunn

Library of Congress Cataloging-in-Publication Data
Names: Smith, Linda J., 1946- , author.
Title: Comprehensive lactation consultant exam review / Linda J. Smith.
Description: Fourth edition. | Burlington, MA : Jones & Bartlett Learning,
  [2017] | Includes bibliographical references and index.
Identifiers: LCCN 2015043495 | ISBN 9781284069273
Subjects: | MESH: Breast Feeding—Examination Questions. |
  Lactation—Examination Questions. | Lactation Disorders—Examination
  Questions. | Patient Education as Topic—Examination Questions.
Classification: LCC RJ216 | NLM WS 18.2 | DDC 613.269076—dc23 LC
record available at http://lccn.loc.gov/2015043495

6048

Printed in the United States of America
21 20 19 18   10 9 8 7 6 5 4

Dedication

This *Fourth Edition* is dedicated to four remarkable women who have greatly influenced my life, my career, and the creation of this edition.

Hannah S. Boswell, my daughter, lived and practiced the principles in this book. As a child, she was the recipient of these principles; she later carried them through expertly into her own mothering. I watched with pride and awe as she nourished and nurtured her daughter Carrie through childhood and beyond. More pertinent to my personal life and the creation of this new edition, she "dropped everything" to come to my rescue during several unexpected health crises, driving hundreds of miles on scant notice to care for me. She expertly used her caregiving and counseling skills when I was recuperating from illness and accident; became a skilled scribe when I broke my arm; and maintained her sense of humor and kind presence as she supported my husband and me in times of crisis. Thank you, Hannah.

K. Jean Cotterman, RNC, IBCLC, was actively helping breastfeeding families literally until the day she died on June 11, 2014, at age 83. She and I spoke and consulted on many occasions, and she regularly lectured in my Exam Preparation courses. Her family gave permission to use many of her clinical photographs in this edition. Her deep and thorough investigation into the role of intravenous fluids on postbirth breast edema bore fruit after her death as the publication of a remarkable peer-reviewed article on the topic: Kujawa-Myles, S., Noel-Weiss, J., Dunn, S., Peterson, W., & Cotterman, K. (2015). Maternal intravenous fluids and postbirth breast changes: A pilot observational study. *International Breastfeeding Journal, 10*(1), 18.

Chris Mulford, RN, IBCLC, FILCA, was a role model and mentor since before the birth of this profession. Chris was a professional musician, La Leche League Leader, avid gardener, nurse, and IBCLC. She devoted many wise and collaborative hours to the development of global and U.S. national policies in breastfeeding. Chris and her husband, George, were frequent guests at my home on their way to yearly vacations in the Rocky Mountains before Chris's unexpected death in 2011. Every time I reference the *Healthy People 2020* Goals or a WABA initiative, I fondly remember Chris's gentle ways and expansive wisdom. A favorite publication of Chris's was Mulford, C. (1995). Swimming upstream: Breastfeeding care in a nonbreastfeeding culture. *Journal of Obstetric, Gynecologic, & Neonatal Nursing, 24*(5), 464–474.

Nikki L. Rogers, PhD, CPH, CKC, continues to profoundly influence my work. As an anthropologist, she invited my collaboration on a research project in Ethiopia, studying colostrum avoidance. As a faculty member in the public health program in the Boonshoft School of Medicine at Wright State University, she continues to steer MPH students toward collaborating with me on their Culminating Experience projects related to breastfeeding. She volunteers many hours in support of the Ohio Lactation Consultant Association. Her curiosity, academic rigor, enthusiasm, creativity, energy, and friendship have been invaluable resources as she continues to successfully and skillfully weave breastfeeding solidly into the academic medical school and public health world by connecting medical and public health graduate students with this body of knowledge and community, both locally and internationally. Nikki literally became my right arm and hand (after I broke my arm), enabling me to finish editing the last few hundred questions in this edition.

Contents

Acknowledgments

This edition would not have been possible without the expertise and contributions of many skilled and talented people. I am again grateful to my husband, Denny Smith, for building, refining, and repairing (sometimes at short notice and at inopportune times) the elegant relational database that keeps my growing collection of questions organized. I am especially grateful to the late Jean Cotterman's family, the late Mary Kroeger, Laura Atkinson, Maya Bolman, Kimarie Bugg, Melissa Courts, Carole Dobrich, Jerene Fleming, Ashley Frantz, Catherine Watson Genna, Cammie Jo Goldhammer, Mona Lisa Hamlin, Marilyn, Hildreth, Kay Hoover, Sarah Hung, Mudiwah Kadeshe, Heather Spada, Yuwen Ren, Kathy Kendall-Tackett, Virginia (Ginny) Kooyman, Carol Narigon and Sophie Holquist, Erika Nehlsen, Greg Notestine, Cathy Norris, Katherine Shealy, Ann Witt, Barbara Wilson-Clay, and colleagues for many new pictures and concepts. Thank you to Lois Arnold, Elizabeth Brooks, Judy Campbell, Carol Chamblin, Hillary Flower, Katrina Hennessey, Audrey Inouye, Dee Kassing, Laura Knisley, Evelyn Landry, Teresa Pittman, Elisabeth Sterken, Diana West, Diane Wiessinger, and several people who wish to remain anonymous—your case reports have greatly enriched this book. I'm always awed by and grateful for my sister Nancy Dahlstrom's artistic vision and expertise, particularly her insights into the cover design of this edition. And without Nikki Rogers' expertise, curiosity, kindness, and physical support when I shattered my right arm, this edition might have been delayed many more weeks.

I'm also thankful for the patient expertise of the editorial and production teams at Jones & Bartlett Learning who guided the production of this book: Teresa Reilly, Amanda Clerkin, Lauren Vaughn, Rebecca Humphrey, Wes DeShano, and others whom I've inadvertently omitted or never met in person. Thank you!

About the Author

Linda J. Smith, MPH, IBCLC, FACCE, FILCA, is a lactation consultant, childbirth educator, author, and international consultant on breastfeeding and birthing issues. She was a founder of IBLCE, founder and past board member of ILCA, and serves on the United States Breastfeeding Committee. Her diverse background spans four decades of direct education and support for pregnant and breastfeeding women in nine cities in the United States and Canada. She has worked in hospital systems and local and state public health agencies, and supported colleagues with service on related associations' boards. Linda is an Adjunct Instructor in the Boonshoft School of Medicine at Wright State University in Dayton, OH, and has represented ILCA to the World Health Organization's biannual meetings of BFHI Country Coordinators from Industrialized Countries since 2006. Linda is also a consultant to Baby-Friendly USA and INFACT Canada/ IBFAN North America. She is currently the owner and director of Bright Future Lactation Resource Centre (BFLRC), whose mission is "Supporting the People Who Support Breastfeeding" with lactation education programs, consulting services, and educational resources. BFLRC is on the Internet at www.BFLRC.com. She is the author of four professional textbooks on birth and breastfeeding and co-author of *Sweet Sleep* by La Leche League International. She has lectured in 19 countries; her presentations have been translated into 12 languages including Chinese, Russian, and Inuktitut. She has presented her key research areas to international health experts at the World Health Organization meetings. Her Lactation Management/Exam Preparation Course is the longest-running course of its kind, the first to be based on the IBLCE Exam Blueprint, and has been presented to thousands of students for over 23 years.

Introduction

The lactation consultant profession celebrated its 30th anniversary in 2015. We've come a long way since 250 candidates took the first exam simultaneously in Melbourne, Australia, and Washington, DC in 1985. The 30th administration of the IBLCE exam took place in 159 sites in 40 countries on 5 continents in 17 languages and was administered to more than 4,000 candidates. As of this writing, more than 45,000 candidates have taken the exam and 27,450 IBCLCs now practice in 101 countries.

The *Fourth Edition* of *Comprehensive Lactation Consultant Exam Review* expands on the previous 3 editions with 950 practice questions, 20 case studies with questions, and more than 300 clinical photos. Every question has been reviewed, sometimes revised, referenced, and reassigned to the *2016 Detailed Content Outline* (formerly called the Exam Blueprint). This book is designed to give exam candidates practice in answering multiple-choice questions typical of the questions found on the examination administered by the International Board of Lactation Consultant Examiners (IBLCE). None of these questions have been submitted to IBLCE for possible use, and all were created by the author or an IBCLC contributor.

Preparing for the IBLCE Exam includes information about the exam layout, successful study and preparation strategies, and an expanded set of clinical exercises based on the *2016 Detailed Content Outline*. The clinical exercises for each discipline help the student explore a variety of aspects of lactation consultant practice. Some research suggests that candidates who complete clinical exercises and analyze the effects on their practice of doing the exercises may perform better on the exam. My experience is that students who use the exercises to explore a wide variety of lactation consultant activities are enriched, enhanced, and excited by the process.

Chapters 1–11 are practice questions based on the chronological periods in the *2016 Detailed Content Outline*. Even though most of the textbooks in our field are arranged by topic (discipline), effective support of the breastfeeding dyad is usually based on the baby's age, which determines the stage of lactation; the mother's progress in maternal role acquisition; nutrition, growth, and development of the mother and child; changes in milk biochemistry and immunology; and more. There may be overlap in some of the chronological periods. Many clinical situations involve more than one discipline. In this book, each question has been assigned to only one period, one discipline, and one of the seven taxonomy categories, which are identified in the answer sections. The IBLCE exam uses the sophisticated Nedelsky technique to establish the passing grade. Each question also has a "degree of difficulty" rating based on how close the incorrect answers approximate the correct answers. Choices that every candidate should reject are easy to eliminate; choices that only well-prepared candidates will reject are more difficult to distinguish from the correct answer. The difficulty rating is calculated from the mix of "obviously wrong" choices and "wrong-but-close" choices: the higher the difficulty rating, the harder the question. In general, the higher the percentage of difficult questions that are asked in a given year's exam, the lower the passing score that year. The average passing grade over many years has been approximately 65%.

Chapter 12 presents 20 clinical case studies with several multiple-choice questions based on each case. This format allows more in-depth analysis of the body of knowledge required to help the mother and baby in each case and more closely simulates situations encountered in actual practice. All of the clinical case studies in this book are actual situations contributed by lactation consultants, with identifying details changed to maintain client confidentiality.

The online interactive testing program has two complete practice exams with pictures. The distribution and number of questions in each discipline and chronological period are balanced to conform to the *2016 Detailed Content Outline*, which is derived from an analysis of skills, knowledge, and abilities of practicing lactation consultants. Common functions and activities of lactation consultants were examined for frequency of use in practice and criticality of that function or activity to breastfeeding success. Knowledge, skills, and abilities that are used more frequently or are more critical to lactation success are more heavily weighted in the exam content outline. Therefore the number of questions per discipline and chronological period on the practice exams are based on the relative importance of that topic or period in actual clinical practice.

Every attempt has been made to include questions that relate to the wide body of knowledge that is tested on the IBLCE exam. All questions have been referenced to the published professional literature, and an extensive bibliography is included in the appendix.

When studying, use the most current editions of widely available texts and research articles published in relevant professional journals. If one reference appears to contradict another, look carefully for the common ground, or examine the primary research on the topic. The exam will test the most critical and frequently used principles of supporting breastfeeding families, not esoteric trivia. Some research articles can be downloaded in their entirety from the online version of peer-reviewed journals for free or a fee. In other cases, the abstract is available for free online. Most medical libraries provide public access to a wide selection of the journals cited.

- Knowledge areas are found in the suggested readings and bibliographies.
- Skills are learned through experience, preferably supervised, and indirectly tested by the questions with accompanying photographs.
- Attitudes are difficult to test with a paper-and-pencil (or computerized) multiple-choice examination, yet are central to effective breastfeeding care. Listening to mothers' concerns and experiences is vital to understanding the supportive attitudes that emerge in the sample questions. The clinical exercises will help develop skills and deepen your understanding of each discipline, especially the exercises that involve interviewing or observing mothers and babies.

The practice questions may include signs and symptoms of various diseases, therapeutic treatments including antibiotics and other prescription medications, and other information related to the overall health or medical condition of the lactating mother or breastfed child. Inclusion of this information does not imply that the lactation consultant, on the basis of IBCLC certification alone, is qualified or legally allowed to diagnose medical conditions or recommend, prescribe, or determine medical treatments of the mother or child.

Although this book is intended to help candidates prepare for the IBLCE exam, no guarantees of passing the IBLCE exam are expressed or implied. This book is intended to augment lactation management or exam preparation textbooks and courses, not replace them. Students in lactation management courses often find that coursework focuses their study, validates existing knowledge, and identifies weak areas. The book can be used as a guide for self-study, the formation of study groups, or to supplement academic courses.

Until recently, all lactating/breastfeeding adults were referred to as mothers or women. This was not intended to diminish the relevance or existence of individuals who were assigned male gender at birth and transitioned to being female nor individuals who were female at birth and transitioned to being male; some of these individuals may be breastfeeding parents. Nor was there any intent to assume that the partner of the breastfeeding person is necessarily of the opposite gender or whether a partner is involved with the breastfeeding person at all. Gender pronouns (he or she) referring to the baby or babies in the cases or questions were randomly selected, or reflect the actual child or children in the question or photograph.

Finally, I made every attempt to include questions that cover the depth and breadth of topics that might be tested on the IBLCE exams. This book may over- or under-represent some topics tested on a given year's exam. New research will inevitably be published after this book is released that expands, deepens, or even replaces earlier understandings. Therefore, this book's questions, references, and exercises should be considered a guide and starting point for study, not the final word on any topic or concept. I am grateful to readers who contact me with comments, possible corrections, and suggestions. My email is lindaj@bflrc.com.

For more information and update, regarding IBLCE certification, contact www.iblce.org/about-iblce/worldwide-offices.

IBLCE International Office
703-560-7330
IBLCE in the Americas and Israel
703-560-7330
IBLCE in Europe, the Middle East, and North Africa
+43 (0) 2252 20 65 95 (within Austria) or
+43 2252 20 65 95 (outside Austria)
IBLCE in Asia Pacific and Africa
07 5529 8811 (within Australia) or
+61 7 5529 8811 (outside Australia)

Preparing for the Exam:
Study and Exam Preparation Strategies

The IBLCE examination tests a broad and diverse body of knowledge, skills, and attitudes important to two individuals with interrelated physiology and needs: the mother–baby breastfeeding dyad. The WHO/UNICEF *Global Strategy for Infant and Young Child Feeding* states elegantly and eloquently that "Mothers and babies form an inseparable biological and social unit; the health and nutrition of one group cannot be divorced from the health and nutrition of the other."

It is wise to develop a study plan well in advance of the exam that fits your personality, study habits, and available time. The *Core Curriculum for Lactation Consultant Practice, Third Edition*[1] and IBLCE's *Detailed Content Outline* are useful guides for a study plan. Although no single book covers all the material that could be tested on the IBLCE exam, the most recent editions of core textbooks are excellent places to start your review.

Personal study preferences and learning styles will affect your preparation. For example, I'm an extrovert and learn better when I'm with a group of peers. When I am preparing to take or retake the exam, I invite local colleagues to study sessions at my home. A schedule of dates and topics is circulated; each person is invited to pick a topic or month to lead the group discussion; and we all bring research articles, dolls, breast models, equipment, videos or DVDs, textbooks, pictures and slides, and snacks to share. I have learned that groups containing individuals from different backgrounds work well, because a nurse will have different areas of expertise from that of a dietitian, and a mother-support group leader will bring experiences that are different from those of a midwife or speech therapist. A kinesthetic learner might want to take copious notes or even make flash cards to study. Those who spend significant time driving or riding on public transportation may find listening to recorded conference presentations to be an effective way to study. I also learn better from in-person instruction and interactive activities than I do from online learning opportunities. With that in mind, I developed and continue to offer the Lactation Consultant Exam Preparation course sponsored by Bright Future Lactation Resource Centre www.BFLRC.com, which is the longest-running and the first course of its kind based on the Exam Blueprint (*Detailed Content Outline*).

Do Some Planned "Assignments" or Clinical Exercises

The IBLCE examination is heavily based on practical help for real-life situations. An analysis of courses and candidates' results suggests that doing, and writing up, various clinical exercises is related to higher scores on the exam. Merely doing the exercises is helpful; writing them up and reflecting on what you learned is even better. If your experience in lactation is primarily in

---

[1]http://www.jblearning.com/catalog/9780763798796/

one area (early postbirth, mother-to-mother breastfeeding groups, prenatal education), it is most helpful to concentrate on the areas in which you have the *least* experience.

If you plan to observe lactation care providers, seek permission from the facility, the lactation consultant (LC), and the client being observed. Remember, the facility or LC may welcome you, but the mother may feel uncomfortable with you present. Obey any local protocols (wearing scrubs, etc.). Your role is an observer, not a co-counselor. Seek permission, introduce yourself, and send a thank-you note afterward. During the observation, do not interrupt or attempt to assist the LC or group leader. You may briefly share your own experiences if asked. Take notes on what you have observed. Arrange with the observed party to spend time after the observation period or meeting to talk and ask questions. Be respectful of the LC when asking questions. If you have observed something that you disagree with, tactfully and privately request information on the LC's rationale. You may be surprised to find out that the LC's actions or information was most appropriate for that circumstance regardless of what the books say or what your previous experience dictates. Always thank the client (mother) being observed for her willingness to allow you into her "space." Restrain yourself from exhibiting negative body language in the presence of your hostess or the client. Do not observe on a day when you are sick, distracted, or rushed. Always be courteous, patient, and kind. Thank the LC in person and again with a note. Let her know how she has facilitated your education and about the positive things you experienced and saw. Everyone likes a "pat on the back" for a job well done. (Be genuine, don't fabricate. You can always find something to compliment!)

Challenge Yourself with the Questions in Chapters 1–11

Each chronological period in this book represents a chronological period in the *Detailed Content Outline*. The age of the baby determines the care and solutions specific to that child's developmental stage, the stage of lactation of the mother, unique developmental tasks of the dyad, and far more. The IBLCE exam includes general principles, prenatal development and details of the mother–baby breastfeeding relationship extending beyond the first 12 months of the child's life, because breastfeeding for at least 2 years is a global recommendation. The answers for all the chronological-stage questions follow each exam's questions and include the correct answer, an explanation or rationale, the discipline and period, whether which taxonomy best applies to the concept tested, and the degree of difficulty.

Read the Clinical Case Presentations and Questions (Chapter 12)

Each of the cases describes a real mother and baby who contacted a lactation consultant for help. The associated questions explore the knowledge, skills, and attitudes needed to resolve the mother and baby's breastfeeding situation. IBLCE now includes case presentation–format questions on the exam, although the format may differ from those in this book. The answers to each case's questions follow the questions for that case and include the correct answer, an explanation or rationale, the discipline and period, which taxonomy best applies to the concept tested, and the degree of difficulty.

Before the IBLCE Exam

- Review your knowledge and skills several days before the exam. Then, put away all books and references until after the exam. **Do not cram!** Cramming does not help and increases anxiety. Cramming can even lower your actual test scores.

- Do something relaxing and fun during the 2 days prior to the test. Ideally, get some fresh air and a change of pace on the day before the test. Go for a walk, clean the closets, bathe your dog, paint the fence or a picture, go to a movie or play or picnic—in other words, do anything *other* than obsess about the exam.
- Allow sufficient travel time to the exam site to avoid feeling rushed. Get a good night's sleep, and follow your normal routine as closely as possible. Wear comfortable clothes in layers.
- Eat normally and emphasize protein-rich foods that will help you stay alert and focused. Drink water, which facilitates brain and nerve function.
- Trust yourself. Give yourself positive affirmations and trust your knowledge of mothers and babies; for example, "I know how to help breastfeeding mothers and babies," and "I am a good test taker."
- Use calming or centering techniques that have served you well in the past, such as taking a deep breath, closing your eyes, meditating, or focusing on your breathing. Visualize recalling all the wealth of your knowledge, passing the exam, and receiving your excellent score report.
- Anxiety isn't always a bad thing. Allow yourself to feel any anxiety that arises—it will pass, just as a labor contraction does, and you will feel normal afterward. A slight rise in adrenal hormones may sharpen your focus and concentration, even as the same hormones have the unpleasant side effect of making you feel "testy."
- Carefully examine each question (and image, if there is one) before answering. Read each question, especially the stem, very carefully before you answer.
- Never change an answer unless you are absolutely, positively *sure* the first answer was clearly wrong. If you are unsure, rely on your best guess and first hunch.
- Allow yourself to miss a few questions. Nobody has yet achieved a score of 100% in the 30 years that this examination has been administered around the world. Review the Candidate's Guide and IBLCE resources one more time, paying attention to the structure and format of test items.

Be Patient and Calm While Waiting for the Exam Results

During any breaks and after the exam, resist the temptation to discuss your answers with other candidates. This is a sure recipe for self-doubt and increased anxiety! Remember that you only have to *pass*. If the worst happens and you don't get a passing grade, you can take the exam again in the next cycle. Use your score report to focus on areas of weakness. Take additional formal and informal educational courses, arrange mentoring experiences, and use the time to reflect on long-term goals and aspirations.

Celebrate and Network

Keep reading to stay up to date, whether or not you pass the exam. New information is constantly appearing that will either confirm or change existing practices. Avail yourself of as many resources as possible, especially new texts and reference books. Many publishers schedule textbook revisions approximately every 5 years.

Plan your budget to purchase several new books and attend at least one major breastfeeding conference each year. Attend continuing educational programs in breastfeeding and related fields. Read the *Journal of Human Lactation, Breastfeeding Medicine, International Breastfeeding Journal,* and *Breastfeeding Review*, and as many resources as you can find or afford. Search the Web frequently for pertinent information.

Use your new credential proudly! Join ILCA and national, state, provincial, or local affiliates or chapters and participate as time allows. Continue building a support network for yourself as a lactation consultant. Just like the mothers you work with, lactation consultants need a support system, too!

Clinical (Field) Exercises

Clinical (field) exercises help the LC experience the full depth and breadth of breastfeeding in real-life situations. They add a practical, dynamic and multidimensional aspect to the course material. The IBLCE examination is highly based on practical help for real-life situations, and an early analysis of courses and candidates' results suggests that doing, *and writing up*, various clinical exercises is related to higher scores on the exam. Merely doing the exercises is helpful; writing them up and analyzing what you learned is even better. If your experience in lactation is primarily in one area (early postbirth, mother-to-mother breastfeeding groups, prenatal education), it is most helpful to concentrate on the areas in which you have the least experience.

Instructions

Complete several exercises in areas that are different from your routine daily work and in different categories/disciplines. The goal is to expand your view of lactation beyond your current setting. Describe (write up) what you learned from doing the exercise, focusing on new insights, application of new information, and how the exercise broadened or expanded your understanding of breastfeeding & human lactation. Merely describing the situation is not enough; you need to include a reflection of how the experience changed your knowledge, attitudes, or understanding of the "world of breastfeeding."

- *Recommended for everyone:* At least one exercise that involves listening to mothers tell their own stories.
- *Recommended for those without mother-support experience:* at least one exercise that involves attending or observing a community breastfeeding support group.
- *Recommended for those without in-hospital experience:* at least one exercise that involves observing or following a hospital-based clinician or explores in-hospital breastfeeding management.
- *Recommended for those without experience in managing breastfeeding problems past the early postbirth period:* at least one exercise that involves working with breastfeeding techniques or equipment and/or breastfeeding into toddlerhood

Shadowing/Observation Guidelines

- Seek permission from the facility, LC, group leader or other professional, and the client being observed. Remember, the facility or LC may welcome you, but the mother may feel uncomfortable with you present. Obey all local protocols (wearing scrubs, etc.).
- You are an observer, not a co-counselor. Seek permission, introduce yourself, and say a thank you. During the observation, do not interrupt or attempt to assist the LC or professional. You may briefly share your own experiences if you are invited to do so.

- Take notes on what you've observed. Arrange with the observed party to spend time after the observation period or meeting to talk and ask questions.
- Be respectful of the LC or professional when asking questions. If you've observed something that you disagree with, tactfully and privately request information. You may be surprised to find out that the LCs or professional's actions or information was most appropriate for that circumstance regardless of what the books say or what your previous experience dictates.
- Always thank the client (mother) being observed for her willingness to allow you into her "space".
- Restrain yourself from exhibiting telltale negative body language in the presence of your hostess and of the client.
- Do not observe on a day when you are sick or distracted. Always be courteous, patient, and kind.
- Thank the LC or professional in person and again with a note. Let her know how she has facilitated your education and about the positive things you experienced and saw. Everyone likes a "pat on the back" for a job well- done. (Be genuine, don't fabricate. You can always find something to complement!)

Online Resources for Literature Searches

- U.S. National Library of Medicine (PubMed): www.nlm.nih.gov
- World Health Organization e-Library of Evidence for Nutrition Actions (eLENA): www.who.int/elena/en
- Cochrane Library: www.cochranelibrary.com
- Centers for Disease Control and Prevention: www.cdc.gov

Overview of Lactation Consultation

1. Interview three or more practicing lactation consultants in a variety of settings. Ask the LCs how they bring the concepts of "protection, support, and promotion" into their work; their philosophy of care; how they integrate therapy into their practice; how they view their role.
2. Write an analysis of the breastfeeding content in your own academic or professional training. Compare this with your personal experience with breastfeeding and information learned from informal sources. Include your feelings about how your formal training affected your personal experiences with breastfeeding. Describe how both kinds of learning have been helpful or harmful in your clinical practice.
3. Write up/prepare at least two case studies of actual breastfeeding situations, changing the names of the families for privacy. Write at least two multiple-choice questions based on the factors in each case that could be used on a lactation exam. The questions should include a stem, four possible answers, and an explanation of why the correct answer is correct and the incorrect answers are wrong, and a reference. (Request the question-writing template if you elect this exercise.)

I. Development and Nutrition

A. INFANT

1. Read at several research articles or text sections on the infant mouth, which could include palate shape, tongue and other structures, size and jaw configuration, maturity, anomalies, and/or defects. Discuss the influence on breastfeeding on different aspects of infant oral anatomy, and influence of infant oral anatomy on breastfeeding.

2. Examine at least two different sources for recommendations on complementary feeding of breastfed babies. Include the age recommended for starting solids, the order and texture of foods presented, and mother–baby interactions involved in feeding. Compare the recommendations with PAHO's *Guiding Principles for Complementary Feeding of the Breastfed Child*.

3. Observe five babies at breast for two consecutive complete feeding episodes. The babies should be of different ages. Estimate the total volume of milk obtained based on quality and quantity of feeding. Perform pre- and post-feed weighs on a gram-sensitive scale to verify your estimates.

4. Select one to three long-term or chronic health issues that are affected by breastfeeding. Investigate support groups, Internet sites, and educational resources on those issues to see how much information on breastfeeding is (or is not) included in easily available resources. You could contact one organization dedicated to a long-term health issue affected by breastfeeding, and find out how breastfeeding could be inserted into their educational and support programs.

5. Research the causes and risk factors of low infant birth weight and implications for breastfeeding. Use at least two to three sources.

6. Describe at least five differences between nutritional requirements for preterm infants and term infants, with implications for breastfeeding.

7. Research preterm development and growth compared with growth of term infants. Include common concerns raised by parents and professionals related to breastfeeding a premature infant. You could interview a parent of a preterm infant or a professional who regularly works with preterm infants for this exercise. Include references in your write-up.

8. Describe signs of normal and abnormal skin tone, muscle tone, and reflexes that would affect breastfeeding. Discuss breastfeeding management for at least one infant with abnormal findings, including the impact for the mother.

9. Go to a local shopping mall, park, or other public place and watch 5–10 mothers and babies under the age of 3 years interacting. Estimate the age of the child based on its behavior, then verify the child's age by asking the mother. At least half the sample should include breastfeeding dyads.

10. Describe at least five uses for banked pasteurized donor human milk for babies with serious illnesses, metabolic deficiencies, or other pathological conditions. Include any political, cultural, or social controversies related to donor human milk.

11. Ask three breastfeeding mothers to record feeding frequency and duration of all feeds for three consecutive days. Select infants of different ages. Compare the patterns of the mother–baby pairs with those in popular parenting books. Discuss with the mothers why they did or did not read or follow these books' advice.

12. Carefully examine the 2006 WHO Growth Standards and compare them with older growth-monitoring documents, including anthropometric data. Investigate why the selection sites were chosen and how the mothers and families were supported. Investigate how the WHO standards data are being used in your community.

B. MATERNAL

1. Compare ultrasound studies of the lactating breast by Donna Ramsay Geddes and other authors with those in books or references published prior to 2010. Describe differences in structure and function, and the implication of these differences on breastfeeding management, techniques, and education of parents.

2. Compare the protein, fat, immune factors, and vitamin content of colostrum, preterm milk, mature milk, and milk produced after 12 months of lactation; (2) influence of fatty acids in human milk in relation to brain development; and (3) effect of maternal diet on the fat, protein, carbohydrates, minerals, fat-soluble, and water-soluble vitamins in her milk. Discuss why these components are important.
3. Select one to three immune components in human milk and research the function of those components. Describe any variations in these components over time, and during heating or freezing and storage. Include short-and long-term implications of immune components in human milk.
4. Read several sources on nipple structure and variations, and discuss implications of various configurations on the course of breastfeeding. If you are able to photograph any mothers with unusual nipple/breast structures, obtain written permission and include a photo in your write-up.
5. Interview a mother who had any type of breast surgery about her experiences with breastfeeding. OR read a publication designed to support breastfeeding women who have had breast surgery.
6. Interview a mother who has unusual nipple structure (inverted, bifurcated, large, small, flat, etc.) and her experience on breastfeeding. OR, read a publication with photos of normal and unusual nipple structure and variations related to breastfeeding.
7. Research the impact of maternal malnutrition and obesity on the mother's ability to lactate normally. This exercise could include global initiatives, policies and practices, or clinical implications for breastfeeding.
8. Do a literature search on maternal and hormonal disorders and their effect on lactation (thyroid, polycystic ovary syndrome, etc.).
9. Investigate the relationship between maternal autoimmune disorders and lactation. This could include lupus, Graves' disease, myasthenia gravis, etc.

II. Physiology and Endocrinology

1. Interview three women who are using the Lactational Amenorrhea Method (LAM) of family planning. Include feeding patterns, night-feeding arrangements, reasons the mothers are using this method, drawbacks or obstacles they encountered, return of menstruation, and effect of this method on other health behaviors in their families.
2. Read several sources or protocols on relactation and induced lactation. Design a basic management protocol to support these processes with rationales and references. If possible, design your plan for a specific mother you have met.
3. Interview a mother who breastfed or is breastfeeding twins, triplets, or quadruplets. Include in your interview the following questions: When did you first learn you were having twins? How did you feel? How did your family react to the news? What is the easiest part about breastfeeding twins? The hardest part? What would you want another mother expecting twins to know? What are the unique features of having multiple babies instead of one at a time? Write up your observations.
4. Investigate tandem nursing by interviewing a mother whose children tandem-nursed and/or by reading *Adventures in Tandem Nursing* and/or checking into any social media site on tandem nursing. Explore the physiology of lactation when the mother is pregnant again, and after the new baby is born.
5. Read several resources and/or policy statements on newborn hypoglycemia. Compare what you've read with any policy or practices in your community. Include a list of acceptable medical reasons for supplementation.

6. Discuss the course of pregnancy, birth and lactation for women with type 1 and type 2 diabetes. Try to interview at least one woman with diabetes who breastfed her child, and include her experiences. Provide some references.

7. Read several sources about the relationship between infertility and lactation, including warning signs and management considerations.

8. Prepare a timeline of normal stooling of the breastfed child from birth through 2 years of age.

III. Pathology

A. INFANT

1. Interview at least two mothers whose children are allergic. Describe the strategies and resources used by the mothers to confirm and manage the allergens that affect their child, and any modifications made by the mother and rest of the family.

2. Interview two mothers whose babies were premature or ill at birth. Explore how breastfeeding was affected by their baby's condition and how they managed to maintain lactation and assist the baby to breastfeed directly during their baby's hospitalization.

3. Read several sources on at least two of the following conditions: nipple and oral thrush; congenital abnormality or structural defect; or endocrine irregularity in the mother or infant. If possible, interview at least one mother whose baby has that condition.

4. Read several professional organizations' position papers and policies on jaundice and/ or hypoglycemia. Compare these resources with current research articles on these topics, and discuss the differences and any contradictions or controversies.

5. Tour a neonatal intensive care unit (NICU) or interview a staff member who works in a NICU at a hospital other than where you work. Ask some of the following questions: Which babies are most likely or least likely to be breastfed? What is your policy on giving donor human milk to babies? What are your criteria for determining which milk is usable or unusable? How do mothers obtain breast pumps and attachment kits? What is the recommended pumping regimen? At what point do mothers begin to breastfeed their babies? What kind of breastfeeding support is provided for breastfeeding families? Under what circumstances do you not recommend breastfeeding? Write up your impressions, comparing the answers with current best practices.

6. Read about tongue-tie (ankyloglossia) as it affects the infant and breastfeeding mother. If possible, interview a professional who is skilled in treating tongue-tie and/ or a breastfeeding mother whose baby was affected by ankyloglossia.

7. Investigate causes, treatments, and impact of cleft lip and palate on the course of breastfeeding.

8. Investigate the impact of congenital anomalies (cardiac, GI, respiratory, orthopedic, sensory) of the mother or baby on the course of breastfeeding. Choose one or two to focus on, and if possible interview a mother whose family is affected by a congenital anomaly.

9. Describe the prevalence, causes, treatments, and implications of gastroesophageal reflux (GERD) in breastfeeding infants. Read both parent-oriented and professional resources for this exercise.

10. Explore at least three acute infant diseases (bacterial, fungal, viral, and systemic) that may affect the breastfed baby, with implications for management.

11. Interview a mother whose infant has any neurological disability. How was this identified in her infant? Who was especially helpful or unhelpful in helping her breastfeed? What are the implications of breastfeeding to this child, and the impact of the condition on breastfeeding and maternal-infant attachment?

12. Describe the impact of SGA (small for gestational age) or LGA (large for gestational age) on the course of breastfeeding, taking into account the mother's reactions and baby's behavior and unique needs.

B. MATERNAL

1. Interview at least two mothers who experienced mastitis or breast abscess. Ask each about the history leading up to the condition, the actions of professionals who interacted with her, and how she felt about the help she received or failed to receive. Read and cite at least two references in your write-up.

2. Look into normal, overactive, and impaired milk-ejection reflex. What factors influence milk ejection? What hormones influence timing, length, and intervals of milk ejection? What can someone observe during a breastfeed during the milk-ejection reflex?

3. Explore at least three acute maternal diseases (bacterial, fungal, viral, and systemic) that may affect the nursing mother, with implications for management. If possible, interview at least one mother who had a severe acute illness during breastfeeding.

4. Read several sources on a chronic maternal illness/condition and its effect on breastfeeding, and the course of breastfeeding for a mother with this condition. The condition could be diabetes, multiple sclerosis, epilepsy, dwarfism, schizophrenia, sensory or orthopedic impairments, etc. If possible, interview at least one mother with a chronic condition regarding her pregnancy and breastfeeding experiences.

5. Contact a mother with a disability or chronic illness. Interview her and ask what accommodations she has made to care for herself and her baby. on pregnancy, birth, breastfeeding, and caring for her baby. Include a list of several references that address that condition and its impact on lactation.

6. Meet with a healthcare professional who works in an emergency department or urgent healthcare center. Investigate the department's policies and practices for treating/managing a nursing mother who presents with any acute illness or trauma. Compare what you learned with any published resource on acute maternal illness or traumatic injury in a nursing mother.

7. Describe the causes, consequences to breastfeeding, and treatments for pre-eclampsia (pregnancy-inducted hypertension) or postbirth hemorrhage. If possible, interview at least one mother who experienced one or both of these complications of pregnancy and the breastfeeding outcomes.

8. Compare the differences between nipple trauma, nipple infections, and non-infectious nipple or breast pain, citing several references. Include causes, treatments, and prevention strategies.

9. Write up a case study of a mother with chronic *low* milk production. Include prenatal signs, labor and birth, postbirth experiences, and remedies/solutions attempted. How did she feed her baby? What was her emotional reaction to chronic low milk production? What strategies worked well, and which were not helpful? Cite several references in your write-up.

10. Write up a case study of a mother with chronic *high* or over-production of milk. Include any prenatal signs, labor and birth, postbirth experiences, and remedies/

solutions attempted. How did she feed her baby? What was her emotional reaction to chronic high milk production? What strategies worked well, and which were not helpful? Cite several references in your write-up.

11. There is growing interest in providing "encapsulated placenta" to postbirth women in some groups. Investigate this practice in your community, including any adverse effects that have been reported. Describe the hormonal influences on lactogenesis, and comment on this practice related to human placenta and lactation physiology.

IV. Pharmacology and Toxicology

1. Write a case study of two breastfeeding women taking a prescription drug. Include the specific drug and reason why she is taking it, any instructions given to the mother by her physician, nurse, or counselor; rate or amount of passage of drug into milk; implications for the baby; any alternatives.

2. Pick at least five common over-the-counter and prescription medications. Using at least two references, discuss the compatibility of the drug to breastfeeding.

3. Investigate the history of galactogogues and lactation suppressants, including "folk" remedies and cultural beliefs, prescription drugs, and herbs. Describe any research available on the safety and effectiveness of at least one of these on milk production and on the infant.

4. Investigate the influence of hormonal methods of family planning (contraception) on lactation, using several sources. Develop a chart or handout that could be used use in a prenatal clinic or postbirth breastfeeding class, or prepare a brief presentation on this topic.

5. Do an Internet or PubMed search on nipple creams/ointments, and read several sources. What are the alleged reasons for their use? How are these products tested and regulated? Where can a mother report an adverse experience with a nipple cream or nipple-care product?

6. Research medicinal herb use during lactation, using several sources. Develop a list of evidence-based resources on medicinal herbs during lactation.

7. Follow any social media source for new mothers, and track "can I take XX while breastfeeding?" discussions. Compile a list of evidence-based resources on prescription, over-the-counter, and drugs of abuse use during lactation.

8. Research the prevalence and outcomes of alcohol and tobacco (and marijuana) use during lactation. Compile some teaching points that could be used in prenatal and postbirth clinics or classes, with references.

9. Contact someone working with pregnant women addicted to drugs of abuse. What are the local policies and practices to help her breastfeed safely? What happens in your community if a newly delivered mother's toxicology screen reveals opiates or other drugs abuse? Investigate programs or protocols that support breastfeeding mothers during treatment for drug abuse.

V. Psychology, Sociology, and Anthropology

1. Interview two women who have had childbirth experiences different from what they expected, or negative experiences. You may include yourself as one of the mothers. Ask them what they didn't like, what they would have done differently, what they wanted others to have done differently, and how this experience affected their sense of self as a parent and their breastfeeding relationship with their child. Caution: Be an active

listener. Do not attempt to justify or rationalize the behavior of others. Stay focused on the mother's feelings.

2. Observe at least one complete hospital-based labor and birth episode. Focus on the mother's knowledge and use of non-drug and pharmacologic pain relief techniques and coping techniques and their effect on mother and baby. Describe the status of breastfeeding one week after birth.

3. Interview at least two breastfeeding mothers who have more than one child, and discuss how the mothers manage nighttime feeds and sleep. Gently inquire why they do, do not, or sometimes share a bed with their nursing infant and/or older children, where the children nap during the day and sleep at night, and how these decisions were made in their family. Caution: Just listen with curiosity. Write up your observations and how the families' practices align with or differ from current recommendations.

4. Attend two different meetings of La Leche League or other breastfeeding mother-support group. Observe variations in mother–infant breastfeeding interactions related to individual differences in infant behavior, infant age, and maternal response. Listen to the comments and concerns that mothers raise during the meeting and during breaks. Write up your observations and compare them to what you've heard in your professional role.

5. If you have breastfed, write an essay describing your thoughts on being pregnant, attitudes about labor and birth, feelings about being a mother, and the impact of the attitudes of your immediate family on your becoming a mother. Focus on what surprised you emotionally. If you have not breastfed, interview two mothers concerning the above topics and write an essay on their comments and your reactions to their discussion of their feelings.

6. Investigate local or cultural beliefs about foods that should be eaten or avoided during breastfeeding. Are there biological rationales for these beliefs? How do mothers maintain breastfeeding when on restricted diets for religious or cultural reasons?

7. Investigate at least one cultural or religious group in your community different from your own culture. Who supports the mother during pregnancy and breastfeeding? Whom does the mother trust (or distrust)? What is the father's typical role and engagement in early parenting? Are grandparents involved, and in what way? Are any spiritual advisors especially influential in the course of pregnancy, birth, or breastfeeding?

8. Create a directory of breastfeeding resources in your community, including warm lines, equipment depots, breastfeeding care providers and support groups, etc. Consider making it available widely.

9. Investigate at least one maternal mental/emotional health condition that affects pregnancy and breastfeeding (depression, anxiety, bipolar, history of abuse, ADHD, autism). Compile a bibliography of evidence-based information on that condition that could be made available in your community or workplace. If your workplace has such a directory of resources, compare that with what you find in referenced breastfeeding resources.

10. Describe how you would assist and support a mother with a psychological or cognitive impairment. Would you do anything differently, and if so, why? If possible, interview someone who has worked closely with a breastfeeding mother with cognitive impairment.

11. Read at least one book or watch a DVD or YouTube video clip on safe bedsharing for breastfeeding families. Describe how that resource differs from (or is consistent with) local public health messages about safe sleep, and your personal or professional experiences related to "safe sleep" issues.

12. Compare global recommendations for breastfeeding for two or more years to any two mothers you've encountered. When did the mothers' babies wean? Did the baby nurse longer than she initially intended, or shorter, and why? What were the best and most challenging aspects of weaning?

13. What does "cultural competency" mean to you? How does that concept apply to your current or future practice?

VI. Techniques

1. Interview two mothers whose babies had sucking or feeding problems after full-term births. Discuss the problem's impact on breastfeeding, as well as the impact of breastfeeding on the baby and/or the problem.

2. Interview or observe at least two mothers who experienced breastfeeding problems in the first few days after giving birth. For each, write brief summary of the problem and discuss how the problem should or could have been prevented or handled at a lower level of intervention. Include interactions of other professionals, whether by omission or commission.

3. Watch at least two videos or DVDs on immediate skin-to-skin contact after birth, Kangaroo Mother Care or general skin-to-skin care contact. Discuss your personal or professional experiences with either or both, and include some references and resources.

4. Observe at least three babies at breast for two consecutive complete feeding episodes. The babies should be of different ages. Estimate the total volume of milk obtained based on quality and quantity of feeding. Perform pre-and -post feed weighs on a gram-sensitive scale to verify your estimates.

5. Read or watch at least two sources on hand expression of milk. Practice the motions on a breast model, or if possible with some experienced mothers who are willing to let you practice on them.

6. Compile a list of conditions when babies might have difficulty latching onto the breast. Include at least one strategy for overcoming a problem, and provide references.

7. Perform breast exams and nipple assessments of three different women in different stages of lactation. If possible, include prenatal, lactating, and post-weaning breasts. Write a description of each, including the implication of each situation on the breastfeeding dyad.

8. Investigate the what and how of medically indicated supplementation of the breastfed baby, including WHO recommendations and research-based protocols.

9. Examine the policies and protocols that apply to the first hour after birth in any health facility (including your own). Describe documentation, training, and reactions of families. If your hospital has changed practices recently, describe staff and family reactions to the new practices.

10. Examine at least three different devices or products for breast or nipple care or therapy. What are the indications and drawbacks of each? You could include nipple shields, breast shells, thermal treatments, everters, bra pads, etc.

11. Test several brands of breast pumps with a pressure gauge or balloons, and compare what you find.

12. Test-weigh several common objects using a scale used for weighing babies, and compare with the weight listed on the object (bag of sugar, etc). Then, weigh several babies before and after a feed, estimate how much milk they transferred during the feed, and compare with the scale's results.

VII. Clinical Skills

A. EQUIPMENT AND TECHNOLOGY

1. Examine and measure several infant-feeding devices (teats, pacifiers, tubes) and/or devices used inside the infant mouth (nipple shields, bulb syringes, gavage tubes). Compare the length, diameter, and flexibility (texture) of these devices and the dimensions of the infant mouth, and discuss the implications to breastfeeding.

2. Do a literature search on handling and storage of human milk. Then do one of these: (1) Create an easy-to-read handout (with references) that could be used by breastfeeding mothers in your setting. OR, (2) find at least three handouts for parents on handling and storing human milk, and evaluate them for consistency with evidence-based guidelines that you researched in the first part of this exercise.

3. Examine several different devices or products for nipple care or therapy. What are the indications and drawbacks of each? Include nipple shields, breast shells, and everters. Provide at least two references.

4. Dig into the research on pacifiers, both drawbacks and possible indications. You can include policy statements and position papers, Internet sources and parents' experiences, and the impact on duration of breastfeeding.

5. Follow an International Board Certified Lactation Consultant on hospital or clinic rounds for at least 3 hours. Discuss with the LC what you observed, including all equipment used by mothers or babies during that period. Observe the dynamic interaction between the mother and the LC as much as the clinical problem. In your write-up, discuss any new concepts you observed being used, why you might (or might not have) done things differently, the baby's responses, and how the LC documented the interaction.

6. Test at least five devices for assisting breastfeeding. Milk-removal devices can be tested using a vacuum gauge or balloons. Or, interview several women who have used several different kinds of equipment to assist breastfeeding. Discuss the advantages and drawbacks of these devices or techniques including cost, comfort, and the effect on the mother–baby relationship.

7. Locate at least two different scales used to weigh babies, and check the accuracy of these with standard weights or common objects with verified weights. Investigate the history of weighing babies, including a discussion on why the weight of a newborn is deemed important.

8. Look into several ways that smartphones, Skype, electronic medical records, text messaging, and social media are used (or abused) by mothers and healthcare providers. Write up a description of at least one successful program that uses modern communication technology.

9. Using the *Score Sheet for Evaluating Breastfeeding Educational Materials*, evaluate the content of a handout, video clip or website. Submit a summary of your evaluation and recommendation. (See http://www.bflrc.com/ljs/documents/ScoreChart2010.pdf and http://www.bflrc.com/ljs/documents/EvalBF_EducMaterials.pdf.)

B. EDUCATION AND COMMUNICATION

1. Attend Level I of LLLI's Communication Skills program or, if not available, a workshop or class in non-violent or compassionate communication or motivational interviewing. Practice the active listening skills at work and at home for at least a week or two. Describe others' general responses to you when you use these techniques.

2. For each chronological stage on the *Detailed Content Outline* (http://iblce.org/wp-content/uploads/2013/08/IBCLC-Detailed-Content-Outline-for-2016-for-Publication.pdf), prepare a list of about 8–10 key breastfeeding issues to expect during that stage.

3. Examine several sample care plans that might be given to a mother at a postbirth breastfeeding consult. OR, interview several mothers who have been helped by a breastfeeding care provider, and ask about the care plans that were communicated to them by the provider. Were the plans realistic and effective? What could have been included or omitted to make the plan more useful?

4. Review some lactation consultant assessment forms or electronic charting screens. Comment on the strengths and weaknesses of each, and any changes you would make. OR, design a set of assessment and reporting forms for use in your setting. Discuss what you learned by doing this exercise.

5. Attend at least two meetings (preferably a full four-meeting series) of La Leche League or other organized mother support group. Observe the communications and group dynamics techniques in use at the meetings. Meet with the leaders afterward, and ask how they manage the group logistics, direct discussion, and handle uncomfortable questions or silence. Write up your observations.

6. Attend and observe at least one breastfeeding class taught in a facility other than where you are currently employed, such as at a WIC clinic, hospital, community center, physician or midwife's office, or other setting. Pay attention to the structure and timing of the class, reaction of participants, and how the instructor handled questions and challenges. In your write-up, discuss the topics and information presented and whether these concepts were (or were not) effective or helpful to the participants.

7. Attend a lecture or presentation on breastfeeding that is at least 1 hour long. Comment on the published objectives, accuracy of the content, effectiveness of the teaching/presentation methods, and the speaker's comfort.

8. Examine at least two resources for educating professionals. These could include books, pamphlets, courses, online programs, DVDs, etc. If possible, interview professionals who have attended or used these products, and discuss how they reacted to the program's content and presentation effectiveness.

9. Talk to several women whose baby or babies' breastfed longer than 1 year. What factors helped or hindered their breastfeeding relationship? How did their family, health-care providers, and others react to their nursing child as the child continued to nurse past infancy? Listen with curiosity and an open mind. Ideally, find a situation where you can observe nursing toddlers and their mothers.

10. Write a self-reflection on what "emotional support" means to you. You could describe a situation when someone provided important emotional support in a crisis or a situation where you wanted and needed emotional support but none was available. The "facts" of the situation are less important to describe than the emotions involved. How does this relate to your role as a lactation professional?

11. Investigate opportunities for group support for breastfeeding mothers in your local community. You could include WIC, online groups, La Leche League, faith-based groups, breastfeeding cafés or clubs, etc. Prepare a listing or series of Web links that could be distributed widely.

C. ETHICAL AND LEGAL ISSUES

1. Research laws and policies that protect breastfeeding in public places. OR, search the Internet or news outlets for stories of women who were harassed for breastfeeding

their babies in public places. OR, search for stories of protests or nurse-in demonstrations that occurred in response to mothers who were told they couldn't nurse their babies in public places.

2. Read IBLCE's Clinical Competencies (http://iblce.org/wp-content/uploads/2013/08/clinical-competencies.pdf), and evaluate yourself as of today. Reflect on your areas of strength, and where you seek improvement. Keep a copy, to compare your self-evaluations now and in the future.

3. Download and read IBLCE's Scope of Practice and Code of Professional Conduct documents (http://iblce.org/resources/professional-standards). Reflect on these concepts and how you do or will apply these in your practice.

4. Read several sources for principles of confidentiality in healthcare setting in your country or jurisdiction, including IBLCE's policy on exam confidentiality (http://iblce.org/wp-content/uploads/2013/08/confidentiality-policy.pdf). Reflect on these principles and how they are (or are not) applied in your personal experience. Do not identify any places of employment or individuals in your reflection.

5. Read at least two sources related to copyright and intellectual property rights. You could interview an attorney specializing in intellectual property rights for this assignment. Discuss how copyright law and intellectual property rights apply to lactation consultant education and practice.

6. Collect resources on Universal Precautions and how these apply to lactation consultant settings. Include references on the handling of human milk.

7. For each of the following scenarios, decide whether the behavior is ethical or not, give a thorough rationale for your decision, and include any relevant references to support your point of view.
   a. Scene 1: The LC sees every patient of the doctor for whom she works. When asked by clients what to take to the hospital to facilitate their breastfeeding experience, the LC sells them a package of breastfeeding aids (shells, lanolin, manual breast pump, bra pads, a book.). The LC keeps 100% of the profit.
   b. Scene 2: The LC teaches all the breastfeeding and childbirth classes in a hospital. Mrs. A attends the childbirth class and later calls the LC for help. She needs more help than can be provided by phone. The LC arranges a home visit and charges the mother for this service. There is no other breastfeeding care provider in this community.
   c. Scene 3: The LC is working with a baby who has an obvious short frenulum, which severely inhibits breastfeeding. The doctors in this community refuse to acknowledge the need for treatment for short frenulum and recommend cessation of breastfeeding if it causes a problem. The LC tells the baby's mother about a dentist in the neighboring community who can diagnose and treat the short frenulum; the LC does not ask permission from the primary care physician to make the referral.
   d. Scene 4: As a hospital-based LC, you have been tasked with providing in-service education on breastfeeding to the entire professional staff—doctors, nurses, etc. You have been offered funds from two sources: Abbott-Ross Laboratories and Procter & Gamble. Your supervisor tells you to use the Abbott funds to pay for the in-services because the representative recently donated a new photocopier to the unit.

8. Prepare a collection of resources related to ethical and legal aspects of breastfeeding. This could include divorce/custody issues, workplace accommodations, and/or breastfeeding in public places.

9. Interview someone who works in a Baby-Friendly (BFHI) designated hospital. Ask about the ease or difficulty of making changes to achieve BFHI designation, parents' responses, impact of BFHI designation on other hospitals in the community, and what the person likes best (or least) about working in a BFHI-designated facility.

10. Go on a treasure hunt at your workplace, the Internet, or any healthcare facility in your community, looking for advertising of infant formula, bottles and teats, pacifiers to the public. If possible, collect samples or take digital photos of the products, noting where you spotted them. Write up your observations and comment on any violations of the International Code of Marketing of Breast-milk Substitutes, conflicts of interest, or ethically questionable ads.

D. RESEARCH

1. Write a critique of a research report (article) related to any aspect of breastfeeding from a recent (within 2 years) primary source. Consider submitting this critique to a journal or other source. Note any significant flaws in the research, with implications for your practice.

2. Write a review of videotape, book, or teaching aid pertinent to any aspect of breastfeeding. Follow the rules for reviews from a professional journal. Consider submitting it to a professional journal for publication.

3. Prepare an annotated bibliography of any clinical aspect of breastfeeding that is relatively new to you using primary and secondary references.

4. Read at least one resource on evaluating research, such as *How to Read a Paper* by Trisha Greenhalgh. Then select any recent research article (you can ask your instructor for suggestions) and analyze that article for weaknesses and strengths.

5. Describe the concept of "levels of strength of evidence" and give an example of a policy with levels of evidence cited.

6. Investigate the history of evidence-based medicine (EBM), including its roots, development, etc. How is EBM applied at your workplace, or in a healthcare facility familiar to you?

7. Choose any published policy from a professional association related to breastfeeding. Read the policy, look through the references, and reflect on whether the policy supports, protects, and promotes breastfeeding adequately.

E. PUBLIC HEALTH AND ADVOCACY

1. Interview at least three LCs who work in different practice settings. Compare and contrast their role, commenting on the similarities and differences.

2. Do ONE of the following: (1) Find a list or compendium of laws protecting breastfeeding, and propose a new law with protections for breastfeeding. (2) Prepare testimony designed to convince your local legislators to protect breastfeeding in some way in your community. (3) Prepare a draft breastfeeding support policy for your workplace, school, or other institution.

3. Using the BFHI Self-Evaluation Criteria, evaluate some aspect of your work setting for "friendliness" to breastfeeding. Devise at least one short-term and long-term strategy for improving breastfeeding management that you personally could implement where you work.

4. Establish a breastfeeding coalition, consortium, or network in your community. Hold at least one meeting and write up what your goals are to promote, support, and protect breastfeeding in your community.

5. Interview someone who has worked at the national or state level in some aspect of breastfeeding promotion. Discuss how they became involved, what obstacles or resistance they have encountered, what progress they have seen, and their vision for the future.

6. Contact your local emergency preparedness agencies and investigate their policies and staff training related to care of pregnant women, breastfeeding mothers, and young children in emergencies and disasters. Extra bonus points: compile local, national, and international resources on infant feeding in emergencies.

7. Read the entire International Code of Marketing of Breast-milk Substitutes and relevant World Health Assembly Resolutions. Here is one concise source: http://ibfan .org/the-full-code. Reflect on any aspect of the Code or Resolutions that you find especially important or interesting.

CHAPTER 1

Prenatal Questions

1.1 **A mother wants to continue breastfeeding her 18-month-old child during a subsequent pregnancy. A neighbor told her to wean the child so that the toddler's breastfeeding does not trigger premature labor. Your BEST response is to:**

a. suggest she immediately wean the older baby.

b. tell her breastfeeding during a normal pregnancy is not harmful to either child.

c. suggest she use lanolin during the pregnancy to prevent nipple pain.

d. recommend that she discontinue sexual relations so that uterine contractions do not jeopardize the pregnancy.

1.2 **A mother who is pregnant for the second time asks, "Will I be able to breastfeed my second child if I was unable to breastfeed my first baby?" Which of the following should be your FIRST response to her?**

a. You are wise to be asking these questions now, during pregnancy.

b. Yes, most second babies breastfeed better than first babies.

c. The answer depends on the reason you had problems the first time.

d. No, because your breasts have insufficient glandular tissue.

1.3 **A researcher is studying breastfeeding incidence in two neighboring community prenatal clinics. In one clinic, a new videotape is used to teach breastfeeding; the other clinic continues to use an older videotape. At the follow-up, both clinics report similar increases in breastfeeding initiation. The MOST LIKELY reason for this is:**

a. that all instructional videotapes are equivalent.

b. the Hawthorne effect.

c. that changing the videotape had no effect.

d. the Nedelsky effect.

1.4 **Which technique is MOST LIKELY to help this mother and baby achieve a comfortable and effective nursing session?**

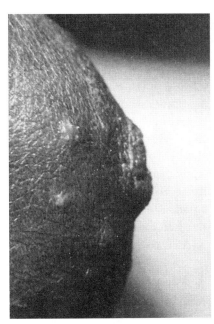

See color plate 1.

Courtesy of K. Jean Cotterman.

a. Suggest the mother pull and stretch her nipple before trying to nurse.

b. Have mother apply cold cloths or ice cubes to her nipple before trying to latch.

c. Start the feed with a silicone nipple shield, then remove it after a few minutes.

d. Have the mother semi-recline, and put the baby prone skin-to-skin on her chest and see if the baby will self-attach.

1.5 **A well-balanced diet with sufficient calories accompanied by early and regular prenatal care significantly reduces the incidence of:**
   a. infants with diabetes.
   b. low birth weight.
   c. maternal gestational diabetes.
   d. lactation failure.

1.6 **A health care provider wants to encourage pregnant women to choose breastfeeding. Which statement is MOST SUPPORTIVE of breastfeeding?**
   a. Are you considering breastfeeding?
   b. What have you heard about breastfeeding?
   c. Are you going to breastfeed or bottle-feed?
   d. You are not thinking about breastfeeding, are you?

1.7 **You are working with a 3-month-old infant with persistent feeding difficulties. Although the mother's milk production is abundant, the child shows poor coordination at breast and with several feeding devices and is gaining weight very slowly. You notice that the baby's upper lip is thin, the space under her nose is noticeably flat, and her eyes are relatively small. What should you NEXT ask the mother about her pregnancy?**
   a. Did you have a high fever more than once during your pregnancy?
   b. Was there a time during your pregnancy when you got very drunk?
   c. Was you home ever tested for ground radiation or radon levels?
   d. Were you responsible for emptying your cat's litter box during your pregnancy?

1.8 **When does the mammary secretory glandular tissue develop?**
   a. During puberty
   b. Some development occurs with each menstrual period.
   c. In the first trimester of pregnancy
   d. During pregnancy and the early weeks postbirth

1.9 **This woman is in her third trimester of pregnancy. What is the MOST IMPORTANT action you could take to help her prepare to breastfeed?**

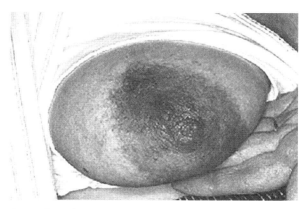

See color plate 2.

   a. Teach her good positioning and latch-on technique, using a doll as a model.
   b. Provide her with breast shells to wear several hours a day.
   c. Teach her Hoffman's techniques to prepare her nipples.
   d. Instruct her to rub her nipples with a towel several times a day.

1.10 **Which of the following actions is MOST LIKELY to improve this pregnant mother's breastfeeding experience?**

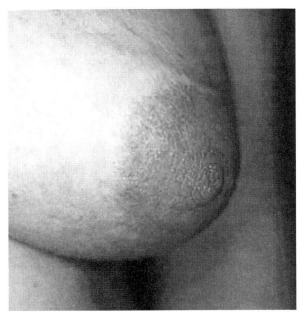

See color plate 3.

    a. Wearing breast shells several hours a day for a few weeks during her pregnancy

    b. Learning nonpharmaceutical methods of pain relief for labor

    c. Vigorously pulling and stretching her nipples several times a day

    d. Immediate and uninterrupted skin-to-skin contact at birth allowing the infant to self-attach

1.11 **A pregnant woman is worried about giving birth prematurely because of hypertension. Which strategy is MOST LIKELY to prevent or reduce the risk of pregnancy-related hypertension?**

    a. Well-balanced diet with sufficient protein

    b. High-carbohydrate diet

    c. Drinking at least 2 liters of milk every day

    d. Prenatal vitamin supplements

1.12 **A 27-year-old woman will birth her first baby in about 3 weeks. She asks if she will be able to breastfeed after having a breast reduction with her nipple auto-transplanted at the age of 19. Your BEST response is:**

    a. There will be no problem breastfeeding.

    b. It may be possible for the first 3 months.

    c. You may not be able to breastfeed.

    d. Try it and see what happens.

1.13 **Which is the MOST COMMON site of placental implantation in the uterus that could affect the baby's intrauterine position and cause labor complications?**

    a. Anterior side, cervical region

    b. Anterior side, fundal region

    c. Posterior side, cervical region

    d. Posterior side, fundal region

1.14 **A mother wants to know how soon she will return to her prepregnancy weight after her baby is born. Which is the BEST of the following responses?**

    a. Most breastfeeding mothers lose 2 to 3 pounds (0.9 to 1.4 kg) per week.

    b. Making milk uses 1000 calories a day from your diet.

    c. Gradual weight loss preserves your health and energy.

    d. Restrict your food intake to 1500 calories a day.

1.15   **What is this mother MOST LIKELY doing?**

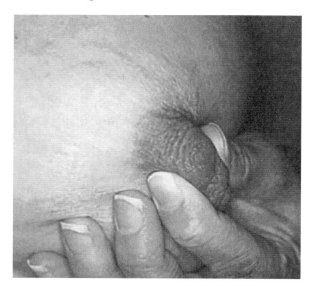

   a.   Expressing colostrum
   b.   Performing the pinch test
   c.   Everting her retracting nipple
   d.   Nipple rolling to firm the tip

1.16   **Which prenatal breast condition is MOST LIKELY to affect lactation?**
   a.   No leaking of colostrum by the third trimester
   b.   Flat nipples
   c.   No change in pigment of the nipple and areola
   d.   No change in breast size during pregnancy

1.17   **A pregnant woman is worried that her milk may not come in with her second baby. She said she never actually made milk after her first baby's birth and never became engorged. Which of the following birth complications is MOST RELATED to delayed onset of lactogenesis?**

   a.   Cesarean birth
   b.   Retained placental fragment
   c.   Premature birth
   d.   Episiotomy

1.18   **A pregnant woman taking an antiseizure medication was advised to not breast-feed her first two children because of the medication. She is being encouraged to breastfeed this third child by her neurologist. What is the MOST SUPPORTIVE information you should share with her now?**
   a.   Your neurologist must know what he's talking about, so following his advice is wise.
   b.   Your milk has many components that foster and support brain growth, even if some medication is in the milk.
   c.   You followed the best advice at the time with your other children, so do not feel guilty.
   d.   Your milk's nutritional properties are not changed by the medication that might be present.

1.19   **What process is primarily responsible for the increase in breast size (volume) during pregnancy?**
   a.   Increase in fatty stores in the breast
   b.   Development of the duct system
   c.   Growth of secretory epithelial cells
   d.   Growing uterus triggers ribcage expansion

1.20   **A defect in which structure may cause gastroesophageal reflux?**
   a.   Esophagus
   b.   Trachea
   c.   Small intestine
   d.   Large intestine

1.21 How would you BEST document this pregnant woman's breasts?

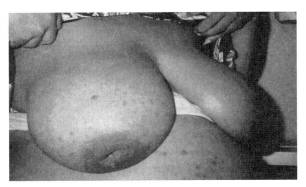

Courtesy of K. Jean Cotterman.

   a. Saggy
   b. Apparent inverted right nipple
   c. Insufficient glandular tissue
   d. Hyperpigmented areola

1.22 A pregnant woman who has type 1 diabetes expresses interest in breastfeeding. Your BEST response is:

   a. You may need to adjust your insulin dosage if you breastfeed.
   b. You may need to eat a snack before you breastfeed.
   c. It will be more difficult to control your blood sugar if you breastfeed.
   d. Breastfeeding may reduce your baby's risk of developing diabetes.

1.23 This mother is 36 weeks pregnant. Your BEST recommendation would be:

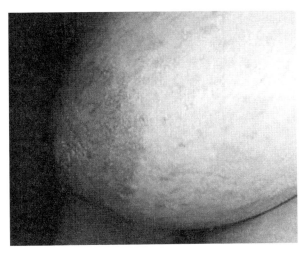

See color plate 4.

   a. Rub your nipples with a towel twice a day.
   b. Be sure to breastfeed in the first hour postbirth.
   c. Pull and roll the nipple to stretch it.
   d. You will not be able to breastfeed.

1.24 You are asked to teach formula feeding and breastfeeding to expectant parents. Which approach is MOST SUPPORTIVE of breastfeeding?

   a. Refuse to teach formula feeding and refer students to other resources.
   b. Teach breastfeeding in the class and offer a separate 1:1 session on formula feeding on request.
   c. Teach both during the group sessions, and offer additional information on breastfeeding separately.
   d. Schedule separate classes for breastfeeding and formula feeding.

1.25 This pregnant mother is concerned about the appearance of her nipples. Your BEST response is:

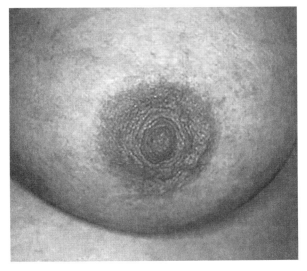

See color plate 5.

   a. You probably have a thrush infection.
   b. A bacterial infection is a possibility.
   c. Do not breastfeed until the herpes lesion heals.
   d. Your breast appears normal.

1.26 **A pregnant woman follows a vegan diet and intends to breastfeed. She should be informed that :**
   a. Her milk supply may be compromised by her diet.
   b. She should take a vitamin B$_{12}$ supplement.
   c. Her baby will need a multivitamin supplement.
   d. She will have to change her diet if she wants to breastfeed.

1.27 **What is the MOST LIKELY use of milk donated by mothers whose baby died?**
   a. Support adults with IgA deficiencies or receiving solid-organ transplants
   b. Research on milk properties, storage, or other factors
   c. Dispensed on prescription to sick or premature babies
   d. Extract human stem cells for research purposes

1.28 **During a prenatal consult, a pregnant woman shows you her left nipple and says it is very sensitive to any touch. Based on what you see in the photograph, what is your BEST next action?**

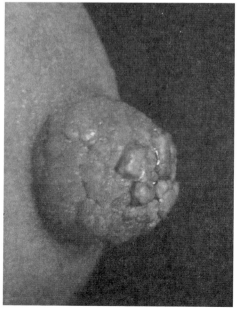

Courtesy of K. Jean Cotterman.

   a. Share your observations with her primary care provider
   b. Provide her with sterile gauze to clean her nipple
   c. Reassure her that nipple pain is normal during pregnancy
   d. Teach her how to roll and stretch her nipple to reduce tenderness

1.29 **Which hormone involved in lactogenesis is absent and cannot be provided artificially when a mother is inducing lactation and has never been pregnant?**
   a. Estrogen
   b. Progesterone
   c. Prolactin
   d. Placental lactogen

1.30 **Your client is a pregnant 38-year-old woman who had breast reduction surgery through use of the inferior pedicle technique 10 years ago, after having breastfed two children for about 1 year each. She had low milk production with each of the children. What is the likelihood of a full milk production for the new baby?**
   a. High because of the surgical technique used
   b. High because of her two previous lactations
   c. Unlikely because of the type of breast reduction surgery
   d. Unlikely because of length of time since reduction

1.31 **A pregnant woman reports seeing a sticky greenish discharge come from her nipple during a bath. The MOST LIKELY cause of this discharge is:**
   a. Intraductal papilloma
   b. Breast abscess
   c. Infected Montgomery tubercle
   d. Mammary duct ectasia

1.32 **A pregnant woman with many allergies asks about infant feeding. Your BEST response is:**

a. A baby is never allergic to his mother's milk, but he may be sensitive to foods in the mother's diet.

b. Because many allergic tendencies are inherited, there is nothing you can do to reduce your baby's chances of being allergic.

c. The hypoallergenic formulas will prevent any allergic reaction in your baby.

d. Whether or not you breastfeed, you should delay solid foods until 6 months or later to help your baby avoid allergies.

1.33 **A pregnant woman is hesitant to breastfeed because she has heard that she needs to eat a high-calorie, nutrient-rich diet during lactation. Your BEST response is to:**

a. inform her that women living under a wide variety of circumstances are capable of fully nourishing their infants by breastfeeding.

b. refer her to a supplemental food program to ensure adequate nutrient intake.

c. provide her with a multivitamin-and-mineral supplement.

d. discourage her from breastfeeding, as her current circumstances make it doubtful that she is eating adequately.

1.34 **A 4-year-old girl was hurt in an auto accident, and as part of her treatment, a chest tube was placed between her ribs below and distal to her right nipple. What is the MOST SIGNIFICANT effect that this surgery might have on her future ability to breastfeed?**

a. Damage to the ductal structure

b. Damage to the blood vessels supplying the breast

c. Severed nerve pathways to the nipple

d. Cut blood vessels to the breast

1.35 **Which structure supports the breast on the chest wall?**

a. Bandl's fibers

b. Cooper's ligaments

c. Mammary ligaments

d. Myoepithelial tissue

1.36 **The MOST IMPORTANT action in helping this mother breastfeed is to:**

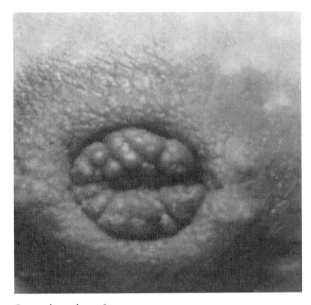

See color plate 6.

Courtesy of K. Jean Cotterman.

a. Put the baby on her bare chest, skin-to-skin, immediately after birth for at least an hour or until after the first feed.

b. Recommend that she wear breast shells for several hours every day during the last trimester.

c. Teach her how to hand-express her milk and use a breast pump until her baby can latch directly.

d. Refer the mother to her primary provider to investigate the nipple configuration for pathology.

1.37 **A pregnant woman had surgery to drain a breast abscess during a previous lactation and asks about consequences to breastfeeding this time. Which aspect of the surgery is MOST LIKELY to negatively affect breastfeeding?**
   a. The circumstances leading up to the abscess
   b. How long ago the surgery was performed
   c. Location of the incision relative to milk ducts and nerves
   d. Stage of lactation when the surgery was done

1.38 **Which fetal structure may remain open or be reopened by excessive infant crying?**
   a. Ductus venosus
   b. Ductus arteriosus
   c. Foramen ovale
   d. Portal sinus

1.39 **A breastfeeding mother is also pregnant. She asks what it takes to "eat for three" while she's pregnant. Which of the following is the best response by a lactation consultant (LC)?**
   a. You need to wean; breastfeeding while pregnant will rob the fetus of needed nutrients.
   b. Check with a nutrition professional for specific recommendations.
   c. Make sure you are gaining weight within the same parameters as if you were pregnant and not breastfeeding.
   d. Do you ordinarily have special dietary needs (for example, do you avoid dairy, causing you to need alternative sources of calcium)?

1.40 **This pregnant and breastfeeding mother calls and complains of tender nipples and lower milk supply. Your BEST response is:**

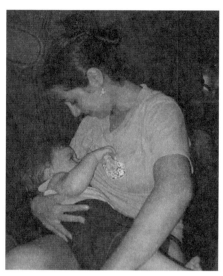

Courtesy of Sarah Hung.

   a. It's best if you start weaning your daughter; she's nursed long enough already.
   b. See your primary care provider about the sudden-onset nipple pain – it might be thrush.
   c. Drink fenugreek tea to increase your milk supply.
   d. What you are experiencing is common for women who are pregnant and still breastfeeding.

1.41 **Which is the MOST APPROPRIATE suggestion for a pregnant woman concerned about eating well enough for her own body growth and her developing baby?**
   a. Take prenatal vitamins every day.
   b. Eat fruits, vegetables, and protein-rich food 5 times a day.
   c. Plan your meals and snacks so you eat every few hours.
   d. Plan to gain 25 to 35 pounds (11.4 to 15.9 kg) by the end of your pregnancy.

1.42 **During pregnancy, which characteristic of the breasts is MOST RELEVANT to lactation capacity?**
  a. Breast growth (size change) during pregnancy
  b. That one breast is markedly different in size from the other
  c. That colostrum can be expressed from the breasts
  d. Tubular shape of the breasts

1.43 **A pregnant woman and the baby's father both have many allergies. She asks whether there is anything she can do to reduce her child's risks of allergic disease. Your BEST response is:**
  a. Avoid common allergens such as cow's milk during your pregnancy.
  b. Exclusively breastfeed for at least 6 months.
  c. Continue breastfeeding to at least 24 months or longer if your child is willing.
  d. Take steroid medications to strengthen your immune system.

1.44 **A breastfeeding mother is also pregnant. She is worried about her bones being depleted of calcium due to the overlap. Which of the following is the MOST APPROPRIATE response by the LC?**
  a. The added burden of pregnancy overlapping with breastfeeding requires an extra 400 mg of calcium a day.
  b. Women aged 19 to 50 need the same amount of calcium regardless of whether they are breastfeeding or pregnant.
  c. An overlap of breastfeeding and pregnancy actually triggers accretion of bone mineral.
  d. You will want to focus on bioavailable calcium sources such as calcium-fortified water and orange juice.

1.45 **A pregnant woman has gestational diabetes. She can reduce her risk of developing type 2 diabetes if she breastfeeds for how long?**
  a. At least 3 months
  b. At least 6 months
  c. At least 12 months
  d. Breastfeeding does not change the risk.

1.46 **Which of the following statements BEST describes fetal nutrition?**
  a. The umbilical cord delivers nutrients directly to the fetal gut.
  b. The fetus swallows and digests amniotic fluid.
  c. The fetus absorbs nutrients from the amniotic fluid through his skin.
  d. The fetus has no digestive enzymes of his own until after 40 weeks.

1.47 **A pregnant mother is HIV positive but otherwise healthy. Breastfeeding is expected in her culture and her family and is her personal strong desire. The FIRST thing you should do is:**
  a. Tell her breastfeeding is contraindicated for HIV-positive mothers.
  b. Tell her breastfeeding is safe for the first 6 weeks only.
  c. Have her talk to her primary care provider and abide by that decision.
  d. Share research results and recommendations of the World Health Organization (WHO) and UNICEF.

1.48 **Which of the following behaviors suggests a woman is having difficulty moving through the normal developmental tasks of pregnancy?**
  a. Wearing maternity clothing in her second trimester
  b. Choosing possible baby names
  c. Discontinuing smoking and consumption of alcohol
  d. Waiting until the third trimester to tell family members of her pregnancy

1.49 **A breastfeeding mother who is 40 years old is also pregnant. She is worried about her bones being depleted of calcium due to the overlap. What is the most helpful response?**

    a. Make sure you are getting the same amount of calcium recommended for adult women.

    b. The more calcium in your diet, the lower is your risk of osteoporosis later in life.

    c. Even with increased dietary calcium, overlapping breastfeeding and pregnancy is likely to result in a long-term loss of bone mineral density.

    d. Focus on plant sources of calcium, like oranges and kale, and reduce your intake of dairy products.

1.50 **A pregnant woman tells you she intends to exclusively pump and bottle-feed. Your FIRST response should be to:**

    a. provide information about effectively pumping to produce an adequate milk supply.

    b. acknowledge her desire to provide good nutrition for her baby.

    c. caution her about how time-consuming this plan can be.

    d. explain the increased risks of her baby needing speech therapy or orthodontia because he was bottlefed.

1.51 **This mother is concerned about breastfeeding her second baby. Her first baby had jaundice and did not thrive until supplements were given. From the picture shown, your FIRST line of inquiry would be:**

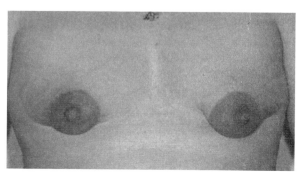

Courtesy of Carole Dobrich.

    a. breast changes during pregnancy.

    b. length of gestation.

    c. age at her first menstrual period.

    d. history of breastfeeding failure in female relatives.

1.52 **A mother asks you to help her write a birth plan that will optimize her success with breastfeeding. Which of the following strategies maximizes achievement of her own birth goals?**

    a. Place of birth where she feels safest

    b. Choice of companions and family members

    c. Access to furniture, hot tub, and equipment that encourages motion and posture changes

    d. Professional attendant who will direct her actions during labor

1.53 **You are conducting a prenatal breastfeeding examination of a mother during her third trimester of pregnancy. Her breasts appear to be small and firm with no visible blue veins on the surface. What is the BEST statement to document your observations?**

    a. Small and perky

    b. Insufficient glandular tissue

    c. Tanner stage 3

    d. Normal development

1.54 **This mother calls you to find a solution for sudden and persistent sore nipples that have not responded to standard remedies. She had a menstrual period 10 weeks ago but has not had once since. Your FIRST comment should be:**

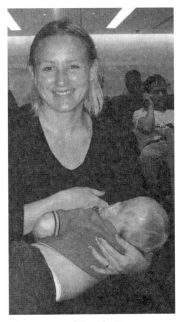

Courtesy of Sarah Hung.

a. You will need to wean your toddler because continued breastfeeding might cause a miscarriage.

b. The tenderness is probably because of pregnancy hormones. How much of a problem is this for you?

c. Is your toddler teething? His saliva may be irritating to your nipples now.

d. Have you or he recently taken an antibiotic?

1.55 **Pregnant vegan mothers would need to supplement their plant foods–only diet by taking:**

a. Vitamin B_{12}

b. Calcium

c. Fat-soluble vitamins (A, D, E, and K)

d. Iron

Answers for Prenatal Questions

1.1 **The answer is b.** Unless the pregnancy is very high risk, there is no documented harm to either the fetus or the older child by continuing to breastfeed. Nipple pain during a subsequent pregnancy is hormonally based and may be unavoidable. (Difficulty: 4; Discipline: Physiology; Taxonomy: Goals)

1.2 **The answer is a.** Supporting the mother's decision to explore the reasons for her previous unsuccessful breastfeeding experience is the best FIRST response, because that technique helps build her confidence. After an empathetic response, providing a problem-solving answer would be appropriate. (Difficulty: 4; Discipline: Clinical Skills; Taxonomy: Goals)

1.3 **The answer is b.** The Hawthorne effect means that observing a population for a specific behavior change often produces the desired change, independent of the intervention being studied. (Difficulty: 2; Discipline: Clinical Skills; Taxonomy: Evaluate)

1.4 **The answer is d.** Self-attachment and skin-to-skin contact are now known to be successful and effective strategies for helping babies and mothers achieve comfortable and effective breastfeeding, even when the mother's nipple is flat. Choice a may help a little. Choice b is irrelevant and an outdated idea. Choice d is an inappropriate use of a nipple shield for the condition shown in the photograph. (Difficulty: 4; Discipline: Techniques; Taxonomy: Plan)

1.5 **The answer is a.** A healthy maternal diet during pregnancy significantly reduces the incidence of low-birth-weight infants. Diet may have a relationship to the development of gestational diabetes. Maternal diet does not directly affect infants with diabetes or lactation failure. (Difficulty: 3; Discipline: Clinical Skills; Taxonomy: History)

1.6 **The answer is b.** Open-ended questions are the most supportive statements and are designed to explore the mother's preconceived ideas about breastfeeding. (Difficulty: 3; Discipline: Clinical Skills; Taxonomy: Collaboration)

1.7 **The answer is b.** The child's facial appearance, slow growth, and feeding difficulties are common manifestations of fetal alcohol spectrum disorder (FASD) (fetal alcohol syndrome [FAS]), so a request for a full pediatric evaluation should be made. High fever during pregnancy, radon or ground radiation, and toxoplasmosis transmitted from cat feces can also cause birth defects. The pattern of facial characteristics in this situation is most due to FASD/FAS. (Difficulty: 3; Discipline: Pathology; Taxonomy: Assessment)

1.8 **The answer is d.** Lactocytes (mammary secretory cells, also called glandular tissue) develop on the basement membrane of the duct structure starting during pregnancy. Growth continues for several weeks post-birth. (Difficulty: 5; Discipline: Development; Taxonomy: Knowledge)

1.9 **The answer is a.** Teaching her how to position her baby for breastfeeding is the most important action. Her nipples are not retracted, so choices b and c are incorrect. Rubbing the skin with rough fabric is inappropriate and can damage areolar structures. (Difficulty: 4; Discipline: Clinical Skills; Taxonomy: Goals)

1.10 **The answer is d.** Immediate skin-to-skin and infant self-attachment ensure an effective start to breastfeeding for the vast majority of mother–baby dyads, even when the nipple is flat. Choice a might be useful; choice b will help as well. Vigorous pulling and stretching have not been shown to improve breastfeeding success for mothers with flat nipples and can actually damage tissue. (Difficulty: 4; Discipline: Techniques; Taxonomy: Plan)

1.11 **The answer is a.** A well-balanced, nutritious diet with sufficient protein may prevent or reduce risk of pregnancy-related hypertension. The other dietary strategies are unlikely to be effective. (Difficulty: 3; Discipline: Development; Taxonomy: Collaboration)

1.12 **The answer is d.** No assumptions can be made about her ability to breastfeed after breast surgery, although she should be followed closely in the first week postbirth because surgery can disrupt ducts and nerve pathways needed for adequate milk synthesis. (Difficulty: 3; Discipline: Development; Taxonomy: Goals)

1.13 **The answer is d.** The most common implantation site is the posterior side of the fundus. This is relevant to breastfeeding because placental implantation affects fetal maturity, position for delivery, and complications during labor including possible cesarean surgery, all of which affect the mother's and baby's ability to breastfeed. (Difficulty: 3; Discipline: Physiology; Taxonomy: History)

1.14 **The answer is c.** Gradual weight loss preserves health and energy. About 500 calories per day are used in making milk. (Difficulty: 4; Discipline: Development; Taxonomy: Goals)

1.15 **The answer is c.** She is attempting to pull the nipple tip outward or forward. This is not an effective motion to express colostrum. (Difficulty: 4; Discipline: Techniques; Taxonomy: Assessment)

1.16 **The answer is d.** No change in breast size during pregnancy can indicate suppressed development of lactocytes (milk-making cells), appearing as breast hypoplasia. Secreted colostrum may not appear at the nipple until after birth, when oxytocin levels are high. Nipple shape and protractility often change in pregnancy. Pigmentation changes of the nipple and areola have not been researched related to lactation. (Difficulty: 4; Discipline: Development; Taxonomy: History)

1.17 **The answer is b.** A retained placental fragment is the most likely factor associated with delayed onset of lactogenesis. Cesarean surgery may also delay the onset of lactogenesis. (Difficulty: 3; Discipline: Pathology; Taxonomy: History)

1.18 **The answer is b.** Brain growth in infants is the most common concern when mother is taking any psychoactive medication, and antiseizure medications are considered compatible with breastfeeding. Choice a is incorrect because information was requested, not an opinion, even if the neurologist's opinion is consistent with evidence. Choice c is inappropriate because implying feeling is not providing information. Choice d is accurate but less supportive than choice b. (Difficulty: 4; Discipline: Clinical Skills; Taxonomy: Collaboration)

1.19 **The answer is c.** Growth of the secretory epithelial cells (lactocytes) is the primary factor causing breast growth during pregnancy. (Difficulty: 5; Discipline: Development; Taxonomy: Knowledge)

1.20 **The answer is a.** Reflux may be caused by an esophageal defect at the upper sphincter, where the esophagus meets the stomach. (Difficulty: 2; Discipline: Pathology; Taxonomy: Knowledge)

1.21 **The answer is b.** This woman's breasts are large and pendulous; the right nipple appears inverted. The amount of glandular tissue cannot be determined by visual examination alone. "Saggy" is not an appropriate term. Her visible areola is darker than the surrounding skin, as would be expected in a pregnant woman. (Difficulty: 4; Discipline: Clinical Skills; Taxonomy: Document)

1.22 **The answer is d.** Babies who are breastfed have a reduced risk of both type 1 and type 2 diabetes. Mothers with diabetes often have improved blood sugar levels and need less insulin during lactation. Mothers with type 1 diabetes can have low blood sugar while breastfeeding; they should monitor their blood sugar levels closely and may need to eat a snack before breastfeeding. (Difficulty: 4; Discipline: Physiology; Taxonomy: Plan)

1.23 **The answer is b.** Immediate and uninterrupted skin-to-skin contact and early breastfeeding are the most important actions when a mother has flat nipples or, for that matter, for all mothers. Prenatal "nipple preparation" has not been shown to significantly improve flat nipples. (Difficulty: 3; Discipline: Pathology; Taxonomy: Plan)

1.24 **The answer is b.** Breastfeeding can and should be taught in a group setting and with one-to-one instruction. Formula feeding should be taught individually only to those mothers who will not breastfeed for various reasons. (Difficulty: 2; Discipline: Clinical Skills; Taxonomy: Plan)

1.25 **The answer is d.** This appears to be a normal breast. The person in the photograph is near the end of her pregnancy. (Difficulty: 4; Discipline: Development; Taxonomy: Goals)

1.26 **The answer is b.** A vegan diet includes no animal sources and thus is deficient in vitamin B_{12}. A supplement taken by the mother will provide adequate B_{12} to the baby through her milk. Ensuring adequate maternal nutrition, especially the B vitamin complex, is an important part of prenatal care and can affect B vitamin levels in mother's milk. (Difficulty: 4; Discipline: Development; Taxonomy: Plan)

1.27 **The answer is b.** Bereavement milk is most likely to be used for research purposes. Occasionally it may be pasteurized and used for lower-risk babies or adults. Bereavement milk is usually not given to the most vulnerable newborns because the mothers were not screened before donating. (Difficulty: 4; Discipline: Clinical Skills; Taxonomy: Collaboration)

1.28 **The answer is a.** This rare condition is pregnancy-related keratosis, a thickening of the skin of the nipple. Evaluation by a credentialed provider is the only reasonable option, since this condition does not look like any lactation-related condition that would fall into a LC's scope of practice to manage. (Difficulty: 2; Discipline: Pathology; Taxonomy: Collaboration)

1.29 **The answer is d.** Placental lactogen is the most important lactogenic hormone, deriving from the placenta. In induced lactation, it cannot be provided artificially. The other key lactogenic hormones can be provided with medications. (Difficulty: 3; Discipline: Physiology; Taxonomy: History)

1.30 **The answer is b.** Each pregnancy develops more lactocytes. Hormonal stimulation during menstruation recanalizes milk ducts following surgery. Choices a and b are incorrect because the surgery is a risk factor for milk production. (Difficulty: 4; Discipline: Pathology; Taxonomy: Evaluate)

1.31 The answer is d. Mammary duct ectasia is the most likely cause of nipple discharge in pregnancy. The other conditions do not cause greenish discharge. Her primary provider should be notified, although this is usually a benign occurrence during pregnancy. (Difficulty: 4; Discipline: Pathology; Taxonomy: Knowledge)

1.32 The answer is a. Exclusive breastfeeding for about 6 months is the best strategy to reduce the baby's risk. The mother's avoidance of known allergens during pregnancy may also reduce the baby's risks of allergy. It is more important that the mother exclusively breastfeed for about 6 months than other actions she should be considering at this time. Delaying solid foods does not address the baby's more likely early exposure to cow's milk and soy proteins, which are very common allergens in humans. (Difficulty: 3; Discipline: Pathology; Taxonomy: Knowledge)

1.33 The answer is a. A well-balanced diet with adequate calories is important for the mother's overall health. Most milk components are not substantially related to the mother's dietary intake. (Difficulty: 4; Discipline: Development; Taxonomy: Goals)

1.34 The answer is c. Severing nerve pathways would be the worst consequence for lactation. The fourth intercostal nerve has a major role in lactation, and is located approximately where the tube was placed. (Difficulty: 5; Discipline: Development; Taxonomy: History)

1.35 The answer is b. Cooper's ligaments support the breasts. Softening or stretching of these ligaments during pregnancy may contribute to sagging as the woman ages. (Difficulty: 3; Discipline: Development; Taxonomy: Knowledge)

1.36 The answer is a. Research has confirmed that most babies will move to the breast and begin breastfeeding within about an hour of birth, regardless of the mother's nipple structure and configuration. Breast shells have not been consistently helpful with retracted or inverted nipples. Choices c and d are incorrect because there is no obvious indication that the baby will have difficulty breastfeeding from this mother's nipple/breast. (Difficulty: 4; Discipline: Development; Taxonomy: Plan)

1.37 The answer is c. The location of the incision is most likely to affect lactation. Incisions that sever the fourth intercostal nerve or many milk ducts are more likely to negatively affect subsequent lactation than are incisions elsewhere in the breast. (Difficulty: 3; Discipline: Development; Taxonomy: History)

1.38 The answer is c. The foramen ovale may remain open or be reopened by excessive infant crying, which produces a Valsalva effect and increases thoracic pressure. This can have significant negative long-term consequences for the person later in life. (Difficulty: 5; Discipline: Development; Taxonomy: Knowledge)

1.39 The answer is c. If a mother is gaining weight within healthy parameters, there is no reason to think that breastfeeding is taking away from the fetus. Choices c and d are appropriate for helping her assess her specific needs. (Difficulty: 4; Discipline: Physiology; Taxonomy: History)

1.40 The answer is d. The LC should help the mother clarify her feelings about continuing to breastfeed and support her decision. The other responses are not appropriate. (Difficulty: 3; Discipline: Clinical Skills; Taxonomy: Plan)

1.41 **The answer is d.** Current recommendations are for pregnant women of normal prepregnancy weight to gain 25 to 35 pounds (11 to 16 kg) during pregnancy. Underweight women and teenagers should gain even more weight to sustain their growing bodies and the developing fetus. (Difficulty: 3; Discipline: Development; Taxonomy: Plan)

1.42 **The answer is a.** Breast growth (size change) indicates the growth of glandular secretory tissue. Growth patterns may vary widely and still be within normal ranges. Different sized breasts are common; expression of colostrum during pregnancy is not expected; and breast shape is rarely relevant to lactation capacity. (Difficulty: 3; Discipline: Development; Taxonomy: Knowledge)

1.43 **The answer is b.** Exclusive breastfeeding is the most effective strategy for reducing the risk of allergic disease. There is evidence supporting choices a and c. Steroids do not reduce the infant's risk of allergy and have other consequences. (Difficulty: 4; Discipline: Pathology; Taxonomy: Goals)

1.44 **The answer is b.** During pregnancy, the body acquires the needed calcium through enhanced uptake. During lactation, calcium taken from the bones is replaced afterwards with no net decrease. Vitamin D aids calcium absorption, so assuring adequate vitamin D may be as important as calcium intake. (Difficulty: 4; Discipline: Physiology; Taxonomy: Plan)

1.45 **The answer is a.** For pregnant women with gestational diabetes, breastfeeding at least 3 months reduces the risk of developing type 2 diabetes. (Difficulty: 4; Discipline: Pathology; Taxonomy: Knowledge)

1.46 **The answer is b.** Amniotic fluid provides protein and other nutrients to the fetus in addition to nutrients present in the cord blood vessels. (Difficulty: 3; Discipline: Development; Taxonomy: History)

1.47 **The answer is d.** WHO, UNICEF, and other authorities support providing the mother with confidential and individualized information to help her make a fully informed decision regarding feeding her baby. The LC's role is to assist the primary care physician and mother by providing appropriate research and other literature on the topic. (Difficulty: 5; Discipline: Clinical Skills; Taxonomy: Assessment)

1.48 **The answer is d.** Telling others of her pregnancy is an early developmental task. Failure to reveal her pregnancy suggests lack of acceptance of the fetus. (Difficulty: 2; Discipline: Psychology; Taxonomy: Collaboration)

1.49 **The answer is a.** Women over the age of 25 need the same amount of calcium regardless of breastfeeding or pregnancy status, and research suggests the same is true for women who are overlapping breastfeeding with pregnancy and tandem nursing mothers. During pregnancy, even for malnourished mothers, extra calcium is excreted with the urine; instead, the body acquires the needed calcium through intrinsic processes such as enhanced uptake. During the exclusive breastfeeding phase, bone mineral density typically dips and then begins to rebound once complementary foods are added to the baby's diet. A study that included a tandem nursing mother showed the same results for her as for other breastfeeding mothers. Research has shown that when breastfeeding and pregnancy overlap, the bones actually "increase" in bone mineral density. Dairy sources of calcium are the most bioavailable. (Difficulty: 5; Discipline: Physiology; Taxonomy: Goals)

1.50 **The answer is b.** Although the mother will need information on effective pumping, she will be most likely to learn the information if she first feels validated for her efforts. Information about risks to baby or disadvantages for mother is unlikely to cause her to change her mind if she does not feel her decision has been accepted. (Difficulty: 4; Discipline: Clinical Skills; Taxonomy: Goals)

1.51 **The answer is a.** This mother's breasts are mildly hypoplastic or underdeveloped and asymmetrical. Both conditions have been linked to limited lactation capacity in some women. (Difficulty: 4; Discipline: Clinical Skills; Taxonomy: History)

1.52 **The answer is b.** Having a companion of the laboring woman's choice has the strongest evidence of positive maternal and infant outcomes. Choices a and c are also effective strategies. The laboring woman is disempowered when others direct her actions during labor. The "take-charge" attitude of the attendant puts her into a passive role, which has been shown to interfere with breastfeeding. (Difficulty: 4; Discipline: Psychology; Taxonomy: Goals)

1.53 **The answer is c.** Tanner described five phases in breast development from puberty until age 15 to 17 years. Stage 3 describes the female breast between the onset of puberty and before the first pregnancy. (Difficulty: 4; Discipline: Development; Taxonomy: Document)

1.54 **The answer is b.** Many mothers experience tender nipples if they become pregnant while breastfeeding. The tenderness is related to high levels of pregnancy hormones and does not respond to the usual remedies. (Difficulty: 3; Discipline: Physiology; Taxonomy: Evaluate)

1.55 **The answer is a.** Women who eat no animal products need a dietary source of vitamin B_{12}. The other nutrients listed can be obtained from plant foods. (Difficulty: 5; Discipline: Development; Taxonomy: Collaboration)

CHAPTER 2

Labor and Birth Questions

2.1 According to the Baby-Friendly Hospital Initiative (BFHI), when will the behavior shown in the image MOST LIKELY occur?

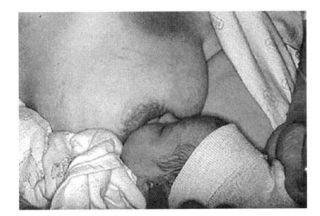

a. Less than 5 minutes after birth
b. Within the first hour after birth
c. Within 6 hours after birth
d. Within 12 hours after birth

2.2 Which hormone is especially high in this mother–baby dyad immediately postbirth?

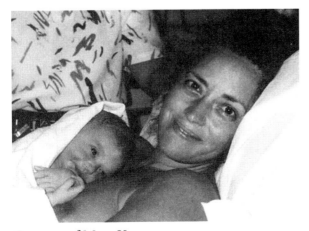

Courtesy of Mary Kroeger.

a. Adrenaline
b. Oxytocin
c. Estrogen
d. Prolactin

2.3 Which conclusion can accurately be drawn from the data presented in this graph?

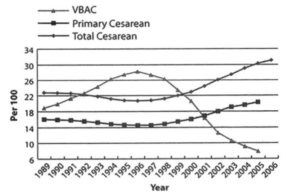

Total cesarean, primary cesarean and vaginal birth after cesarean rates, United States, 1983-2006

Centers for Disease Control and Prevention.

a. The total cesarean rate is increasing faster than the primary cesarean rate.
b. Fear of malpractice lawsuits between 1995 and 1998 changed obstetric practices.
c. More mothers are asking for cesarean delivery instead of going through labor.
d. Vaginal birth after cesarean is more dangerous than a repeat cesarean.

2.4 **Which position for laboring women is MOST LIKELY to reduce blood flow to the uterus and negatively affect the baby's well-being?**

a. Sitting

b. Lying on the left side

c. Lying supine

d. Lying on the right side

2.5 **When a mother is giving birth to twins, which is the MOST LIKELY reason that the second baby might have a problem initiating breastfeeding?**

a. There is a higher likelihood of prolapsed cord.

b. The second baby has longer exposure to labor medications.

c. The mother is busy with the firstborn twin.

d. The second baby is usually the smaller of the two.

2.6 **What would you recommend to this mother to improve initial breastfeeding?**

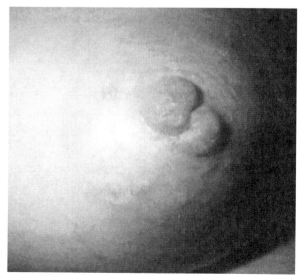

Courtesy of K. Jean Cotterman.

a. Have your baby placed skin-to-skin on your chest immediately after birth.

b. Avoid all labor pain–relief medications including an epidural.

c. Drink several glasses of water every day to keep your skin hydrated.

d. Place a silicon nipple shield over your nipple so baby can latch deeply.

2.7 **Which of the following effects are MOST LIKELY to occur following administration of epidural narcotic drugs given to the laboring woman?**

a. Delayed onset of lactogenesis

b. Longer second stage of labor

c. Increased risk of cesarean birth

d. Increased risk for forceps or vacuum-assisted birth

2.8 **What is the MOST LIKELY outcome from the kind of care being given to this laboring woman?**

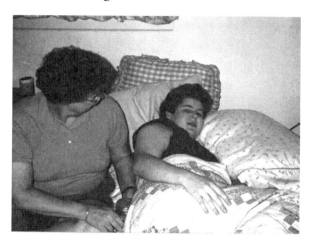

a. Reduced involvement by her husband (partner)

b. Longer duration of breastfeeding

c. Higher risk of poor infant outcomes

d. Shorter postpartum bleeding (lochia)

2.9 Which medication given to this mother a few hours ago is MOST LIKELY to inhibit her baby's initiation of breastfeeding?

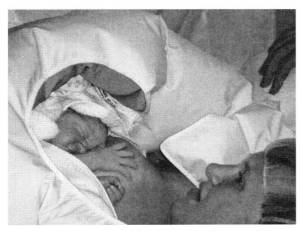

Courtesy of Erika Nehlsen.

    a. Dextrose given intravenously
    b. Nitrous oxide given via mask
    c. Pitocin given intravenously
    d. Fentanyl given via an epidural

2.10 This baby was born about 10 minutes ago. What is the FIRST THING you would say to this mother?

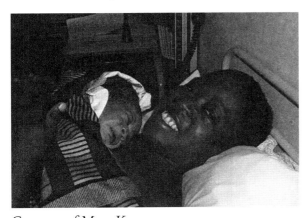

Courtesy of Mary Kroeger.

    a. You and your baby look so comfortable and happy!
    b. When she's ready, I can help you get started with breastfeeding.
    c. We'll give the baby a bath before you try breastfeeding.
    d. Aren't you going to let your partner hold the baby, too?

2.11 Which of the following practices is the MOST APPROPRIATE action professionals should take in the hospital labor and delivery (birthing) area?

    a. Make sure the baby can take formula by bottle before attempting to breastfeed.
    b. Read the hospital policies to the mother before she is admitted in labor.
    c. Deep suction the baby before feeding with oral fluids including breastmilk or colostrum.
    d. Give the baby only the mother's own milk or colostrum unless medically indicated.

2.12 How soon after birth should this activity take place, for a birth facility to comply with BFHI guidelines?

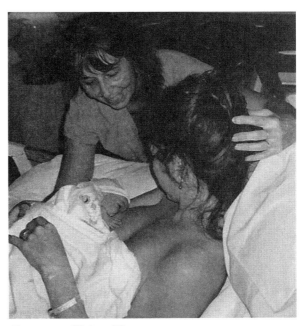

Courtesy of Mary Kroeger.

    a. After the baby has been transitioned in the newborn nursery
    b. After the baby has been examined by a physician or midwife
    c. Within the first few minutes after birth, before any procedures are done
    d. After the baby has been bathed, weighed, and measured

2.13   **The drugs used in this procedure are MOST LIKELY to have which effect on the newborn?**

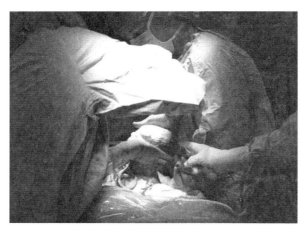

Courtesy of Marilyn Hildreth.

a. Fewer spontaneous kneading movements on mother's chest
b. Depressed respiration in the first 5 minutes postbirth
c. No effect on the infant
d. Transient bradycardia

2.14   **A baby is having difficulty sucking after a long, difficult labor. Which drug administered during labor is MOST LIKELY to cause breastfeeding problems in the baby?**

a. Generic nalbuphine (Nubain)
b. Generic fentanyl (Sublimaze)
c. Generic butorphanol (Stadol)
d. Generic lidocaine (Polocaine)

2.15   **A mother in your prenatal class asks about the impact of labor pain–relieving medications on the baby. What is your BEST response?**

a. Inhaled medications have very little effect on the baby.
b. All pain-relieving drugs affect the baby's breastfeeding-related behavior.
c. The effect of labor pain–relieving drugs on the baby wears off quickly.
d. Epidural anesthetics have no effect on the baby.

2.16   **Which of the following maternal perinatal factors is MOST LIKELY to interfere with initiation of breastfeeding?**

a. Cesarean surgery
b. Magnesium sulfate administered during labor
c. Intravenous hydration during labor
d. History of failed breastfeeding in previous pregnancy

2.17   **A woman received intravenous fluids throughout her long labor. The next day, she says that her breasts are swollen and tender, and her baby is having trouble latching onto her breast. The MOST LIKELY explanation for this is that:**

a. Her breasts are edematous from the intravenous fluids.
b. Her baby is tired from the long labor.
c. Her milk tastes unpleasant because of the fluids given.
d. The fluids diluted the amount of colostrum available, and the baby is frustrated.

2.18   **Which of the following conditions of labor is MOST LIKELY to delay the onset of lactogenesis II (copious milk production)?**

a. Very rapid labor
b. Delivery before 37-weeks'-gestation
c. Long, difficult labor
d. Vomiting during labor

2.19 You are caring for this mother and baby. The baby is 4 hours old and breastfed well about 1 hour after birth. On entering this mother's room, the FIRST THING you should do is:

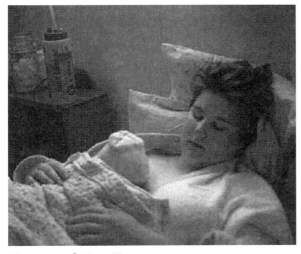

Courtesy of Mary Kroeger.

   a. Attempt to wake the baby for another feeding.
   b. Check the baby's blood glucose by doing a heel stick.
   c. Quietly observe the mother and baby but do not intervene.
   d. Remove the baby to a crib or cot next to the bed.

2.20 A newborn baby, 6 hours old, is awake and alert but having trouble breastfeeding. Which of the following is the MOST likely cause of his difficulty?
   a. Mother received antibiotic treatment for group B *Streptococcus* during labor.
   b. Mother was given epidural anesthesia 3 hours before birth.
   c. Mother received narcotic analgesia less than 30 minutes before birth.
   d. Mother's labor was stimulated by pitocin (oxytocin) given intravenously.

2.21 Which immunofactor in human milk is at its highest level at this point in time?

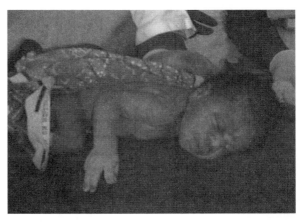

See color plate 7.
Courtesy of Mary Kroeger.

   a. Secretory IgA
   b. Cytokines
   c. Lysozyme
   d. Complement

2.22 To minimize physiologic stress to the infant from this procedure, the BEST strategy would be to:

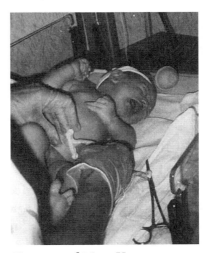

Courtesy of Mary Kroeger.

   a. Warm the room to prevent the infant from becoming chilled.
   b. Delay clamping the cord after it stops pulsing.
   c. Have the mother's partner or helper hold the baby while the cord is clamped.
   d. Perform this procedure while baby is skin-to-skin on mother's body.

2.23 **Pooling or collection of fluid between the skin and cranial bones of the infant's head is called:**

a. caput succedaneum.

b. cephalhematoma.

c. periosteal swelling.

d. hydrocephalus.

2.24 **The likelihood that this mother and baby will enjoy a successful start to breastfeeding is:**

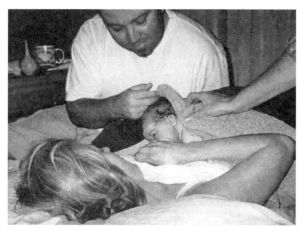

Courtesy of Mary Kroeger.

a. decreased, because new mothers prefer to do for themselves.

b. decreased, because the mother is likely to be confused by so many different people.

c. increased, because many people are supporting the mother.

d. increased, because family members can take over night feedings while she rests.

2.25 **Which prenatal or birth practice is MOST LIKELY to result in higher iron stores for the exclusively breastfed infant's first 6 months?**

a. Mother takes prenatal iron supplements.

b. Delay clamping of the umbilical cord until pulsing stops.

c. Mother eats foods high in iron for the first 6 months.

d. The baby is supplemented with iron-fortified formula.

2.26 **A pregnant woman has heard that letting epidural anesthesia wear off prior to delivery will avoid anesthesia-related breastfeeding problems. Which of the following is the MOST IMPORTANT thing you should tell her?**

a. Drugs can take much longer to clear the baby's system, so there is still possible breastfeeding risk with this approach.

b. The combination of drugs used in epidural anesthesia makes it difficult to determine which medications cause breastfeeding problems.

c. Epidural anesthesia has minimal or no effect on the baby regardless of how long before delivery it is administered.

d. Epidural anesthesia increases the likelihood of other birth interventions that can affect breastfeeding.

2.27 **Your job at a hospital includes determining what items patients are given on discharge. A formula company representative is pressuring you to include their "breastfeeding" bag, which contains samples of powdered formula, coupons for more samples, and pictures that idealize that company's product. What is your BEST course of action?**

a. Accept the bags as generous gifts because some mothers may need the supplement.

b. Accept the bags, but remove the samples and coupons before distributing them.

c. Refuse the bags because giving samples violates BFHI Step 6 and the International Code of Marketing of Breastmilk Substitutes.

d. Accept the bags and a competing company's bags so mothers will have a choice.

2.28 Which birth practice results in the MOST IMMUNE protection for the baby?

a. Cesarean surgery under sterile conditions

b. Lying down with a clean cloth or sheet under the mother's pelvic area

c. Assisting the mother to birth in a supported squatting position

d. Administering an enema to remove any feces from the lower bowel

2.29 This mother has not completed Stage III of her labor. Her baby is healthy. The NEXT action you should take is to:

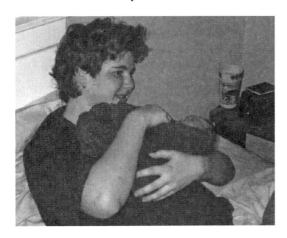

a. get her to a hospital.

b. help the mother put the baby to breast.

c. give her oxygen for her exhaustion.

d. have her assume a supine position.

2.30 A mother was given high doses of pain-relieving drugs during labor. When the baby's cord blood is tested for the presence of drugs, none are found. The MOST LIKELY explanation is that:

a. pain-relieving drugs are lipid soluble and sequester in the infant brain.

b. pain-relieving drugs do not cross the placenta.

c. the mother's body metabolizes most drugs before birth.

d. pain-relieving drugs have a very short half-life.

2.31 After an unmedicated labor and birth, how soon is a baby MOST LIKELY to be able and ready to breastfeed?

a. Within the first 5 minutes

b. Within the first hour

c. At approximately 6 hours

d. By 12 hours

2.32 A mother has recently been diagnosed with gestational diabetes. Following the birth of her infant, which of the following is MOST LIKELY?

a. The infant is more at risk of hypoglycemia and hyperbilirubinemia.

b. Onset of copious milk secretion may be delayed about 24 hours.

c. Breastfeeding may help protect the infant against type 2 diabetes.

d. Lactation will increase the mother's chance of developing adult-onset diabetes.

2.33 During a difficult birth, a baby sustained damage to the hypoglossal nerve. What is the MOST LIKELY effect on breastfeeding? The baby would be:

a. unable to maintain latch at breast.

b. unable to move tongue to collect milk.

c. unable to swallow.

d. unable to grasp breast with mouth/lips.

2.34 A mother required multiple units of blood by transfusion after a difficult birth. By postpartum day 7, her milk has not yet "come in." What is the MOST LIKELY cause of her delayed lactogenesis?

a. Long, difficult labor

b. Sheehan syndrome

c. Separation from her baby

d. She did not start expressing or pumping soon enough.

2.35 **Which part of the infant skull MOST OFTEN presents during birth?**
   a. Occipital bone
   b. Parietal bone
   c. Frontal bone
   d. Sphenoid bone

2.36 **A pregnant woman contracted chicken-pox a short time ago. The lesions are now completely crusted over, and she is in labor. The MOST APPROPRIATE action to take when she gives birth is to:**
   a. separate her from the baby until she is noninfectious.
   b. allow her to hold but not breastfeed her baby.
   c. separate her from the baby but feed her expressed milk to the baby.
   d. help her breastfeed immediately after birth with 24-hour rooming-in.

2.37 **According to the WHO/UNICEF "Ten Steps to Successful Breastfeeding" (BFHI), what should the mother do after giving birth?**
   a. Remain in the hospital with her baby for 48 hours after delivery.
   b. Express colostrum or milk within 6 hours after birth.
   c. Place her baby skin-to-skin immediately after birth.
   d. Keep her premature baby skin-to-skin as many hours as possible.

2.38 **Local perineal injection of an anesthetic drug prior to performing an episiotomy is MOST LIKELY to:**

   a. not affect the infant in any way.
   b. alter the baby's breastfeeding-related behaviors.
   c. suppress the baby's sucking response.
   d. reduce the duration of the second stage of labor.

2.39 **Which is the MOST SIGNIFICANT outcome from using this device?**

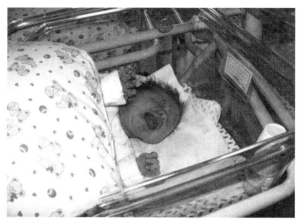

Courtesy of Erika Nehlsen.

   a. Increase in stress hormones in the baby
   b. Neonatal hypothermia
   c. Facilitates thorough examination of infant
   d. Increased infant crying

2.40 **Separating babies from their mothers shortly after birth and caring for them in separate rooms is MOST LIKELY to result in which of the following?**
   a. Improved sleep-wake patterns in infants
   b. Increased infant stress hormones
   c. More rest for the mother
   d. Improved infection control practices

2.41 **Which of these practices MOST SUPPORTS the baby's actions shown in the photograph?**

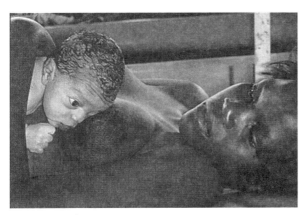

Courtesy of Mary Kroeger.

a. Avoiding washing off the amniotic fluid from baby's hands
b. Bathing the mother immediately so her perspiration does not offend the baby
c. Giving narcotics by epidural during the labor so the mother is pain free at this stage
d. Suctioning the baby to clear his airway of mucus

2.42 **Which action is MOST LIKELY to support the baby's ability to start breastfeeding?**

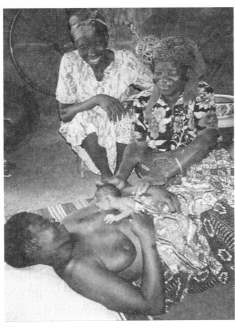

Courtesy of Mary Kroeger.

a. Lift the mother's breast into the baby's mouth.
b. Ask the mother to sit up and bring her baby to breast.
c. Observe the baby while he crawls to the mother's breast.
d. Have the mother compress her breast and tickle the baby's lips.

2.43 **Why is this position for birth beneficial for the newborn's health?**

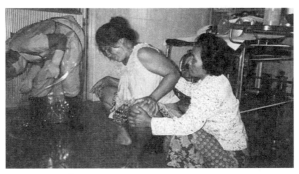

Courtesy of Mary Kroeger.

a. Grandmother can be the first to view the baby, thus enhancing bonding.
b. Attendant cannot pull on the newborn's head, thus avoiding head and neck trauma.
c. Mother can lift the baby out of her body herself, thus empowering her.
d. Baby is exposed to mother's normal gut flora in her feces, thus colonizing with beneficial bacteria.

2.44 **A mother's psychological and emotional reactions to birth are MOST LIKELY to be affected by:**
a. the mother's age and marital status.
b. whether this pregnancy was planned.
c. how she was treated and nurtured during labor.
d. the temperament and health of her baby.

2.45 **Which medication given to a laboring woman is MOST LIKELY related to newborn sucking problems?**

a. Magnesium sulfate
b. Fentanyl
c. Propofol
d. Penicillin

2.46 **During the first 24 hours, about how much fluid volume of colostrum does the average normal newborn consume per breastfeeding session?**

a. 90 mL (3 oz)
b. 60 mL (2 oz)
c. 30 mL (1 oz)
d. 7 mL (0.2 oz)

2.47 **What is the MOST LIKELY consequence of a cesarean birth to the breastfeeding mother–baby dyad?**

a. Less postpartum bleeding for mother
b. Need for maternal pain medications
c. Early onset of lactogenesis II
d. More separation of mother and infant

2.48 **Which statement regarding the timing of lactogenesis II is MOST ACCURATE?**

a. It begins 30 to 40 hours after delivery of the placenta.
b. It may initially go unnoticed by mother.
c. It may be delayed 36 to 48 hours if mother has diabetes.
d. Timing is dependent on breast stimulation by the baby.

2.49 **Why would you want to discourage this practice in the first few hours postbirth?**

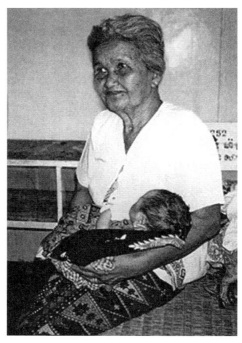

Courtesy of Mary Kroeger.

a. The grandmother might drop the baby or fail to support its head sufficiently.
b. The clothing used to wrap the baby may be unclean or unsterile, risking an infection.
c. It is more important that the baby's father and grandfather be the first to hold the baby.
d. The grandmother's bacterial flora is foreign to the baby and prevents colonization with the mother's flora.

2.50 **A pregnant women asks about the effect of epidural drugs on the mode of birth, because she wants to hold her baby and breastfeed immediately afterward. Which of these statements is MOST ACCURATE?**

a. There is no known relationship between epidural medications and mode of delivery.
b. Epidural drugs increase the risk of emergency cesarean surgery.
c. The epidural will help you relax and have a natural (unassisted) birth.
d. Your labor will be shorter and easier if you have epidural medication,

2.51 Compared with mature milk, colostrum is higher in:
   a. lactose.
   b. immunofactors.
   c. volume.
   d. hormones.

2.52 A woman in the active phase of labor complains of a severe backache. This is MOST LIKELY caused by:
   a. a weak back due to lack of exercise.
   b. a herniated disk in the lumbar spine.
   c. the fetus being in an occiput posterior presentation.
   d. tetanic contraction of uterus.

2.53 What is the MOST IMPORTANT reason to support a mother using an upright position to birth?
   a. Her feces will colonize her baby with normal beneficial bacterial flora.
   b. Her milk will change from colostrum to mature milk sooner.
   c. Her support person will be able to hold the baby immediately.
   d. The baby will rotate to an easier position for birth.

2.54 Which birth practice is MOST LIKELY to negatively affect the initiation of breastfeeding?
   a. Malpresentation
   b. Breech birth
   c. Cesarean surgery
   d. Induction of labor

2.55 Which feature of a mother's birth plan is MOST LIKELY to optimize breastfeeding success?
   a. Birth takes place in a major hospital.
   b. Mother has a supportive companion of her choice.
   c. Mother may move around freely during the first stage of labor.
   d. Medications for pain relief are available early in labor.

2.56 Twelve-hour-old Rose was born after 15 hours of hard labor and pushing, with forceps and vacuum extractor, deep suctioned for meconium above the cords, and molded cranium and puncture mark from an internal monitor probe. Her mother is anxious to bond and breastfeed within the first hour after delivery. Your FIRST intervention should be to:
   a. bring Rose horizontally to her mother's breast level.
   b. rub Rose's face with a cold washcloth.
   c. pull Rose's chin down for a latch-on.
   d. place Rose skin-to-skin with her mother and turn down the lights.

2.57 You are assisting this family during the mother's labor and birth. To fully implement Step 4 of the BFHI, what is the NEXT action that should be taken by the medical staff?

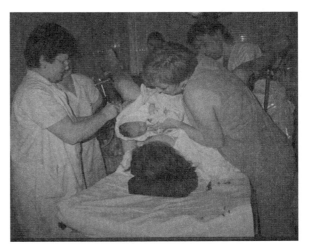

Courtesy of Erika Nehlsen.

   a. The wrapped baby should be placed in the father's arms.
   b. The baby should be unwrapped and placed on mother's bare chest.
   c. The baby should be moved to the radiant warmer wearing a hat and blanket.
   d. The staff should hold the baby until the mother is in the recovery area.

2.58 **If you were assisting this family during the baby's birth, what is the next MOST IMPORTANT action you should take?**

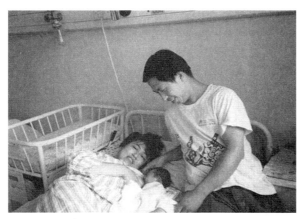

Courtesy of Mary Kroeger.

a. Remove the baby if the mother starts to fall asleep.

b. Ask the man to hold the baby so the mother can wash up.

c. Suggest that the professional attendant move the baby for a better examination.

d. Encourage mother to keep her baby skin-to-skin at least until after the first feed.

2.59 **A mother experiences a severe hemorrhage postpartum. She is at risk for which of the following conditions?**

a. Retained placental fragments

b. Anemia

c. Sheehan syndrome

d. Eclampsia

Answers for Labor and Birth Questions

2.1 **The answer is b.** Babies placed skin-to-skin will usually begin breastfeeding within the first hour. (Difficulty: 4; Discipline: Techniques; Taxonomy: Knowledge)

2.2 **The answer is b.** Oxytocin is especially high in the immediate postbirth period, which helps mother and baby develop trust in one another. (Difficulty: 4; Discipline: Physiology; Taxonomy: Knowledge)

2.3 **The answer is a.** Total cesarean rate is increasing in the United States faster than the rate of increase in primary cesarean rate. The graph does not provide any information about the cause(s) of these rate changes. (Difficulty: 4; Discipline: Clinical Skills; Taxonomy: Evaluate)

2.4 **The answer is c.** In the supine position, the uterus can compress the inferior vena cava, causing maternal hypotension and reduced blood flow to the uterus. This is relevant to breastfeeding because a long, difficult labor can delay the onset of copious milk production. (Difficulty: 3; Discipline: Psychology; Taxonomy: Knowledge)

2.5 **The answer is b.** The second-born twin is exposed to more maternal anesthesia than is the firstborn twin. (Difficulty: 2; Discipline: Pharmacology; Taxonomy: History)

2.6 **The answer is a.** Immediate skin-to-skin after birth is the most important action regardless of mode of delivery, medications used, or mother's breast or nipple configuration. This mother's bifurcated nipple is within the range of normal and may pose no challenge to her baby . Choice b is wise but less important than immediate skin-to-skin contact. Normal oral hydration is sufficient, and a nipple shield is not indicated. (Difficulty: 3; Discipline: Development; Taxonomy: Assessment)

2.7 **The answer is a.** All labor pain–relief drugs have been shown to delay onset of lactogenesis, as reported in a 2014 study by Lind et al. Epidural narcotic or anesthetic drugs cross the placenta and appear in cord blood. Epidurals are also documented to lengthen the second stage of labor and increase the likelihood of operative birth. (Difficulty: 5; Discipline: Pharmacology; Taxonomy: Evaluate)

2.8 **The answer is b.** The continuous presence of a companion of the mother's choice during labor (doula care) extends the duration of breastfeeding, shortens labor, reduces cesarean births, and results in less infant asphyxia. Doula care can enhance the husband's (partner's) involvement in the birth. (Difficulty: 4; Discipline: Psychology; Taxonomy: Evaluate)

2.9 **The answer is d.** Fentanyl appears to alter a newborn's instinctive behavior in the early hours after birth. Dextrose intravenously may result in overhydration. Nitrous oxide is metabolized quickly by the baby. Pitocin has no documented effect on newborn breastfeeding. (Difficulty: 5; Discipline: Pharmacology; Taxonomy: Collaboration)

2.10 **The answer is a.** Supporting the mother is always the FIRST response, especially when she is as happy as the mother in the photograph. Choice b would be appropriate after you've complimented the mother. The other two responses are not appropriate. (Difficulty: 3; Discipline: Clinical Skills; Taxonomy: Goals)

2.11 **The answer is d.** Direct breastfeeding is the norm. All other feeding methods are considered interventions with known and unknown consequences. The BFHI Step 6 requires documentation of medically acceptable reasons for supplementing a breastfed baby. (Difficulty: 3; Discipline: Clinical Skills; Taxonomy: Collaboration)

2.12 **The answer is c.** The newborn should be placed at breast immediately postbirth and assisted (if needed) to begin breastfeeding within the first hour. The BFHI and other policies suggest that all non–life-saving procedures be delayed until after the first effective breastfeed. (Difficulty: 2; Discipline: Psychology; Taxonomy: Collaboration)

2.13 **The answer is a.** Research shows that locally injected lidocaine and other medications used for labor pain relief alter the newborn's spontaneous ability to crawl to the breast, explore the breast with hands, and latch effectively to the breast. (Difficulty: 4; Discipline: Pharmacology; Taxonomy: Evaluate)

2.14 **The answer is b.** Fentanyl, especially in higher doses, is related to breastfeeding problems and early weaning. (Difficulty: 5; Discipline: Pharmacology; Taxonomy: History)

2.15 **The answer is b.** All labor pain medication cross the placenta and have documented effects on the baby's motor and neurobehavioral scores. Choices a and c are stated in ways that would make it difficult for the mother to make an informed decision.

Choice d is incorrect. (Difficulty: 4; Discipline: Pharmacology; Taxonomy: Plan)

2.16 **The answer is a.** Cesarean surgery is associated with breastfeeding difficulties in several research studies, regardless of the reason for the cesarean. Magnesium sulfate is suspected of causing problems—likewise for intravenous hydration. A history of failed breastfeeding could be from numerous causes, including infant factors. (Difficulty: 4; Discipline: Psychology; Taxonomy: Knowledge)

2.17 **The answer is a.** Overhydration during labor may cause breast, nipple, and areolar edema, making latch-on difficult for the baby. New research suggests that the total amount of intravenous fluids given, the flow rate per hour, and even any intravenous fluids may affect breast swelling/firmness and edema. (Difficulty: 5; Discipline: Pharmacology; Taxonomy: History)

2.18 **The answer is c.** Delayed lactogenesis (onset of copious milk production delayed past 72 hours) is most likely associated with long, difficult labor. Specific factors and interventions of long, difficult labors may also play a role. Rapid labor, premature delivery, and vomiting during labor are not known to be related to the timing of onset of lactogenesis II. (Difficulty: 3; Discipline: Pathology; Taxonomy: Knowledge)

2.19 **The answer is c.** This mother and baby are content, safe, and warm. Keeping the mother and baby in skin-to-skin contact is ideal for stabilizing the baby's systems. Preserving the mother–baby relationship is a primary responsibility of the lactation consultant (LC). Continue observing the dyad; the baby will likely wake to feed soon. The baby's hat is not necessary because the mother's body is keeping the baby in thermal stability. (Difficulty: 2; Discipline: Psychology; Taxonomy: Plan)

2.20 **The answer is b.** All pain relief drugs given to the mother reach the baby within seconds to minutes. Drugs given more than 30 minutes or less than 4 hours prior to birth appear to have more effect on the infant than those given at other times. The effect is dose related. (Difficulty: 4; Discipline: Pharmacology; Taxonomy: Evaluate)

2.21 **The answer is a.** Secretory IgA in milk/colostrum is 10 times higher on the first postpartum day than at any other time during lactation. (Difficulty: 4; Discipline: Development; Taxonomy: Knowledge)

2.22 **The answer is d.** Skin-to-skin contact is calming and soothing for the infant. Most procedures can be done while the baby is resting skin-to-skin on mother's body. (Difficulty: 5; Discipline: Psychology; Taxonomy: Plan)

2.23 **The answer is a.** Caput succedaneum is the collection of fluid between the skin and cranial bone of the newborn, often associated with the use of vacuum extraction devices. Any head injury or insult may affect the infant's ability to breastfeed. (Difficulty: 3; Discipline: Pathology; Taxonomy: Knowledge)

2.24 **The answer is c.** Social support increases the likelihood of successful breastfeeding. The importance of labor support (Difficulty: 3; Discipline: Psychology; Taxonomy: Knowledge)

2.25 **The answer is b.** Delayed clamping of the umbilical cord until it stops pulsing ensures that the infant receives the normal amount of placental blood. Anemic pregnant or breastfeeding women should increase iron intake for their own health. Supplementation with iron-fortified formula increases risk to the infant and is inappropriate. (Difficulty: 4; Discipline: Psychology; Taxonomy: Collaboration)

2.26 **The answer is a.** Pediatric half-life of labor pain-relief drugs is often much longer than maternal half-life, which is the most important factor to consider. Choices b and d are accurate, as all labor drugs cross the placenta, including those administered in the epidural space. The effect on the baby's ability to breastfeed is dose related. (Difficulty: 4; Discipline: Pharmacology; Taxonomy: Plan)

2.27 **The answer is c.** Discharge bags containing formula samples or coupons violates BFHI Step 6 and the International Code. Discharge bags are a marketing tool that has been clearly found to undermine breastfeeding. Furthermore, powdered formula is not sterile, which could put babies at risk and therefore your hospital at legal risk. (Difficulty: 3; Discipline: Clinical Skills; Taxonomy: Collaboration)

2.28 **The answer is c.** According to Dr. Lars Hanson, "Human babies, like all mammals, are delivered next to their mother's anus. This ensures exposure to the mother's normal and beneficial intestinal bacteria." All the other procedures listed actually reduce the baby's immune protection because the infant is exposed to other bacteria in the environment, instead of the mother's beneficial gut bacteria. (Difficulty: 5; Discipline: Psychology; Taxonomy: Knowledge)

2.29 **The answer is b.** Putting the baby to breast will help the uterus expel the placenta and reduce bleeding. Skilled birth attendants carry medications to aid uterine contractions for emergency situations. (Difficulty: 5; Discipline: Physiology; Taxonomy: Plan)

2.30 **The answer is a.** Pain-relieving drugs influence the central nervous system and therefore are highly lipid soluble and sequester in the infant brain. The other answers are incorrect. (Difficulty: 3; Discipline: Pharmacology; Taxonomy: Knowledge)

2.31 The answer is b. The BFHI Step 4 is interpreted as "Place babies in skin-to-skin contact with their mothers immediately following birth for at least an hour and encourage mothers to recognize when their babies are ready to breastfeed, offering help if needed." Some babies get to breast and are nursing well in the first 5 to 10 minutes. Many babies born to unmedicated mothers are nursing well by 30 minutes, while some babies take an hour or longer to accomplish their first feed. (Difficulty: 4; Discipline: Development; Taxonomy: Knowledge)

2.32 The answer is b. Delayed onset of lactation is a major consequence of maternal diabetes. Delayed onset of copious secretion is not a reason to supplement with bovine or soy-based formula because those are both triggers for diabetes in susceptible infants. Choices a and c are also true. (Difficulty: 4; Discipline: Pathology; Taxonomy: History)

2.33 The answer is b. The hypoglossal nerve is the primary motor nerve of the tongue; therefore, an inability to move the tongue to gather or collect milk is the most likely result of damage to this nerve. (Difficulty: 5; Discipline: Pathology; Taxonomy: History)

2.34 The answer is b. Sheehan syndrome is the most likely reason for her delayed lactogenesis and may affect her lactation permanently. Severe blood loss related to birth can cause necrosis of all or part of the pituitary gland, which produces prolactin needed for lactogenesis. Long, difficult labor may also delay lactogenesis. Separation from her baby and delay in milk expression can also hinder onset of lactation. (Difficulty: 5; Discipline: Pathology; Taxonomy: History)

2.35 The answer is a. The occiput, or occipital bone, most often presents during a normal vaginal birth. At birth, the occipital bone is in four segments that move to adjust during the birth process. The second most common bone presenting is the frontal bone, which leads in a brow presentation. The frontal bone is in two segments at birth. Babies

have more trouble breastfeeding after a mechanically difficult birth. (Difficulty: 4; Discipline: Development; Taxonomy: Knowledge)

2.36 The answer is d. Chickenpox is no longer contagious when all the lesions are completely crusted over. The mother can breastfeed normally. If she had open lesions on the day of birth, c would be correct. (Difficulty: 5; Discipline: Pathology; Taxonomy: Collaboration)

2.37 The answer is c. BFHI Step 4 states "Place babies in skin-to-skin contact with their mothers immediately following birth for at least an hour and encourage mothers to recognize when their babies are ready to breastfeed, offering help if needed." Research indicates that most babies will begin breastfeeding within the first hour if left undisturbed on the mother's chest/abdomen following birth. The BFHI includes no requirements for length of stay, when expressing milk should begin if the baby cannot breastfeed, or for care of premature babies other than expressing milk for them (Step 5). (Difficulty: 5; Discipline: Clinical Skills; Taxonomy: Collaboration)

2.38 The answer is b. Although perineally injected medications transfer to the infant poorly, pudendal block does affect the newborn's motor skills immediately postbirth. All pain-relieving drugs given to the mother in labor, by any route, reach the infant quickly and affect many aspects of behavior. (Difficulty: 3; Discipline: Pharmacology; Taxonomy: Evaluate)

2.39 The answer is a. Separation from the mother creates psychological and physical stress to the infant, including increased crying, more risk of hypothermia, and elevated stress hormones. Research confirms that any separation except for life-preserving treatments should be avoided. (Difficulty: 5; Discipline: Psychology; Taxonomy: Knowledge)

2.40 **The answer is b.** Research shows that babies separated from their mothers are in a state of higher stress, as measured by salivary cortisol levels and other physiologic markers. (Difficulty: 4; Discipline: Psychology; Taxonomy: Knowledge)

2.41 **The answer is a.** The baby finds his way to the breast partly by smell. Placing the unwashed baby on mother's unwashed body facilitates the baby's ability to self-attach to the breast. The other practices listed would interfere with this natural process. This baby is smelling his hands as he crawls to the breast. (Difficulty: 3; Discipline: Physiology; Taxonomy: Goals)

2.42 **The answer is c.** This baby is capable of crawling to the breast unassisted. Self-attachment suggests that the baby has completed the required behavioral sequencing and will suck normally and effectively. There is no indication that any of the other actions are necessary or even appropriate. (Difficulty: 5; Discipline: Psychology; Taxonomy: Plan)

2.43 **The answer is d.** The newborn is born sterile. Exposure to mother's feces colonizes the infant with her beneficial gut bacteria, which helps avoid colonization with harmful pathogens from the environment. (Difficulty: 5; Discipline: Psychology; Taxonomy: Collaboration)

2.44 **The answer is c.** The mother's treatment during labor strongly affects her sense of accomplishment and self-esteem. The mother's age and other factors are less significant to her experience. (Difficulty: 3; Discipline: Psychology; Taxonomy: Knowledge)

2.45 **The answer is b.** Fentanyl is associated with breastfeeding problems, according to randomized controlled studies of high, low, and none. Propofol is rapidly metabolized and has not been researched for breastfeeding outcomes. (Difficulty: 3; Discipline: Pharmacology; Taxonomy: History)

2.46 **The answer is d.** On the first day, newborns take an average of 7 mL per feed, which matches the physiologic capacity of the newborn stomach at birth. On the first day, total intake ranges from 7 to 122.5 mL (0.2 to 4.1 oz; average 37.1 mL [1.2 oz]). Larger feed volumes overwhelm the newborn. (Difficulty: 3; Discipline: Development; Taxonomy: Knowledge)

2.47 **The answer is b.** Cesarean birth is a surgical intervention, and the mother will need pain relief medications. Postpartum bleeding is not significantly affected by mode of birth. Lactogenesis is likely to be delayed following a surgical birth. BFHI Step 4 requires that babies be skin-to-skin with their mothers even after cesarean birth. (Difficulty: 3; Discipline: Psychology; Taxonomy: History)

2.48 **The answer is a.** Lactogenesis II is triggered by delivery of the placenta and the drop in progesterone. It is not dependent on breast stimulation by the baby and may be initially unnoticed by the mother. If the mother has diabetes, it may be delayed by about 24 hours. (Difficulty: 5; Discipline: Physiology; Taxonomy: Knowledge)

2.49 **The answer is d.** Colonization with the mother's flora sets up the optimal microbial environment for the newborn. When anyone else holds the baby, there is a greater risk of colonization with less-friendly organisms. (Difficulty: 3; Discipline: Psychology; Taxonomy: Goals)

2.50 **The answer is b.** Epidural anesthesia increases the risk of emergency cesarean surgery and vacuum extraction in low-risk first-time mothers, which will make it harder for her to hold and breastfeed immediately after birth. All drugs given for pain relief in labor affect the mother and the fetus/baby; more research is surfacing every year on risks of these. Choice a is incorrect; c is almost never the case; and d is incorrect. (Difficulty: 3; Discipline: Pharmacology; Taxonomy: Goals)

2.51   **The answer is b.** The most important function of colostrum is to protect the baby from pathogens. Colostrum is especially high in secretory IgA and white blood cells. (Difficulty: 3; Discipline: Development; Taxonomy: Knowledge)

2.52   **The answer is c.** Backache in active labor is most likely due to the baby/fetus being in an occiput posterior (OP) presentation. This is relevant to breastfeeding because difficult labors, including OP presentation, may affect the baby's ability to breastfeed. Back pain in labor may also slow labor progress and result in even more drugs for pain relief and other interventions, further affecting the baby's ability to breastfeed. (Difficulty: 4; Discipline: Psychology; Taxonomy: Knowledge)

2.53   **The answer is a.** The newborn is born sterile. Colonization with the mother's normal gut flora by coming in contact with her feces prevents the newborn from being colonized with harmful bacteria in its environment. Some babies will rotate to a more favorable position for birth in this position, but there is little research (at this date) that directly links mother's position at birth with infant outcomes. (Difficulty: 4; Discipline: Psychology; Taxonomy: Plan)

2.54   **The answer is c.** Several research studies have identified cesarean surgery as an important factor affecting breastfeeding initiation. The BFHI recommends immediate skin-to-skin, even after cesarean birth, which can reduce negative consequences of cesarean surgery. Choices a, b, and d may also interfere with normal initiation of breastfeeding. (Difficulty: 5; Discipline: Psychology; Taxonomy: Knowledge)

2.55   **The answer is b.** A supportive companion is the most likely (of these options) to optimize breastfeeding success. Medications to relieve labor pain can significantly interfere with breastfeeding and bonding. Freedom to move about will enhance her comfort and may shorten or ease her labor (Difficulty: 3; Discipline: Psychology; Taxonomy: Plan)

2.56   **The answer is d.** Skin-to-skin contact with reduced sensory stimulation is the FIRST and usually successful intervention. Once that is done, choice a could help. Choice b is harsh and usually unnecessary. Pulling down a baby's chin may cause jaw clenching. (Difficulty: 4; Discipline: Techniques; Taxonomy: Plan)

2.57   **The answer is b.** BFHI Step 2 guidelines are to "Place babies in skin-to-skin contact with their mothers immediately following birth for at least an hour and encourage mothers to recognize when their babies are ready to breastfeed, offering help if needed." Cheek-to-cheek touching is not considered "skin-to-skin." If the mother is unstable or unable to hold the baby due to her own condition, skin-to-skin with the father is appropriate until the mother is stable and able to hold her baby. Radiant warmers are not substitutes for skin-to-skin contact. (Difficulty: 3; Discipline: Clinical Skills; Taxonomy: Plan)

2.58   **The answer is d.** Newborns should remain skin-to-skin with their mothers for at least an hour after birth or until after the first feed. There is no published risk to the baby sleeping on her mother's body or next to her on a firm, clean surface. This photograph was taken about 2 hours after the mother gave birth. The mother is awake and attentive to her baby; nothing else needs to happen at this time. (Difficulty: 5; Discipline: Psychology; Taxonomy: Goals)

2.59   **The answer is c.** Hemorrhage postbirth may trigger Sheehan syndrome, or necrosis of all or part of the pituitary gland. Sheehan syndrome may reduce prolactin levels below that needed for lactogenesis, thus causing primary lactation failure. (Difficulty: 4; Discipline: Pathology; Taxonomy: Evaluate)

CHAPTER 3

Prematurity Questions

3.1 **You are helping a breastfeeding mother of a preterm infant with positioning to optimize her infant's ability to latch and sustain feeding at breast. Which of the following is MOST LIKELY to result in effective breastfeeding for this mother and infant?**
   a. Cradle hold with the baby's head near mother's elbow
   b. Side-lying position on firm bed with pillows behind mother's back
   c. Whichever position is most comfortable for the mother
   d. A cross-cradle hold with the mother's hand behind the baby's upper shoulders

3.2 **A mother is uncertain about providing her own milk for her preterm baby and has been told that her milk helps nerve development. Which sensory system is MOST COMPROMISED by the absence of human milk?**
   a. Olfactory (smell)
   b. Auditory (hearing)
   c. Gustatory (taste)
   d. Visual (sight)

3.3 **A mother delivered a preterm baby at 28 weeks' gestation. Which is the MOST EFFECTIVE strategy to establish and maintain an adequate milk supply?**
   a. Begin expressing or pumping within the first hour following birth.
   b. Express the breasts fully, for 2 minutes after the flow of drops ceases.
   c. Express or pump every 2–4 hours around the clock.
   d. Pump every 2 hours during the day, and get a good night's sleep at night.

3.4 **Which of the following citations is an example of a primary reference or source?**
   a. Anderson GC. Current knowledge about skin-to-skin (kangaroo) care for preterm infants: Review of the literature. Journal of Perinatology 1991; XI: 216–226.
   b. Als H, Lester BM, Tronick E, Brazelton TB. Manual for the assessment of preterm infants' behavior (AFPB). In Fitzgerald JE, Lester BM, Jogman MW, eds. Theory and Research in Behavioral Pediatrics, Vol. 1, New York: Plenum, 1982, 64–133.
   c. Ludington-Hoe SM, Golant SK. Kangaroo Care: The Best You Can Do to Help Your Preterm Infant. New York: Bantam Books, 1993.
   d. Ludington-Hoe SM, Hadeed AJ, Anderson GC. Physiologic responses to skin-to-skin contact in hospitalized premature infants. Journal of Perinatology 1991 Vol. XI, no. 1, p. 19–24.

3.5 **Compared with milk from mothers who deliver at term, milk from mothers who deliver preterm is:**
   a. higher in lactose, vitamins, and minerals.
   b. higher in protein, sodium, chloride.
   c. lower in calcium, magnesium, and phosphorus.
   d. equivalent in immunologic properties.

3.6 **This mother's breast is full with milk. Her baby was born at 36 weeks' gestation and is now 6 days old. What is the MOST LIKELY result when her baby attempts to nurse using the device shown in this photograph?**

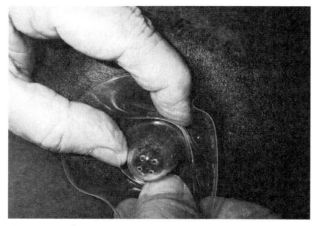

Courtesy of K. Jean Cotterman.

    a. Milk will collect in the tip of the nipple shield, making it easier for the baby to obtain milk.

    b. The baby will imprint on the nipple shield and have difficulty nursing without it.

    c. The nipple shield will block a substantial amount of milk transfer.

    d. The firm tip of the nipple shield will trigger a strong suck response.

3.7 **A mother's labor is being induced at 37 weeks because of high blood pressure. What is the MOST LIKELY consequence to her baby's ability to breastfeed?**

    a. There is no problem; babies have mature sucking responses at 37 weeks of gestation.

    b. The baby's oral muscles are too weak to suck normally.

    c. The baby may have short sucking bursts.

    d. The baby will need to be supplemented after each feed.

3.8 **Mothers of twins are MOST LIKELY to experience which of the following circumstances?**

    a. Premature birth

    b. Cesarean birth

    c. Intrauterine growth retardation

    d. Insufficient milk supply

3.9 **The mother of a premature baby needs to express milk for her baby. She has relatively small breasts. Which expressing pattern is MOST LIKELY to result in abundant supply?**

    a. Six times a day for 30 minutes per breast

    b. Every 3–4 hours for 10 minutes per breast

    c. Every 2–3 hours until the milk flow ceases

    d. Every 1–2 hours during the day and once at night

3.10 **At what gestational age does the swallowing reflex first appear?**

    a. 16 weeks

    b. 22 weeks

    c. 28 weeks

    d. 32 weeks

3.11 **When commencing oral feeds for the preterm infant, which is the MOST IMPORTANT infant factor to consider?**

    a. Cardiorespiratory stability

    b. Toleration of enteral feedings

    c. Ability to suck well on a bottle

    d. Developmental age

3.12 **You are working with the mother of a hospitalized baby born at 30 weeks' gestation. She says her milk supply is low and she cannot keep up with the feeding demands of her infant. She is using a hand-operated single-flange type of breast pump. What is the NEXT suggestion you should make?**

   a. Your pump is adequate, so you are probably making all the milk you can make.

   b. Put your baby to the breast even more often, instead of pumping.

   c. You should begin using a hospital-grade electric pump.

   d. Your current pump is inadequate, so begin taking a galactagogue.

3.13 **In the global context, the MOST IMPORTANT reason to use an open cup for feeding a preterm baby who cannot yet breastfeed is that it:**

   a. is inexpensive and readily available.

   b. has a low risk of fluid aspiration.

   c. fosters appropriate tongue motions.

   d. is easy to clean.

3.14 **Which is the MOST COMMON use for donor human milk worldwide?**

   a. Term babies whose mothers cannot breastfeed

   b. Adopted babies

   c. Premature babies

   d. Babies of mothers who are infected with HIV

3.15 **Which nutrient is most difficult for premature babies to digest?**

   a. Carbohydrates

   b. Proteins

   c. Fats

   d. Minerals

3.16 **A mother has just delivered her baby at 32 weeks' gestation. Which of the following statements is MOST LIKELY to empower her?**

   a. Don't worry dear, your baby is in good hands, we'll take good care of her.

   b. There are a lot of noisy machines that produce "white noise" and that will make your baby calmer.

   c. Your baby seems so much calmer when you're nearby. Please talk and sing to her.

   d. Your milk is so important for your baby. It's really great that you're expressing milk for her!

3.17 **You are assisting a mother of a late preterm infant to latch to the breast. Mother is making sufficient milk with pumping support, but the baby cannot latch and maintain feeding for more than a few moments before slipping off the breast. What should be your NEXT action?**

   a. Tell mom that direct breastfeeding is too tiring to the infant and give her a bottle and teat system.

   b. Urge her to continue pumping until the infant is ready for breastfeeding, approximately her original due date.

   c. Suggest using a thin silicone nipple shield to keep the nipple extended in the baby's mouth during feeds.

   d. Help her use a tube-feeding device to provide extra breastmilk at the breast.

3.18 **Which feeding device is MOST APPROPRIATE if a preterm baby cannot yet breastfeed but can tolerate oral feeds?**

   a. Syringe

   b. Cup

   c. Tube against a finger (fingerfeeding)

   d. Teat

3.19 **Which is the LEAST IMPORTANT reason to use Kangaroo Mother Care (KMC) for premature babies?**
a. Kangaroo Mother Care stabilizes the infant's temperature, breathing, and cardiac rate.
b. Babies breastfeed from a younger gestational age and more frequently.
c. Babies can be discharged to home earlier and more fully breastfeeding.
d. The facility has a shortage of incubators (isolettes).

3.20 **You are working with a mom and a 2-week-old premature baby born at 36 weeks' gestation. Mom is supplementing the baby after every breastfeeding with a bottle of her expressed breastmilk. Baby is currently gaining appropriate weight. What should be your NEXT step in supporting this baby towards exclusively breastfeeding?**
a. Tell mom she no longer needs to use a breast pump, since baby is gaining weight.
b. Discuss with mom how to wean off the bottles and recheck baby's weight in 3–5 days.
c. Tell mom not to give baby any more bottles because she has a good milk supply.
d. Nothing; mom is content with her current situation.

3.21 **Compared with term milk, preterm milk is higher in which component?**
a. Protein
b. Lactose
c. Phosphorus
d. Iron

3.22 **A mother is collecting milk for her ill, premature baby. Which is the BEST container for her milk?**
a. Open plastic cups or bottles
b. Soft plastic polyethylene ("nurser") bags
c. Large containers holding several feeds
d. Glass containers with airtight lids

3.23 **Which milk expression method(s) would be your FIRST recommendation for a mother whose 37-week-gestation baby is hospitalized in a neonatal intensive care unit?**
a. Hand express, starting at 24 hours after birth
b. Hand express within 1 hour then add a hospital-grade pump
c. Double-pump with an adjustable-speed hospital-grade pump
d. Single-pump with a wide-diameter, flexible-flange pump

3.24 **You are working with a late preterm infant (born at 34 to 36 weeks' gestation) who had been in the hospital neonatal intensive care unit (NICU) since birth 10 days ago. The baby falls readily asleep at breast each time you assist mom to latch. Her milk supply is plentiful because of pumping. What is the MOST LIKELY cause for this infant to be unable to sustain his latch at breast?**
a. His suck has low intraoral pressure (vacuum) due to gestational age.
b. Prematurity causes sleepiness at breast until about 40 weeks' gestation.
c. This infant was fed with a bottle during his NICU stay.
d. The mother has delayed lactogenesis resulting from her premature delivery.

3.25 **The MOST IMPORTANT consequence of adding fortifiers to human milk given to premature babies is:**
a. better long-term bone mineralization.
b. increased risk of allergic reaction from bovine protein in fortifiers.
c. increased iron transport.
d. decreased gut transit time.

3.26 **Which of the following developmental processes is MOST INTERRUPTED by premature birth?**

a. Central nervous system development

b. Gut maturation

c. Deposition of fat

d. Hearing and taste

3.27 **Which of the following gastrointestinal illnesses is the MOST SERIOUS condition with artificial (formula) feeding?**

a. Short gut syndrome

b. Diarrhea

c. Necrotizing enterocolitis (NEC)

d. Crohn's disease

3.28 **A 34-week-old premature infant is being sent home after several weeks in the NICU. Which feeding behavior would you MOST EMPHASIZE to the mother?**

a. Express milk after each nursing, as he probably cannot get all your milk.

b. Expect his sucking bursts to be short and irregular.

c. If he does not nurse well, give expressed milk with a slow-flow nipple.

d. Restrict nursing sessions to 10 minutes so he does not tire.

3.29 **You have been working with a mother whose baby was born at 28 weeks of gestation. Today, you learn that her baby has died. The FIRST you should say to her is:**

a. It's OK to stop pumping your milk now.

b. Oh, NO, what a shock! And just when you thought she was improving.

c. I can help you gradually reduce your milk production comfortably.

d. What was your baby's name?

3.30 **Of the following factors, which is the MOST LIKELY reason that a premature baby developed NEC?**

a. The baby received only pumped human milk.

b. The baby received a supplement derived from soy protein.

c. Digested formula can destroy the baby's white blood cells.

d. Exclusive breastfeeding cannot protect an infant from NEC.

3.31 **Of the following, which is the BEST strategy to suggest to this mother to maximize milk production for her 32-week-gestation infant?**

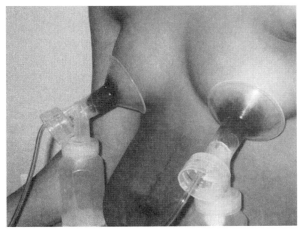

See color plate 8.

Courtesy of K. Jean Cotterman.

a. Massage her breasts during each time she uses this equipment.

b. Drink a glass of milk each time she uses the equipment.

c. Smell a piece of her baby's clothing before using this equipment.

d. Use the smallest-diameter flange available.

3.32 **A mother stopped pumping milk for her premature baby 48 hours ago, and now her breasts are painfully full of milk. Your FIRST action to reduce her discomfort should be to:**

a. suggest she stand in a warm shower to trigger a letdown response.

b. put cold cloths on her breasts to reduce inflammation.

c. help her massage and express some milk.

d. apply a breast binder to suppress lactation.

3.33 Which factor is MOST LIKELY to put a premature infant at risk of evaporative water loss?

a. Lower brown fat reserves

b. Immature thyroid control of metabolic rate

c. Relatively large skin surface area

d. Poor insulin response leading to hyperglycemia

3.34 A baby born very prematurely (weight ≤1500 g) is ready to breastfeed when he:

a. has successfully taken breast milk by bottle.

b. has first fed by spoon or cup.

c. is showing sucking movements.

d. is able to mouth a pacifier.

3.35 Which of the following recommendations would be MOST HELPFUL for a mother who is reducing milk production after her premature baby died?

a. Pump or express only enough milk to soften your breasts when they become full.

b. Bind your breasts tightly with a firm cloth or binder for at least a week.

c. Restrict your fluid intake for the next 2–3 weeks.

d. Ask your doctor to prescribe a medication containing estrogen and progesterone.

3.36 A preterm infant of 1361 g (3.0 lb) has stable cardiac and respiratory systems. Which is the MOST APPROPRIATE feeding strategy?

a. Begin breastfeeding without equipment or devices.

b. Breastfeed with nasogastric tube in place.

c. Cup feed and allow the baby to suck at an empty breast for comfort.

d. Bottlefeed with human milk before breastfeeding.

3.37 Compared with milk from mothers who deliver at term, preterm milk is higher in:

a. macrophages.

b. milk volume.

c. zinc.

d. B vitamins.

3.38 A baby born at 32 weeks' gestation was growing normally for 2 weeks, then his growth began slowing. The MOST LIKELY cause of this sudden slow weight gain is:

a. exclusive use of human milk.

b. respiratory infection.

c. inadequate levels of fat in mother's milk

d. undiagnosed cardiac anomaly.

3.39 Which mineral is particularly difficult for the premature (preterm) infant to absorb?

a. Zinc

b. Iron

c. Sodium

d. Chromium

3.40 You are counseling the mother of a baby born at 36 weeks' gestation who says her infant is quite sleepy. She calls her infant a snacker, which she describes as her infant waking up to feed approximately every 1–2 hours and promptly falling asleep at the breast. What should be your NEXT suggestion for this mother?

a. Apply a cold washcloth to the baby's back during breastfeeding to stimulate him.

b. Keep the baby skin-to-skin, without swaddling blankets, to maintain his temperature during feeds.

c. Follow the infant's cues and breastfeed as often as he requests, including letting him sleep at breast.

d. To break this cycle, pump and feed your expressed milk instead.

Answers for Prematurity Questions

3.1 The answer is d. A position that supports the preterm infant's head and shoulders is most likely to keep the infant's airway aligned for effective feeding. The mother's hand should support the infant's upper back, shoulders, and neck to compensate for relatively weak neck musculature. Cradle hold usually does not provide sufficient support for a preterm infant's upper body. Side-lying position may promote infant sleep instead of facilitating feeding. A position that is comfortable for the mother may not provide sufficient support for a preterm infant to feed effectively. Mothers of preterms should be helped to find positions that are comfortable for the mother and result in effective feeding by the infant. (Difficulty: 4; Discipline: Techniques; Taxonomy: Plan.)

3.2 The answer is d. The visual system is the last sensory system to develop during gestation and therefore the most affected by preterm nutrition. Human milk makes a significant difference in visual development of the preterm infant, partly because of fatty acid profiles. (Difficulty: 2; Discipline: Physiology; Taxonomy: Knowledge.)

3.3 The answer is a. Early, frequent, and thorough removal of milk is essential. Long periods without collecting milk will cause milk stasis, which will suppress lactogenesis II. Expression should begin in the first hour following birth to establish milk production; continuing to express (as in b) is most effective to maintain milk production. (Difficulty: 4; Discipline: Techniques; Taxonomy: Plan.)

3.4 The answer is d. A research article published in a peer-reviewed professional journal is a primary reference. Choice a is a review article, which is a secondary reference. Choice b is a chapter in a book, which is a secondary or tertiary source. Choice c is a book for parents, interpreting other sources in its recommendations. (Difficulty: 4; Discipline: Clinical Skills; Taxonomy: Evaluate.)

3.5 The answer is b. Preterm milk is higher in protein, sodium, and chloride than milk from mothers who deliver at term. (Difficulty: 3; Discipline: Development; Taxonomy: Knowledge.)

3.6 The answer is a. In babies with weak suck, such as premature babies, nipple shields have been shown to improve milk transfer to the baby. The other answers are incorrect. (Difficulty: 5; Discipline: Clinical Skills; Taxonomy: Evaluate.)

3.7 The answer is c. At 37 weeks of gestation, many babies' suck patterns are less organized than at full term even though some babies will breastfeed effectively. Oral muscle strength should be sufficient for breastfeeding by 37 weeks. Supplementation after feeds is often unnecessary. (Difficulty: 4; Discipline: Psychology; Taxonomy: Assessment.)

3.8 The answer is a. Premature birth is the most common of the conditions listed for mothers of twins. Most mothers will produce plenty of milk for several breastfed babies, despite higher risk of early birth-related problems. (Difficulty: 4; Discipline: Physiology; Taxonomy: Evaluate.)

3.9 **The answer is c.** Small breasts usually have less storage capacity than larger breasts, so frequent expression triggers a high rate of milk synthesis. The rate of synthesis is highest when the breasts are emptiest, so expressing until the flow ceases will also maximize the rate of milk synthesis. (Difficulty: 4; Discipline: Techniques; Taxonomy: Plan.)

3.10 **The answer is a.** The infant is able to swallow from about 16 weeks and develops an immature suck pattern at around 26 weeks' gestational age. (Difficulty: 4; Discipline: Development; Taxonomy: Knowledge.)

3.11 **The answer is a.** Cardiorespiratory stability is most important when beginning oral feeds. Skin-to-skin contact and human milk both contribute to cardiorespiratory stability, especially in preterm infants. (Difficulty: 4; Discipline: Development; Taxonomy: Assessment.)

3.12 **The answer is c.** Hospital-grade electric pumps are currently the best devices for compensating for a preterm infant's ineffective suck in supporting milk production. Galactogogues alone will not increase the milk supply. Adequate removal of breastmilk from the breast plus hormonal triggers maintain lactation. Putting a preterm infant with a weak suck to the breast more often will not extract more milk from the breast. (Difficulty: 3; Discipline: Clinical Skills; Taxonomy: Plan.)

3.13 **The answer is d.** Spoons and open cups are easier to clean than other feeding devices. (Difficulty: 4; Discipline: Clinical Skills; Taxonomy: Goals.)

3.14 **The answer is c.** Premature and sick babies are the most common recipients of donor milk. Depending on the local situation and available donated milk, other recipients can include the other choices and more. (Difficulty: 3; Discipline: Clinical Skills; Taxonomy: Knowledge.)

3.15 **The answer is c.** Fats are most difficult for preterms to digest. Human milk fat is released simultaneously with digestive enzymes, making it optimal for preterms. (Difficulty: 4; Discipline: Development; Taxonomy: Knowledge.)

3.16 **The answer is d.** Supporting and validating what the mother is already doing and adding a supportive fact is the best choice. Choices b and c are supportive, but less so than d. validate and support a mother's emotional state and behavior and are thus empowering. The first statement is condescending and disempowering. (Difficulty: 4; Discipline: Psychology; Taxonomy: Goals.)

3.17 **The answer is c.** Of the suggestions listed, a thin silicone nipple shield is most likely to be helpful. The shield compensates for the infant's weak suck and has been shown to lengthen the duration of breastfeeding. Nipple shields may be effective for short-term use until the infant is stronger, and may transfer more milk than direct nursing. Breastfeeding is less tiring for the preterm infant than bottlefeeding. Pumping may be needed for weeks more, but the baby may be feeding effectively before her original due date. Tube-feeding devices do not improve weak suck patterns typical of preterm babies. (Difficulty: 4; Discipline: Techniques; Taxonomy: Plan.)

3.18 **The answer is b.** Cup feeding has been more thoroughly researched than any other alternative feeding device for preterms. Caution should be used to avoid pouring milk down the baby's mouth, and spillage may occur. The baby should be watched closely for signs of stress in all cases. (Difficulty: 4; Discipline: Clinical Skills; Taxonomy: Plan.)

3.19 **The answer is d.** Although a shortage of equipment led to the development of Kangaroo Mother Care, research now supports the other reasons as far more important. (Difficulty: 4; Discipline: Techniques; Taxonomy: Plan.)

3.20 **The answer is b.** Reducing the intake from bottles requires ongoing assessment of baby's weight to ensure proper weight gain and transfer of milk at the breast. The use of a breast pump may be necessary to empty the breasts and preserve mom's milk supply until the premature infant can effectively empty mom's breasts. An adequate (good) milk supply may not mean that the baby can transfer this milk and support weight gain. (Difficulty: 4; Discipline: Techniques; Taxonomy: Plan.)

3.21 **The answer is a.** Preterm milk is higher in protein and similar to term milk in lactose, phosphorus, iron, and most other components. (Difficulty: 2; Discipline: Development; Taxonomy: History.)

3.22 **The answer is d.** Glass is a recommended storage container for mother's own milk. Hard plastic (polycarbonate or polypropylene) containers with lids are acceptable. (Difficulty: 2; Discipline: Clinical Skills; Taxonomy: Plan.)

3.23 **The answer is b.** Expressing or pumping within 1 hour combined with pumping with a hospital-grade pump would be the most likely strategy to maximize milk collection and production. Delaying expression for 24 hours can compromise lactation. A double-pump with adjustable speed may be helpful combined with hand expression. Single-pumping is more time-consuming and does not use milk ejection as well as other strategies. (Difficulty: 4; Discipline: Techniques; Taxonomy: Plan.)

3.24 **The answer is a.** Intensity of suction (intra-oral negative pressure) increases with gestational age. The infant uses suction (negative pressure) to draw the maternal nipple into the oral cavity for effective breastfeeding. However, waiting until infants reach 40 weeks gestation is not best practice. Several interventions effectively achieve transfer of breastmilk at breast prior to 40 weeks. Bottle confusion is unlikely. Infants can sometimes struggle with the different flow rates between bottles and breast, but simply giving bottles in the NICU does not lead to latching problems. Our scenario states that this mom did not experience delayed lactogenesis because her milk supply was preserved with the use of a hospital-grade electric breast pump. (Difficulty: 3; Discipline: Pathology; Taxonomy: Assessment.)

3.25 **The answer is b.** Allergic reactions to fortifiers based on bovine milk are a significant problem for preterm babies. Other serious consequences have been reported. (Difficulty: 2; Discipline: Pathology; Taxonomy: Knowledge.)

3.26 **The answer is a.** Central nervous system development is the most profound process interrupted by premature birth. Choices b and c are also affected by premature birth. Hearing and taste develop early in gestation. (Difficulty: 4; Discipline: Pathology; Taxonomy: Knowledge.)

3.27 **The answer is c.** NEC is the most serious, even lethal, condition associated with formula feeding. Human milk nearly completely protects premature infants from NEC. Formula-fed children are more likely to experience diarrhea and Crohn's disease. (Difficulty: 4; Discipline: Pathology; Taxonomy: History.)

3.28 **The answer is b.** Premature babies often exhibit an irregular and arrhythmic sucking pattern, which improves as they mature. All the other statements are inappropriate. (Difficulty: 3; Discipline: Clinical Skills; Taxonomy: Plan.)

3.29 **The answer is b.** In a highly emotional situation, the consultant should acknowledge the mother's feelings first. Choice b is an example of an empathetic statement. Asking about the baby (choice d) might be a good second response. Clinical help or suggestions can be provided after feelings are acknowledged. (Difficulty: 5; Discipline: Clinical Skills; Taxonomy: Goals.)

3.30 **The answer is c.** Researchers Penn and colleagues reported that "lipase digestion of formula, but not milk, caused significant death of neutrophils (ranging from 47% to 99% with formulas vs. 6% with milk) with similar results in endothelial and epithelial cells." Human milk nearly completely protects premature infants from NEC, whether the milk is pumped and fed or the baby breastfeeds directly. Soy protein may also be a risk for NEC. (Difficulty: 3; Discipline: Development; Taxonomy: Evaluate.)

3.31 **The answer is a.** Breast massage (compression) during pumping increases total milk removal and the proportion of fat in the milk. Drinking milk has no effect on milk production. Smelling the baby's clothing may help trigger a letdown. Small flanges are usually detrimental because they compress the milk ducts. (Difficulty: 4; Discipline: Clinical Skills; Taxonomy: Goals.)

3.32 **The answer is c.** The first strategy is always to help the mother with self-care skills. Gentle hand-expression and massage should help the milk to start moving and require no equipment or devices. A warm shower may help trigger a letdown and is the next best suggestion. There is no indication of inflammation, so cold compresses are inappropriate at best. A breast-binder is likely to increase pain and does not reduce short-term milk synthesis. (Difficulty: 4; Discipline: Techniques; Taxonomy: Goals.)

3.33 **The answer is c.** Preterm and very low birth-weight babies may have higher evaporative water loss because of their relatively large skin surface area. Keeping a baby skin-to-skin and feeding with human milk reduces excess water loss. (Difficulty: 4; Discipline: Development; Taxonomy: Assessment.)

3.34 **The answer is c.** Research has established that a premature baby can go to breast earlier in gestational age than he can feed from devices. (Difficulty: 2; Discipline: Development; Taxonomy: Knowledge.)

3.35 **The answer is a.** Removing some milk but not emptying the breasts will comfortably use the principle of autocrine control of lactation and gradually diminish milk secretion. Breast binding does not suppress lactation and can induce pathology. Fluid intake is unrelated to milk production, and restricting fluids can harm other aspects of mother's health. An estrogen-containing medication will likely suppress milk production, with or without progesterone, but may take several days to be effective. Meanwhile, the mother's milk stasis is painful for her and can trigger other pathology. (Difficulty: 3; Discipline: Techniques; Taxonomy: Goals.)

3.36 **The answer is c.** Cup feeding with non-nutritive sucking at the emptied breast is supported by abundant research. Bottlefeeding has been shown to be stressful for preterm infants and increases the risks of premature weaning. (Difficulty: 4; Discipline: Pathology; Taxonomy: Plan.)

3.37 **The answer is a.** Preterm milk is higher in white cells, especially macrophages, than term milk. Milk volume, zinc, and B-vitamin levels are similar. (Difficulty: 5; Discipline: Development; Taxonomy: Knowledge.)

3.38 **The answer is d.** Once a baby is growing well during breastfeeding, growth should be predictable. Sudden change in growth trajectory often indicates an undiagnosed anomaly or infection. Human milk fat levels show little long-term variance once breastfeeding is established. Effective, exclusive breastfeeding (choice a) does not result in growth faltering. (Difficulty: 4; Discipline: Pathology; Taxonomy: History.)

3.39 **The answer is b.** Preterm infants are often unable to absorb iron effectively. Iron in human milk is more easily absorbed than iron from other sources. (Difficulty: 4; Discipline: Pathology; Taxonomy: Knowledge.)

3.40 **The answer is b.** Late preterm infants may fall asleep if they are slightly chilled, due to inherent thermal instability. Skin-to-skin contact is the best way to maintain thermal stability and maintain alertness. Applying cold is inappropriate. A 1- to 2-hour feeding pattern is normal, but long periods of sleeping at breast may be counterproductive. Pumping and alternate feeding are not necessary. (Difficulty: 3; Discipline: Pathology; Taxonomy: Goals.)

CHAPTER 4

1–2 Days Questions

4.1 This mother just finished pumping her milk. The MOST LIKELY explanation for the condition pictured is:

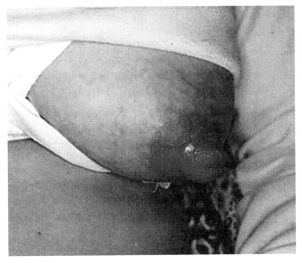

See color plate 9.

    a. Nipple thrush.

    b. Pump flange was too small in diameter.

    c. Reynaud's phenomenon.

    d. Pump has everted her nipples.

4.2 During a home visit on the second postpartum day, you learn that a baby has not yet passed a meconium stool. Your FIRST action should be to:

    a. assess the baby's skin turgor and reflexes, documenting your findings.

    b. inform the baby's primary care provider of your findings.

    c. reassure the parents that delayed passing of meconium is normal.

    d. show the parents how to safely feed infant formula.

4.3 This mother's baby is 20 hours old and has not yet effectively latched on and breastfed. What would be your FIRST strategy to help them?

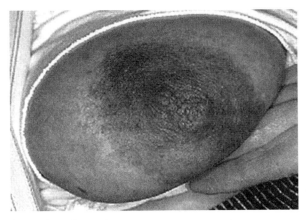

See color plate 10.

    a. Place a silicone nipple shield over her nipples during feeds.

    b. Have the mother pump her breasts to firm and evert the nipple tissue.

    c. Suggest she lean back and place the baby skin-to-skin on her bare chest.

    d. Teach her how to do suck training to coordinate the baby's suck.

4.4 A mother is having trouble keeping her 40-hour-old son awake. The FIRST thing you would suggest is:

    a. Try putting a cool cloth on his face.

    b. Flick his feet with your finger.

    c. Gently massage his back, arms, and legs.

    d. Place him on your chest skin-to-skin.

4.5 **This mother's baby is 4 days old and not feeding effectively. Which is the FIRST suggestion you would make to increase her comfort?**

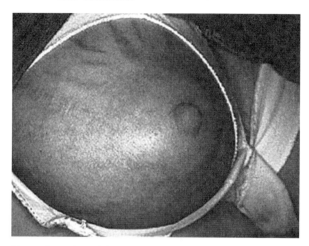

See color plate 11.

 a. Cabbage leaf compresses
 b. Hot compresses
 c. Cold compresses
 d. Gentle massage

4.6 **For optimal breastfeeding, which BEST describes effective positioning at breast?**
 a. The nipple is inside the baby's mouth.
 b. No areola is visible outside the perimeter of the baby's mouth.
 c. The baby's nose lightly touches the mother's breast.
 d. The baby's mouth is open to a wide (>120-degree) angle.

4.7 **A mother had breast reduction surgery when she was a teenager. Now that she has a new baby, she MAY need to use:**
 a. a breast pump to relieve engorgement.
 b. a nipple shield to enhance nipple stimulation.
 c. a feeding tube system because of lactation insufficiency.
 d. breast shells to enhance nipple eversion.

4.8 **After assessing this baby, your FIRST SUGGESTION to the mother should be:**

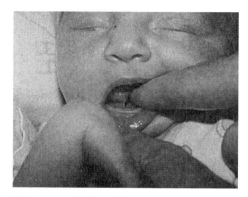

Courtesy of Greg Notestine.

 a. Use a nipple shield during feeds.
 b. Your baby needs an oral surgery consult immediately.
 c. Let's see how your baby does at breast.
 d. Pump your milk and feed with a bottle today.

4.9 **A baby is unable to breastfeed effectively due to a cleft palate. For the best chance to establish an adequate milk supply, the mother should:**
 a. hold her baby frequently and for lengthy periods
 b. pump both breasts with a hospital-grade pump 8–10 times every 24 hours.
 c. allow baby to remain at breast for long feedings so he has plenty of time to draw out enough milk.
 d. avoid pumping at night. Because her baby requires extra care, mother needs more sleep at night so she has plenty of energy.

4.10   **What is the MOST LIKELY cause of the condition shown?**

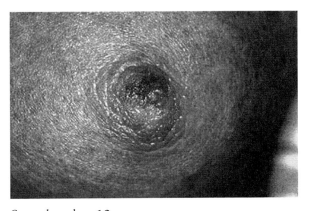

See color plate 12.

Courtesy of Greg Notestine.

    a. Bacterial infection
    b. Allergic reaction from laundry soap
    c. Friction damage from baby's tongue
    d. Mother has fair skin

4.11   **You are working on a policy-development team as your hospital is implementing the WHO/UNICEF Baby-Friendly Hospital Initiative (BFHI). How should your facility address infant formula in its policy guidance?**

    a. No formula or feeding bottles are kept in the hospital; parents must bring their own.
    b. Any formula and bottles must be purchased through regular supply channels.
    c. Only hypoallergenic formula can be kept in the hospital, and they can be given only with a medical order.
    d. Formula and bottles are available only upon maternal written request with informed consent signed.

4.12   **The baby in this photograph is sucking, swallowing, and breathing smoothly, and the mother says breastfeeding is fairly comfortable. Of the following actions, which would be MOST LIKELY to confirm effective breastfeeding?**

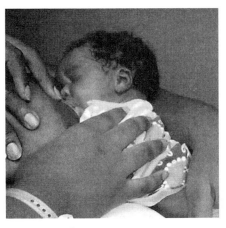

Courtesy of K. Jean Cotterman.

    a. Weigh the baby in the same clothing and diaper before and after her next feed.
    b. Carefully examine her nipple after the baby releases the breast.
    c. Tell the person touching her breast to move away so the baby can move freely.
    d. Ask her to express milk after the baby ends this feed to assess milk production.

4.13   **If a newborn needs to undergo a painful procedure, which pain-management strategy is MOST LIKELY to be effective during the procedure?**
    a. Snug swaddling
    b. Breastfeeding
    c. Skin-to-skin contact
    d. Oral sucrose

4.14   **A mother complains of incision pain following her cesarean birth and requests pain relief medication but is worried about the effect on her baby. Your FIRST response to her should be:**
    a. You can't have any drugs for pain relief while breastfeeding.
    b. Try using patterned breathing like you learned in childbirth classes.
    c. We'll monitor you and your baby closely after you've received pain medication.
    d. Today is the worst; the pain should be less by tomorrow.

4.15 **Which is the LATEST feeding cue that an infant exhibits?**

a. Crying

b. Hand-to-face or hand-to-mouth

c. Grope or mouthing motions

d. Moving into feeding position

4.16 **Even after the baby latched on deeply, the mother's breast is damaged as in the photograph. The MOST LIKELY cause of this nipple wound is:**

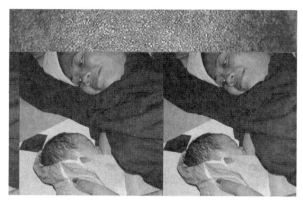

See color plate 13.

Courtesy of Greg Notestine.

a. baby was nursing on the nipple tip.

b. baby is tongue-tied.

c. no nipple preparation during pregnancy.

d. use of a pacifier between feeds.

4.17 **An 18-hour-old baby has not yet success-fully breastfed. He cues to feed but cannot stay on breast. In order to help him suck better, which would be the MOST effective strategy?**

a. Bottle-feed him to help organize his suck.

b. Cup feed him to increase calorie intake.

c. Use a nipple shield to increase sensation to his palate.

d. Have mother rest semireclined with baby on her bare chest.

4.18 **Which of the following suggestions is MOST LIKELY to be helpful for the condition pictured?**

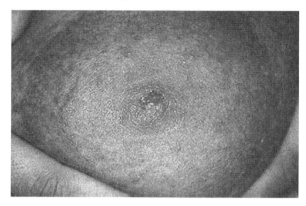

See color plate 14.

Courtesy of Greg Notestine.

a. Air-dry after feedings.

b. Expose the breast to a sunlamp placed about 1 ft (0.3 m) away.

c. Use moist wound healing techniques or preparations.

d. Cover with a breast shell between feeds.

4.19 **This baby is 1 day old. In this picture, what are the white structures in the baby's mouth?**

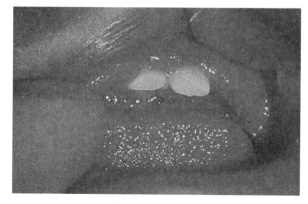

Courtesy of Greg Notestine.

a. Epstein's pearls

b. Natal teeth

c. Incisive papilla

d. Sucking blisters

4.20 At the 6-day visit after a cesarean birth, a baby is still losing weight but is urinating and stooling adequately. The lactation consultant's (LC) FIRST action is to:

a. Ask about medications and intravenous fluids during labor.

b. Directly observe the mother breastfeeding her baby.

c. Supplement the baby with expressed breastmilk.

d. Wait 1 more day because of adequate infant output.

4.21 Which structure in this baby's mouth is MOST LIKELY to cause a breastfeeding problem?

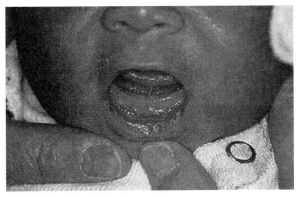

See color plate 15.

Courtesy of Greg Notestine.

a. Alveolar gum ridge

b. Philtrum

c. Lingual frenulum

d. Short tongue

4.22 What event triggers Lactogenesis II (onset of copious milk secretion)?

a. Stimulation from baby at breast

b. Drop in progesterone from placenta separation

c. Rise in oxytocin from uterine contractions

d. Change in blood pH when umbilical cord is cut

4.23 A mother of newborn twins asks whether to feed her babies separately or together. Your BEST response is:

a. Let's see which works best for you and your babies

b. Separately is better so you can focus on one at a time.

c. Together is better to save you time.

d. Feed them together to get their feeding patterns synchronized.

4.24 Of the conditions listed, which is the MOST LIKELY indication for use of the device shown in this photograph?

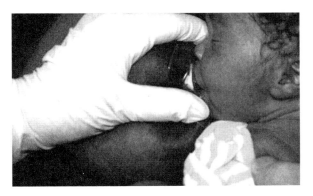

Courtesy of K. Jean Cotterman.

a. Mother has very large breasts and nipples.

b. Baby has anklyoglossia

c. Baby was premature and has a weak suck.

d. Mother is afraid to let baby suck directly.

4.25 **According to the Ten Steps to Successful Breastfeeding, this baby should be:**

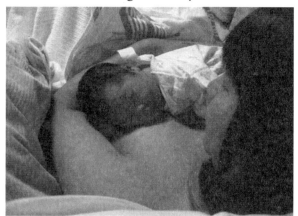

Courtesy of Yuwen Ren.

    a. taken to the admission nursery after 1 hour.

    b. moved to the central nursery only if the mother had a cesarean birth.

    c. given eye prophylaxis after 2 hours of age.

    d. kept with the mother 24 hours a day.

4.26 **Bacterial counts in human milk, expressed 1 hour earlier, are MOST likely to be:**

    a. lower, because the milk is being held at a lower temperature.

    b. lower, because macrophages in the milk are actively phagocytic.

    c. higher, because antibacterial properties of human milk work best at body temperature.

    d. higher, because human milk is a rich medium for bacterial growth.

4.27 **How much milk does a newborn obtain at breast each day during the first week if breastfeeding is on cue (unrestricted)?**

    a. 3–4 oz (90–120 mL) per day of colostrum

    b. increasing amounts each day as milk volume increases

    c. less than needed for adequate hydration until day 5

    d. 25 oz (750 mL) per day from day 2 onward.

4.28 **At which age does this interaction between an adult and a baby begin?**

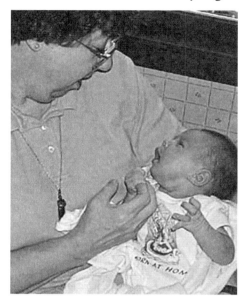

    a. 1 day

    b. 1 week

    c. 2 weeks

    d. 1 month

4.29 **Which statement MOST ACCURATELY describes this baby's oral anatomy?**

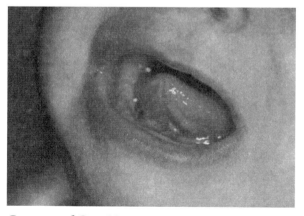

Courtesy of Greg Notestine.

    a. The fat pads are small.

    b. The philtrum is broad.

    c. The lips are thin and tensed.

    d. All visible structures are normal.

4.30 **Which of the following newborn behaviors is MOST LIKELY related to newborn drug withdrawal from maternal opiate use during pregnancy?**

    a. Tremors and hyperreactive reflexes

    b. Coordinated suck-swallow-breathe

    c. Lethargy for several hours after birth

    d. Low muscle tone around the jaw and mouth

4.31 **The adult's hand is MOST LIKELY doing which of these procedures?**

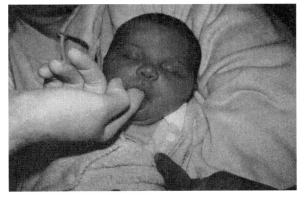

Courtesy of Greg Notestine.

    a. Suck training or reorganization

    b. Digital oral exam or assessment

    c. Finger-feeding

    d. Pacifying a crying/upset baby

4.32 **This mother is experiencing severe nipple pain. The MOST LIKELY explanation is:**

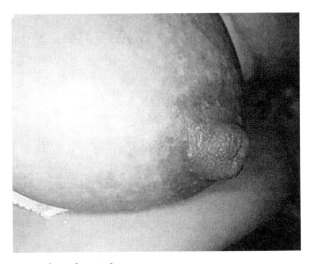

See color plate 16.

    a. inversion in the center of the tip is rubbing on the baby's palate

    b. large, fibrous nipple is being compressed by baby's mouth.

    c. edema of the nipple from baby's vigorous suck.

    d. primary engorgement.

4.33 **Which of the following is the MOST LIKELY condition pictured?**

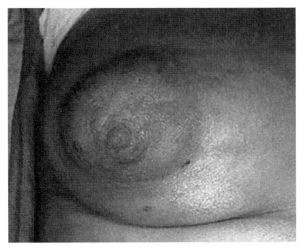

See color plate 17.

    a. Galactocele

    b. Areolar edema

    c. Abscess

    d. Milk stasis

4.34 **Sudden onset of painless bright red bleeding from the nipple of a mother during the first week postpartum indicates the probable presence of:**

    a. breast cancer.

    b. fibrocystic disease.

    c. intraductal papilloma.

    d. nipple tissue breakdown.

4.35 **What is the FIRST thing you would do to support this 5-hour-old baby and her mother?**

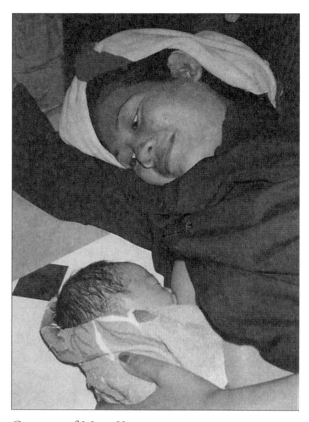

Courtesy of Mary Kroeger.

a. Make sure she and her baby are undisturbed and comfortable in bed together.
b. Raise the side rails of the bed so the baby does not fall out.
c. Monitor the mother every 15 minutes to prevent her rolling onto her baby.
d. Remove the baby at the end of the feed so mother can better rest.

4.36 **This mother is preparing to feed. The NEXT action she should take is to:**

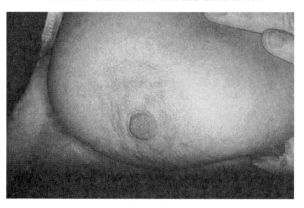

See color plate 18.

a. rub the nipple to make it firmer and more projectile.
b. move the bottom hand closer to the areola to better support the breast.
c. stop pulling back with the top hand.
d. bring the baby onto the breast.

4.37 **During the colostral phase of lactation, drugs taken by the mother can more easily pass into the breastmilk because:**
a. colostrum is more concentrated than mature milk.
b. the intracellular spaces between lactocytes are wide.
c. the mother has a larger blood volume immediately postpartum.
d. the mother's kidneys do not clear drugs as quickly immediately postpartum.

4.38 **You are on a team preparing clinical policies for a maternity unit. Which action is MOST IMPORTANT in preventing postpartum breast engorgement?**
a. Prenatal expression of colostrum
b. Immediate breastfeeding in the first hour or so postbirth
c. If the baby has not breastfed by 12 hours, initiate milk expression
d. Restrict mother's fluid intake in the first 48 hours postpartum

4.39 You have been working with a mother who describes excruciating pain every time her baby's mouth touches her breast, even if he does not latch on and breastfeed. You have ruled out injury, infections, and other causes of nipple pain, and her nipples are not reddened or irritated. You should NEXT consider whether the mother has:

a. a history of any kind of abuse.

b. no interest in breastfeeding.

c. a low pain threshold.

d. allergies.

4.40 What is the MOST serious risk of prelacteal ritual feeds of butter, herbs, etc.?

a. Triggers oversupply of milk

b. Infection with pathogens

c. Alteration of gut flora

d. Reduced availability of colostrum

4.41 This mother and baby are having difficulty breastfeeding. Your FIRST suggestion should be to:

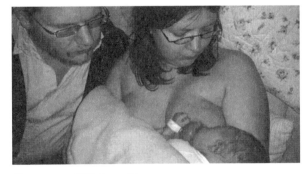

Courtesy of K. Jean Cotterman.

a. Have the mother sit more upright.

b. Lower the hand behind the baby's back so the head can extend slightly.

c. Have her support the breast with her right hand.

d. Swaddle the baby so her hands do not interfere.

4.42 A breastfeeding mother has been diagnosed with postpartum depression. Her physician contacts you to discuss whether she should continue to breastfeed during drug treatment. Your BEST response is:

a. There are several antidepressant medications that are considered compatible with breastfeeding.

b. All medications used to treat mental illness are contraindicated during breastfeeding.

c. Her baby is in great danger and should be kept away from her at all costs.

d. The hormones of breastfeeding will exacerbate her illness.

4.43 After the baby releases the breast after a 20-minute feed, there is a crease across the nipple tip and the nipple appears flattened. The MOST LIKELY cause of this is:

a. normal suck.

b. shallow latch.

c. baby's head is turned away.

d. torticollis in the baby.

4.44 Which of the following statements BEST describes the Babinski reflex?

a. Grasp object when palm is stimulated.

b. Turn mouth toward source of stimulation.

c. Bear partial weight of body while standing on flat surface.

d. Flare toes when sole of foot is stimulated.

4.45 **You are called to help an obese mother with breastfeeding on the second postpartum day. Her baby has not yet breastfed effectively despite several attempts. Your FIRST action should be to:**
   a. put a rolled-up towel under the mother's breast.
   b. compress her nipple and areola to make a breast "sandwich."
   c. demonstrate deep latch with a breast model and doll.
   d. have her sit upright with pillows under her arms.

4.46 **When would a drug given to the mother MOST readily pass into the milk?**
   a. When the mother is collecting milk for a premature baby
   b. In the first 4 days after birth
   c. When the mother has a breast infection
   d. When the drug is given transdermally

4.47 **The MOST IMPORTANT action to take in helping this mother breastfeed is to:**

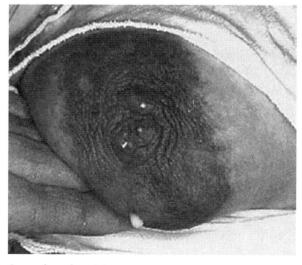

See color plate 19.

   a. have her wear a nipple shield during feedings.
   b. hand-express milk before feeds to soften the large nipple area.
   c. help the baby latch on to the breast deeply.
   d. apply an antifungal preparation to the nipples after every feed.

4.48 **Which of the following approaches will be MOST helpful to assisting a breastfeeding mother who has a hearing impairment?**
   a. Speak to her more slowly.
   b. Talk directly to her interpreter.
   c. Make frequent eye contact with her.
   d. Help her observe the baby's visual cues.

4.49 **The WHO/ UNICEF Ten Steps to Successful Breastfeeding (BFHI) prohibits the use of which devices?**
   a. Tube-feeding devices
   b. Pacifiers (dummies, soothers)
   c. Breast pumps
   d. Open cups or spoons

4.50 **This baby has difficulty latching on to the breast and cannot sustain a sucking pattern for more than a few minutes. Which of the following suggestions would be MOST HELPFUL in assisting baby to breastfeed?**

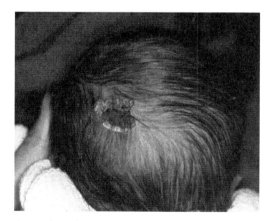

See color plate 20.

   a. Position the baby in a vertical position with his head higher than his shoulders.
   b. Reduce light and sound in the room.
   c. Feed expressed mother's milk with an orthodontic shaped teat (nipple).
   d. Handle the baby gently and slowly as if he has a headache.

4.51 **What should be your FIRST action in helping this baby breastfeed?**

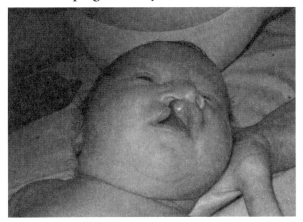

See color plate 21.

Courtesy of Catherine Watson Genna.

    a. Help mother position baby deeply at breast so her breast fills the baby's cleft lip.

    b. Help mother hand-express her milk to feed with an open cup.

    c. Provide an electric breast pump with double collection kit until the baby can latch.

    d. Give the mother a silicone nipple shield to create negative pressure in baby's mouth.

4.52 **What is the FIRST action you would recommend to increase this mother's comfort during breastfeeding?**

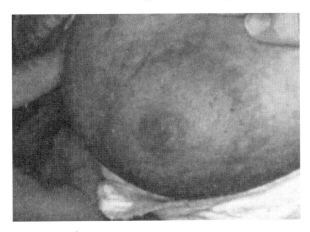

See color plate 22.

    a. Bring the baby more deeply onto the breast.

    b. Use an antifungal cream on her nipples.

    c. Apply lanolin after nursings.

    d. Use a different brand of absorbent bra pad.

4.53 **The behavior shown in this picture is MOST likely to be:**

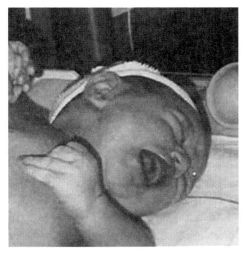

Courtesy of Mary Kroeger.

    a. distress at separation from mother.

    b. an indication of pain.

    c. infant's attempt to manipulate mother.

    d. stressful to the baby's physiology.

4.54 **This mother is worried about her full-term baby's skin color. Your BEST recommendation is:**

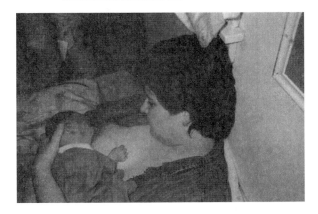

    a. Have the baby's bilirubin checked by the pediatrician.

    b. Adjust her positioning and encourage frequent breastfeeding on cue.

    c. Have her begin supplementing feeds with expressed breastmilk.

    d. Have her give the baby water between breastfeeds.

4.55 **A 12-hour-old baby weighs 2700 g, or 6 lb. Which of the following characteristics of her sucking would lead you to suspect that this child was born slightly preterm (or near term)? The baby:**

a. moves smoothly from rooting behavior to latch-on.

b. sucks, swallows, and breathes in a coordinated rhythm.

c. sucks in short bursts with pauses.

d. begins by sucking rapidly, then slows to a steady rhythm.

4.56 **Which is the MOST IMPORTANT function of colostrum?**

a. Coats the immature gut and prevents adherence of pathogens

b. Provides high-calorie food for energy

c. Blocks transmission of allergens

d. Beta-endorphins reduce infant pain

4.57 **Which hormone's rapid decline after childbirth triggers the onset of lactogenesis II (onset of copious milk production)?**

a. Estrogen

b. Prolactin

c. Oxytocin

d. Progesterone

4.58 **Which of the following statements BEST describes the difference in fat content of colostrum vs. mature milk?**

a. Colostrum has 4–5 g/100 mL, mature milk has 2–3 g/100 mL of fat.

b. Colostrum has 2–3 g/100 mL, mature milk has 4–5 g/100 mL of fat.

c. Colostrum has roughly one-fourth the fat content of mature milk.

d. Colostrum has 10 mL of fat and mature milk has 20 mL of fat.

4.59 **A woman who received intravenous magnesium sulfate during labor to control her blood pressure is having trouble initiating breastfeeding. The MOST LIKELY explanation for this is that :**

a. this medication can cause maternal lethargy, confusion, and muscle relaxation.

b. the medication affected the baby's ability to suck.

c. her milk tastes unpleasant because of the medication.

d. the drug reduced the amount of colostrum available, and the baby is frustrated.

4.60 **An 18-hour-old infant breastfed successfully in the first hour. Since then, he has not fed. The baby is healthy and full term and is not showing any signs of hypoglycemia. To help this baby begin breastfeeding, your FIRST action should be to have the mother:**

a. start using a nursing supplementer at breast.

b. use a nipple shield during feeds.

c. keep her baby skin-to-skin for the next 3 hours.

d. give 2 oz of formula, then try breastfeeding again.

4.61 **The mother in this picture is preparing to breastfeed her baby. Your FIRST suggestion would be:**

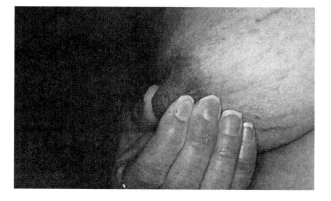

a. Great technique to firm your nipples!

b. Move your hand back behind the areola to support your breast.

c. Place the nipple tip in the baby's mouth.

d. Pinching your nipple can injure the tissue.

4.62 **The MOST LIKELY cause for a mother's nipples to be cracked and bleeding on the second postpartum day is that:**
   a. baby has anklyoglossia.
   b. baby is latching only on to the nipple.
   c. mother has unusually fragile nipple skin.
   d. mother is feeding her baby every 2 hours for 30 minutes each.

4.63 **What might have been a better approach to help this baby latch instead of using the device pictured?**

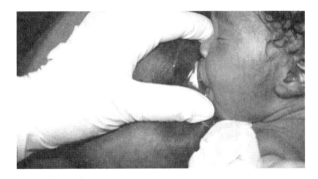

See color plate 23.
Courtesy of K. Jean Cotterman.

   a. Rolling and pulling mother's nipple to make it more extensible
   b. Dripping sweetened liquid or formula over mother's breast to entice baby
   c. Holding the baby in skin-to-skin contact in a quiet environment for several hours
   d. Squeezing the baby's cheeks to make her open her mouth wider

4.64 **The MOST LIKELY gestational age of this baby is:**

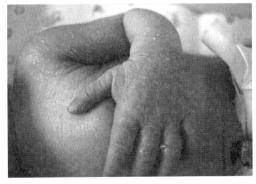

See color plate 24.
Courtesy of Catherine Watson Genna.

   a. 36 weeks.
   b. 38 weeks.
   c. 40 weeks.
   d. 42 weeks.

4.65 **Which situation would have the HIGHEST risk of drug passage into milk?**
   a. Baby was born at 26 weeks' gestation and is now 3 weeks old.
   b. Mother breastfeeds five times a day and supplements with infant formula.
   c. Two days after a cesarean birth
   d. Five-month-old twins, exclusively breastfed

4.66 **What would you do NEXT to help this baby breastfeed?**

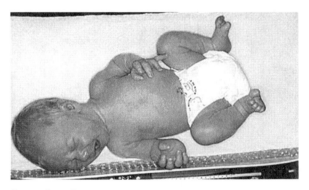

See color plate 25.

   a. Immediately put him to breast while he is alert.
   b. Put him under a radiant warmer for 2 hours to stabilize his temperature.
   c. Put him on his mother's bare chest, with mother slightly reclining.
   d. Swaddle him tightly with a small blanket to contain extraneous movements.

4.67 **After repositioning a 2-day-old baby so he latches more deeply, the mother says her nipples are still creased and painful after a feed. The MOST LIKELY infant-related cause of this continued nipple pain is:**
   a. small for gestational age.
   b. tongue and inner cheeks have a white coating.
   c. labial frenulum is long and elastic.
   d. lingual frenulum is attached at the lower gum ridge.

4.68 Which is the MOST PROFOUND consequence of separating healthy mothers and babies shortly after birth?

a. Increased rates of infection
b. Improved rest for mother
c. Increase in infant stress hormones
d. Difficulty initiating breastfeeding

4.69 A full-term baby 13 hours old has not yet been to breast. Your FIRST CHOICE to feed this baby is:

a. a curved-tip syringe.
b. an open cup.
c. a bottle with preemie nipple(teat).
d. to put the baby to breast.

4.70 Approximately how much milk does a baby of this age obtain at breast?

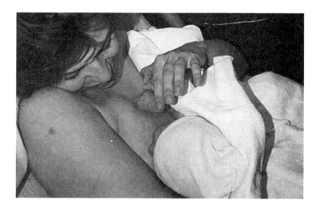

a. The baby gets about 150 mL/day [5 oz/day] of colostrum.
b. The baby gets increasing amounts each day as milk volume increases.
c. The baby needs a supplement until day 5 when mom's supply is sufficient.
d. The baby gets 750 mL/day (25 oz/day) from day 2 onward.

4.71 What is the average normal heart rate of a full-term infant?

a. 80–100 beats per minute
b. 100–120 beats per minute
c. 120–160 beats per minute
d. 160–200 beats per minute

4.72 When a baby is properly latched-on, where is the tip of the mother's nipple located in the baby's mouth?

a. Immediately behind the upper gum ridge
b. At the center of the hard palate
c. Near the juncture of the hard and soft palate
d. At the center of the soft palate

4.73 Lack of eye contact and little talking or caressing of her infant should alert you to the possibility of a:

a. neurologically impaired infant.
b. neurologically impaired mother.
c. developmentally delayed infant.
d. clinically depressed mother.

4.74 A 10-hour-old healthy, full-term baby has a blood sugar level of 36 mg/dL (2 mmol/L). The BEST treatment is to:

a. ask the mother to breastfeed her baby.
b. do nothing; continue to observe.
c. give the baby a bottle of glucose water.
d. give the baby 30 mL (1 oz) of artificial baby milk.

4.75 Which infant disease or condition is incompatible with breastfeeding?

a. Hypothyroidism
b. Down syndrome
c. Phenylketonuria
d. Galactosemia

4.76 **Which infant sleep pattern is MOST LIKELY during the first 2 days after birth? The mother received no drugs or pharmacological pain relief during labor, and the healthy term infant was placed in skin-to-skin contact with mother immediately, without suctioning or separation for any reason.**

   a. 60–90 minutes of sleep at irregular intervals

   b. Absence of rapid eye movement (REM) sleep during daylight hours

   c. 5–6 hours of slow-wave sleep during darkness

   d. Predictable periods of sleep if alone in a crib

4.77 **A 2-day-old baby feeds from one breast for about 25 minutes, then falls asleep and releases the breast. A few minutes later, he wakes and feeds on the second breast for about 10 minutes, then falls asleep and releases the breast. The MOST LIKELY explanation for this behavior is:**

   a. the mother does not yet have enough milk to satisfy the baby.

   b. the baby is not latched deeply on to the breast.

   c. the baby is sleepy and poorly coordinated as a result of labor medications.

   d. this is a normal pattern for this age baby.

4.78 **A mother has treatment-controlled hyperthyroidism. The BEST recommendation is that the baby:**

   a. should not be breastfed.

   b. may be breastfed, but should be monitored for hyperthyroidism.

   c. may breastfeed normally.

   d. will need thyroid medication.

4.79 **Which action or statement would be MOST HELPFUL to this mother?**

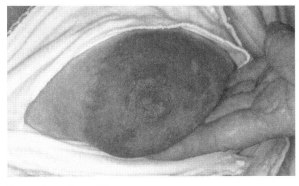

See color plate 26.

   a. Try to get all of your areola into the baby's mouth.

   b. Remove your bra so the baby can get a deep latch.

   c. Support your breast from underneath, between your thumb and first finger.

   d. Center your nipple in the baby's mouth and lean forward to help him latch.

4.80 **Based on this visual assessment, the MOST LIKELY outcome of this breastfeeding session is that:**

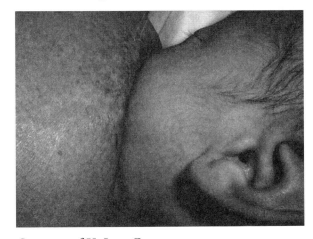

Courtesy of K. Jean Cotterman.

   a. baby will soon release the breast because she cannot breathe.

   b. baby will release the breast in satiation after about 20 minutes.

   c. mom's nipple will be painful, because the baby is latched too deeply.

   d. mother's breasts will remain full because baby's suck was ineffective.

4.81 The parents of a 1-day-old baby born at home without a skilled birth attendant want your help with painful breastfeeding. Your BEST response should be:

   a. I will help only after you've had your baby examined by a physician or skilled professional.

   b. I can talk with you by telephone a few times, off the record.

   c. I charge a fee for home or office visits and can see you later today.

   d. I cannot help, because I am required to work only under a physician's supervision.

4.82 Which technique for helping a mother breastfeed has been found to be offensive to mothers?

   a. Placing the baby skin-to-skin and allowing the baby to self-latch

   b. Grasping the mother's breast and shoving it into the baby's mouth

   c. Showing the mother how to support her breast from underneath

   d. Showing a movie or video of several positions for breastfeeding

4.83 An obese mother's baby weighed 6 lb 12 oz (3.07 kg) at birth; 6 lb 4 oz (2.83 kg) at discharge on day 2, and 6 lb 14 oz (3.12 kg) on a day-4 checkup. She is relieved, because obesity may have which effect on lactation?

   a. Reduced prolactin response to sucking

   b. Overactive letdown response that overwhelms the baby

   c. Suppressed milk synthesis because of excess lipid tissue in the breast

   d. Overproduction because of excess blood glucose

4.84 You are working with a team developing policies for a postpartum (postnatal) unit that support exclusive breastfeeding, ensure safety for all mothers and babies, and facilitate sleep for mothers at risk of postpartum depression. Which practice is MOST LIKELY to facilitate all three factors?

   a. Mother and baby share the same bed unless specific risk factors are present.

   b. Mothers can bedshare when awake or a family member is present.

   c. Babies are placed supine in cots/bassinets in arm's reach of mothers' beds.

   d. Babies are taken to a central nursery while mother sleeps and are returned when mother is awake.

4.85 A mother says that her baby latched on well at first, but now her nipple is painful and "looks flat." Your FIRST action should be to:

   a. carefully observe the baby's behavior at breast during a feed.

   b. have the mother pull the baby's legs in closer.

   c. make sure both upper and lower lips are flanged (rolled) outward.

   d. remove the baby from her breast and re-start the feed.

4.86 On the second postbirth day, an otherwise healthy term baby nurses for 45 minutes, sleeps briefly, then wakes with frantic crying. What is the MOST LIKELY explanation for this pattern?

   a. Normal pattern for day 2

   b. Small for gestational age

   c. Head injury during birth

   d. Shallow latch at breast

Answers for 1–2 Days Questions

4.1   **The answer is b.** The pump flange was too small in diameter for this mother's large, fibrous nipples, causing friction and irritation. A pump flange should be wide enough in diameter to allow the nipple and areola to move back and forth easily. (Difficulty: 4; Discipline: Clinical Skills; Taxonomy: Evaluate.)

4.2   **The answer is b.** The Code of Professional Conduct states that a LC is required to "Inform an appropriate person or authority if it appears that the health or safety of a client or a colleague is at risk." The LC's scope of practice alone does not include a medical assessment of the baby. Meconium should have been passed on day 1. Safe formula feeding may become necessary if other strategies are ineffective. (Difficulty: 4; Discipline: Clinical Skills; Taxonomy: Collaboration.)

4.3   **The answer is c.** Skin-to-skin contact is the FIRST and least interventive of the strategies suggested, and often the most effective. In this case, the mother's nipple and breast configuration are not important. (Difficulty: Discipline: Techniques; Taxonomy: Plan.)

4.4   **The answer is d.** Skin-to-skin contact is the first strategy, followed by massage and other gentle stimulating strategies. Painful stimulation is not appropriate and may even cause the baby to shut down further. (Difficulty: 4; Discipline: Techniques; Taxonomy: Plan.)

4.5   **The answer is d.** This mother's breast is full of milk with milk stasis due to the baby not nursing well. Gentle massage or hand-expression is the best suggestion to get milk flowing and reduce stasis. There is no visual evidence of edema, so choices a and c are inappropriate. Choice b is inappropriate. (Difficulty: 4; Discipline: Techniques; Taxonomy: Plan.)

4.6   **The answer is d.** A wide gap is the most important visible feature of effective positioning and latch. All of the nipple and a portion of the areola should be inside the infant's mouth, but not necessarily all of it, depending on the areola diameter. The nose may lightly touch the breast, or be close to it, not buried in the breast. (Difficulty: 2; Discipline: Techniques; Taxonomy: Evaluate.)

4.7   **The answer is c.** Her breast reduction surgery may have severed the nerves and ducts needed for adequate lactation. Close follow-up is essential. (Difficulty: 3; Discipline: Clinical Skills; Taxonomy: Plan.)

4.8   **The answer is c.** The baby has a short, tight frenulum, which might interfere with effective breastfeeding. However, direct breastfeeding is the ultimate goal and the normative behavior to reinforce. Not all babies with tight frenula will have a problem breastfeeding. If direct breastfeeding is ineffective or painful, options a, b, or d could be considered. (Difficulty: 4; Discipline: Clinical Skills; Taxonomy: Plan.)

4.9   **The answer is b.** Baby cannot produce suction due to the cleft, so extra time at breast is not likely to allow baby to drain the breast. Mother needs to drain the breast well and mimic the average breastfed baby's feeding pattern to induce frequent prolactin spikes to establish full lactation. (Difficulty: 4; Discipline: Pathology; Taxonomy: Plan.)

4.10   **The answer is c.** This is mechanical (friction) damage from a tongue-tied baby. Choices a and b do not cause open wounds. Choice d is an old myth, not consistent with current knowledge and research evidence. (Difficulty: 2; Discipline: Pathology; Taxonomy: Evaluate.)

4.11   **The answer is b.** The BFHI Step 6 requires purchasing of any formula used through normal supply channels. No "free" or low-cost supplies can be solicited or accepted. Acceptable medical reasons for supplementation are available from WHO and updated periodically. (Difficulty: 5; Discipline: Clinical Skills; Taxonomy: Knowledge.)

4.12   **The answer is a.** Weighing a baby before and after a feed, using a sensitive scale and without changing the baby's clothes and diaper, is an accurate assessment of milk transfer. The amount of milk transferred in the first few days is less important than the fact that some milk was taken by the baby. Choice b may be helpful, but does not tell the entire story of the effectiveness of the feed. Choice c might help. Choice d is not necessary, is actually inappropriate, and can discourage the mother. (Difficulty: 3; Discipline: Techniques; Taxonomy: Plan.)

4.13   **The answer is b.** Breastfeeding has been shown to be the most effective pain relief strategy for minor painful procedures. Human milk alone may be pain relieving, even without direct breastfeeding. Skin-to-skin is helpful, even without breastfeeding or breastmilk. Studies on sucrose are mixed; sucrose and a pacifier may be soothing. Swaddling has not been shown to be effective to manage procedural pain. (Difficulty: 4; Discipline: Pharmacology; Taxonomy: Collaboration.)

4.14   **The answer is c.** Pain medications for surgical deliveries are generally compatible with breastfeeding. The LC and nursing staff should monitor the mother and baby for poor or ineffective feeding,

excessive drowsiness, or lethargy. (Difficulty: 2; Discipline: Pharmacology; Taxonomy: Goals.)

4.15   **The answer is a.** Crying is a late sign of hunger and occurs after all other cues have been ignored. Babies should be fed when they exhibit early feeding cues. (Difficulty: 2; Discipline: Development; Taxonomy: Evaluate.)

4.16   **The answer is b.** This wound was caused by a baby whose lingual frenulum was short and tight (tongue-tied). (Difficulty: 4; Discipline: Pathology; Taxonomy: Evaluate.)

4.17   **The answer is d.** Of the options listed, d is most likely to be successful, triggering the baby's innate responses. (Difficulty: 5; Discipline: Clinical Skills; Taxonomy: Plan.)

4.18   **The answer is c.** Moist wound healing is most effective. Choice d is the second-best response. Choices a and b are not helpful strategies because they dry the skin surface and retard healing. (Difficulty: 4; Discipline: Pathology; Taxonomy: Plan.)

4.19   **The answer is b.** The white structures in this newborn's mouth are natal teeth. Rarely do these interfere with breastfeeding. (Difficulty: 3; Discipline: Development; Taxonomy: Assessment.)

4.20   **The answer is b.** It is always best to evaluate breastfeeding problems in person, because you can weigh the baby, observe the breastfeeding, and more. (Difficulty: 4; Discipline: Techniques; Taxonomy: Collaboration.)

4.21   **The answer is c.** This baby's lingual frenulum, the string-like tissue between the tongue and the floor of the mouth, is short and tight and likely to restrict tongue motion needed for effective feeding. (Difficulty: 3; Discipline: Development; Taxonomy: Assessment.)

4.22 **The answer is b.** Lactogenesis II is triggered by the withdrawal of progesterone when the placenta separates from the uterus. (Difficulty: 4; Discipline: Development; Taxonomy: Knowledge.)

4.23 **The answer is a.** Each mother–baby system will develop unique feeding patterns. The LC supports any and all patterns that meet the mother's and babies' needs. (Difficulty: 5; Discipline: Psychology; Taxonomy: Goals.)

4.24 **The answer is b.** This baby was tongue-tied, which quickly damaged mother's nipples. The nipple shield provided temporary protection to the nipple while frenotomy was arranged. In a premature baby, a nipple shield can improve milk transfer, but this baby is clearly not premature. Large breasts or nipples are not necessarily an indication for use of a nipple shield. The last option is speculative. (Difficulty: 3; Discipline: Pathology; Taxonomy: Plan.)

4.25 **The answer is d.** Twenty-four-hour rooming-in from birth onward is Step 7 of the Ten Steps to Successful Breastfeeding (BFHI). (Difficulty: 4; Discipline: Clinical Skills; Taxonomy: Collaboration.)

4.26 **The answer is b.** Macrophages and possibly neutrophils and T-lymphocytes actively kill microbes by phagocytosis. (Difficulty: 4; Discipline: Development; Taxonomy: Knowledge.)

4.27 **The answer is b.** On days 1–3, the baby gets about 30 mL/day of colostrum. As lactogenesis II occurs, baby obtains more per day as milk volume rapidly rises to ≥600 mL/day on day 5. (Difficulty: 4; Discipline: Development; Taxonomy: Knowledge.)

4.28 **The answer is a.** An infant can imitate the adult's facial expressions shortly after birth. This baby is 4 days old and clearly is imitating the woman's expression. (Difficulty: 4; Discipline: Development; Taxonomy: Assessment.)

4.29 **The answer is d.** This baby's oral anatomy is normal. (Difficulty: 3; Discipline: Development; Taxonomy: Document.)

4.30 **The answer is a.** Tremors and hyperreactive reflexes are typical of newborn abstinence syndrome, which can significantly affect the infant's ability to feed. The infant may have seizures, high-pitched crying, and ineffective feeding. Low tone and lethargy are unlikely. Coordinated suck-swallow-breathe patterns are unlikely. (Difficulty: 4; Discipline: Pathology; Taxonomy: Knowledge.)

4.31 **The answer is b.** An oral exam can be part of a lactation assessment. Suck training is considered an advanced therapy and is rarely needed. During fingerfeeding, a thin tube is held against the adult's finger. The baby in the picture is being held and appears asleep; therefore, choice d is unlikely. (Difficulty: 5; Discipline: Techniques; Taxonomy: Assessment)

4.32 **The answer is b.** This mother's large, fibrous nipple was being compressed by her baby's small mouth and shallow palate. (Difficulty: 2; Discipline: Pathology; Taxonomy: Evaluate.)

4.33 **The answer is a.** The bulge on this woman's areola at the 10:00 position was a galactocele and caused her no discomfort or difficulty breastfeeding. (Difficulty: 4; Discipline: Pathology; Taxonomy: Assessment.)

4.34 **The answer is c.** Intraductal papilloma is the most likely cause of painless bright red bleeding in the early postpartum period. If the bleeding continues, a professional should be consulted for further evaluation. (Difficulty: 4; Discipline: Pathology; Taxonomy: Collaboration.)

4.35 **The answer is a.** Mothers and babies thrive when 24-hour rooming-in with safe bedding-in is practiced. This mother is on a firm surface, awake and alert, and holding her baby at breast in a protective position. The other actions are unnecessary or inappropriate. (Difficulty: 4; Discipline: Psychology; Taxonomy: Plan.)

4.36 **The answer is d.** The hand positions shown are adequate. The next appropriate action is bringing the baby to the breast. (Difficulty: 5; Discipline: Techniques; Taxonomy: Plan.)

4.37 **The answer is b.** The concentration of colostrum does not affect how chemicals enter the colostrum. A larger blood volume actually leads to a more dilute concentration of drug in the mother's plasma. In healthy mothers, the kidneys function normally after birth. (Difficulty: 3; Discipline: Pharmacology; Taxonomy: Knowledge.)

4.38 **The answer is b.** Immediate effective breastfeeding in the first hour or so, followed by 24-hour rooming-in and feeding on cue are the most important strategies. Prenatal expression of colostrum is just now being researched. If the baby cannot breastfeed, milk expression should begin soon after birth. Restricting mother's fluids is inappropriate and dangerous. (Difficulty: 4; Discipline: Clinical Skills; Taxonomy: Collaboration.)

4.39 **The answer is a.** Extreme nipple pain in the absence of visual symptoms may indicate a deeper problem such as prior history of abuse. (Difficulty: 5; Discipline: Pathology; Taxonomy: History.)

4.40 **The answer is b.** Prelacteal ritual feeds increase the risk of infections and illnesses and interfere with breastfeeding. Choices c and d are also correct but usually less critical.

(Difficulty: 4; Discipline: Pathology; Taxonomy: Knowledge.)

4.41 **The answer is b.** The hand on the baby's back should be slightly lower, allowing the baby to extend her head for easier coordination of suck-swallow-breathe. Supporting the breast might help if the first suggestion is ineffective. (Difficulty: 3; Discipline: Techniques; Taxonomy: Plan.)

4.42 **The answer is a.** Many of the antidepressant medications are compatible with breastfeeding. Continuing to breastfeed may help her recover from her illness. (Difficulty: 4; Discipline: Pharmacology; Taxonomy: Collaboration.)

4.43 **The answer is b.** Shallow latch is the most likely reason that the mother's nipple is flattened after a feed with a crease across the nipple tip. Position of the baby and torticollis are possible explanations to explore after the depth of attachment is corrected. Normal suck should not crease, flatten, or damage the mother's nipple. (Difficulty: 4; Discipline: Pathology; Taxonomy: Evaluate.)

4.44 **The answer is d.** The Babinski reflex, flaring of the toes, is triggered when the sole of the foot is stimulated. This reflex is not central to a baby's ability to breastfeed, but if any reflex appears to be abnormal, a thorough pediatric exam should be conducted. (Difficulty: 4; Discipline: Development; Taxonomy: Knowledge.)

4.45 **The answer is c.** Deep attachment is key to comfortable, effective breastfeeding. Demonstrating with model and a doll empowers the mother and develops her own skill in holding and positioning her baby effectively. The other techniques may be helpful if the next attempt at latching is unsuccessful. (Difficulty: 5; Discipline: Techniques; Taxonomy: Plan.)

4.46 **The answer is b.** Drugs more readily pass into milk in the first few days postbirth because the junctures between mammary secretory cells are open at this point, permitting passage of medications and other substances into the alveolar lumen. (Difficulty: 4; Discipline: Pharmacology; Taxonomy: Knowledge.)

4.47 **The answer is c.** Ensuring proper positioning and latch is always the first action. This mother's bifurcated nipple was fully functional, and the baby fed from this breast easily and effectively. (Difficulty: 2; Discipline: Clinical Skills; Taxonomy: Plan.)

4.48 **The answer is d.** Mothers with hearing (auditory) impairments are generally very familiar with visual and tactile communication. Breastfeeding may be easier for her than artificial feeding. (Difficulty: 4; Discipline: Psychology; Taxonomy: Goals.)

4.49 **The answer is b.** The BFHI Step 9 is "Give no artificial teats or pacifiers (also called dummies or soothers) to breastfeeding infants." This step also includes the prohibition of feeding bottles. Bottles that are attached to breast pumps are not addressed because they are considered collection containers (Difficulty: 2; Discipline: Clinical Skills; Taxonomy: Knowledge.)

4.50 **The answer is a.** With an injury on the head, the baby is likely to be more comfortable in a more vertical position, Birth injuries such as this wound from a vacuum extractor may cause head pain in the baby. Direct breastfeeding should be tried first; if unsuccessful, other methods could be explored. Choice b may help. (Difficulty: 4; Discipline: Techniques; Taxonomy: Plan.)

4.51 **The answer is a.** Direct breastfeeding is always the first choice. This baby was able to feed directly at breast because the mother's soft breast filled the cleft lip. The other strategies might be appropriate if direct breastfeeding was ineffective.

(Difficulty: 5; Discipline: Techniques; Taxonomy: Goals.)

4.52 **The answer is a.** Correcting positioning and latch represent the most important strategy to increase nipple comfort during breastfeeding. In this mother's case, deeper attachment significantly reduced pain; treating the mild thrush infection removed the remaining discomfort. (Difficulty: 5; Discipline: Techniques; Taxonomy: Plan.)

4.53 **The answer is d.** Crying is extremely stressful to the baby. Babies cue or signal for their needs to be met. Crying is an indication of pain, abandonment, fear, and a LATE sign of hunger; it is also a sign that the baby has exhausted all other resources in getting his needs met. (Difficulty: 4; Discipline: Development; Taxonomy: Evaluate.)

4.54 **The answer is b.** The baby's skin is slightly yellow, suggesting hyperbilirubinemia. Ensuring frequent, effective breastfeeds is the most appropriate strategy to use at this point. (Difficulty: 4; Discipline: Pathology; Taxonomy: Plan.)

4.55 **The answer is c.** Short sucking burses with pauses is an indicator of immaturity. The other patterns are indicators of a mature infant. (Difficulty: 3; Discipline: Development; Taxonomy: Assessment.)

4.56 **The answer is a.** Its protective role appears to be even more important than its role in providing calories to the infant. Beta-endorphins in colostrum are natural pain relievers. Colostrum is rich in anti-infective and anti-inflammatory properties. (Difficulty: 4; Discipline: Development; Taxonomy: Knowledge.)

4.57 **The answer is d.** Delivery of the placenta causes a sudden drop in levels of progesterone, triggering the onset of lactogenesis II. (Difficulty: 3; Discipline: Physiology; Taxonomy: Knowledge.)

4.58 **The answer is b.** Colostrum has 2–3 g/100 mL, mature milk has 4–5 g/100 mL of fat. (Difficulty: 3; Discipline: Development; Taxonomy: History.)

4.59 **The answer is a.** Magnesium sulfate can cause maternal drowsiness and lethargy. The American Academy of Pediatrics considers this medication compatible with breastfeeding. (Difficulty: 5; Discipline: Pharmacology; Taxonomy: History.)

4.60 **The answer is c.** Skin-to-skin contact helps babies initiate breastfeeding. None of the other actions are appropriate or backed by current evidence. (Difficulty: 3; Discipline: Techniques; Taxonomy: Plan.)

4.61 **The answer is a.** This mother is gently and correctly rolling her retracted nipples to firm them before feeding. (Difficulty: 4; Discipline: Techniques; Taxonomy: Assessment.)

4.62 **The answer is b.** Most early cracked nipples are caused by poor breastfeeding technique and/or sucking problems. The length and/or frequency of breastfeeds are far less important causes of nipple damage than maternal skin conditions or the baby's ability to suck correctly. (Difficulty: 4; Discipline: Pathology; Taxonomy: Evaluate.)

4.63 **The answer is c.** Many babies will self-latch, even after difficult births and initial problems, if placed skin-to-skin on mother's bare chest for several hours. There is no evidence that mother's nipple is not already everted. Dripping fluids onto the breast to entice the baby is inappropriate. Never try to manipulate the baby's mouth to force a latch, which can trigger aversive behavior. (Difficulty: 3; Discipline: Techniques; Taxonomy: Evaluate.)

4.64 **The answer is d.** This baby was born at 42 completed weeks of gestation, which is considered the late end of normal gestation. Peeling skin is one visual clue to a baby nearing postterm gestational age. Breastfeeding difficulties are associated with preterm and sometimes postterm birth. (Difficulty: 4; Discipline: Development; Taxonomy: Assessment.)

4.65 **The answer is c.** The risk of drug passage into milk is highest in the early postpartum period when the junctures between the mammary secretory epithelial cells (lactocytes) are open. After the first week or so, the tight junctures between cells inhibit most drugs from passing into milk. (Difficulty: 4; Discipline: Pharmacology; Taxonomy: Knowledge.)

4.66 **The answer is c.** Immediate skin-to-skin contact is an effective strategy to calm and warm a baby in preparation for breastfeeding. If the mother is slightly reclining, this strategy is even more likely to be effective. Choice a would be the second-best strategy. Choices c and d are not helpful. (Difficulty: 4; Discipline: Clinical Skills; Taxonomy: Plan.)

4.67 **The answer is d.** A short and/or tight lingual frenulum, or one that is attached near the lower gum ridge and/or tongue tip, is the most likely infant condition listed to cause persistent nipple pain. Small gestational age is not likely related to nipple pain. The white coating is likely oral candidal infection, which can be painful but unlikely to cause nipple distortion. The upper lip (labial) frenulum as described is normal. (Difficulty: 3; Discipline: Pathology; Taxonomy: Evaluate.)

4.68 **The answer is c.** Separation destabilizes infants and elevates cortisol levels in mother and infant and disrupts early prefeeding behavior. Research shows mothers rest better when mothers and babies are kept together following birth. (Difficulty: 5; Discipline: Physiology; Taxonomy: Collaboration.)

4.69 **The answer is d.** Direct breastfeeding should be tried first. Devices should only be considered when direct breastfeeding is impossible. (Difficulty: 3; Discipline: Clinical Skills; Taxonomy: Plan.)

4.70 **The answer is b.** On days 1–3, the baby gets about 30 mL/day (1 oz/day) of colostrum. As Lactogenesis II progresses, the baby obtains more per day as milk volume rapidly rises to about 600 mL/day (20 oz/day) or more by day 5. (Difficulty: 5; Discipline: Development; Taxonomy: Assessment.)

4.71 **The answer is c.** Normal newborn heart rate is 120–160 beats per minute. Tachycardia (fast heart rate) or bradycardia (slow heart rate) can interfere with the baby's ability to breastfeed. The LC works closely with the baby's primary care provider especially when cardiac differences are present. (Difficulty: 5; Discipline: Development; Taxonomy: Evaluate.)

4.72 **The answer is c.** The nipple tip extends to or close to the juncture of the hard and soft palates during normal latch and positioning. (Difficulty: 4; Discipline: Clinical Skills; Taxonomy: Evaluate.)

4.73 **The answer is d.** Lack of eye contact and little talking or caressing of her infant may be signs of postpartum depression. The LC should report these signs to the mother's primary care provider immediately. (Difficulty: 4; Discipline: Psychology; Taxonomy: Assessment.)

4.74 **The answer is a.** Colostrum is the treatment of choice for asymptomatic hypoglycemia. A small amount of colostrum stabilizes blood sugar. Some methods of testing blood sugar are not accurate. Direct breastfeeding is always the first and best course of action. A newborn normally breastfeeds every 1–3 hours in the first 24 hours, and nothing in this question indicates when, if ever, the baby had previously been fed.

(Difficulty: 4; Discipline: Pathology; Taxonomy: Plan.)

4.75 **The answer is d.** Babies with galactosemia cannot metabolize lactose, which is in high amounts in human milk. If the inability to metabolize lactose is complete, the baby should not have any breastmilk at all. (Difficulty: 4; Discipline: Pathology; Taxonomy: Knowledge.)

4.76 **The answer is a.** Newborn sleep cycles are approximately 60–90 minutes in irregular patterns throughout the first few months. REM sleep and slow-wave sleep are part of sleep cycling. Babies cannot sleep long periods until at least 6-9 months of age. Solitary sleep results in less sleep for the infant and parents. (Difficulty: 2; Discipline: Development; Taxonomy: Evaluate.)

4.77 **The answer is d.** This is a normal pattern on day 2. The baby's appetite, interest, and ability to feed will determine whether one or both breasts are taken at a given feeding. This pattern would be described as a "paired" breastfeed. (Difficulty: 5; Discipline: Development; Taxonomy: Evaluate.)

4.78 **The answer is c.** The baby may breastfeed normally. Maternal thyroid disease that is properly treated is compatible with breastfeeding. (Difficulty: 3; Discipline: Pathology; Taxonomy: Collaboration.)

4.79 **The answer is c.** Supporting this soft breast from underneath is the MOST helpful suggestion. Other techniques may be even more helpful, including allowing the baby to self-attach. This mother's areolae are very large and may not be fully covered by the baby's mouth. Removing the bra is probably irrelevant, as much of the breast is available. Leaning forward is usually uncomfortable at best. (Difficulty: 4; Discipline: Techniques; Taxonomy: Goals.)

4.80   **The answer is b.** This baby is deeply latched to the breast with both upper and lower lips nearly invisible. The nose is lightly touching the mother's breast, and the chin is well into the breast. Without any other data, one would expect a comfortable feed for mother and baby. (Difficulty: 2; Discipline: Techniques; Taxonomy: Evaluate.)

4.81   **The answer is c.** A LC can ethically provide postpartum consults in a client's home or in an office, providing the fees are discussed first. The other choices are not appropriate. All client consults, by phone or in person, or electronically, must be documented, and the lactation consultant must be in contact with the family's care provider(s). (Difficulty: 5; Discipline: Clinical Skills; Taxonomy: Collaboration.)

4.82   **The answer is b.** Mother do not like for staff members to grab their breasts or push the baby onto their breasts, and may be too intimidated to express their displeasure. Demonstrating with a doll or with a video may be more helpful. Choice a, self-attachment, is usually very helpful and effective. Supporting the breast from underneath may compress some surface milk ducts. (Difficulty: 3; Discipline: Techniques; Taxonomy: Goals.)

4.83   **The answer is a.** Obesity is associated with reduced prolactin response to suckling in the early days of lactation. Prolactin response to suckling is more important for milk production in the first postpartum week than it is later in lactation.

(Difficulty: 2; Discipline: Physiology; Taxonomy: Goals.)

4.84   **The answer is a.** Bedsharing on a firm mattress facilitates exclusive breastfeeding, results in mothers getting more sleep, and maintains normal hormone and stress levels in mothers and babies. If maternal or infant risk factors are present, for example maternal medication that affects alertness, then a side-car device attached to her bed provides more safety for the infant and still facilitates breastfeeding. Separating the mother and baby increases stress hormones in both, results in less rest and sleep for the mother, and undermines breastfeeding. (Difficulty: 4; Discipline: Psychology; Taxonomy: Evaluate.)

4.85   **The answer is a.** The LC should observe a full feed before suggesting any changes. The other actions or suggestions might be appropriate, depending on what is observed. (Difficulty: 5; Discipline: Techniques; Taxonomy: Assessment.)

4.86   **The answer is d.** Shallow latch and/or weak suck is the most likely explanation for this pattern in a healthy term infant. A normal pattern is in the range of 10-30 minutes of effective sucking, followed by a longer sleep stretch. Frantic crying suggests inadequate milk transfer during the feed. While choices b and c are possible, choice d is the MOST likely explanation for this infant's behavior. (Difficulty: 4; Discipline: Development; Taxonomy: Evaluate.)

CHAPTER 5

3–14 Days Questions

5.1 **If you see the pictured condition on a lactating breast, during the first postpartum week, what should be your FIRST action?**

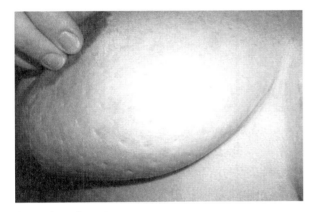

See color plate 27.
Courtesy of Catherine Watson Genna.

    a. Refer the mother to a physician specializing in breast disease.
    b. Help her learn to express her milk by hand.
    c. Suggest that she put cool cloths on the breast.
    d. Warn her to avoid feeding the baby from that breast.

5.2 **What is the MOST LIKELY reason this mother is using this device to feed her baby?**

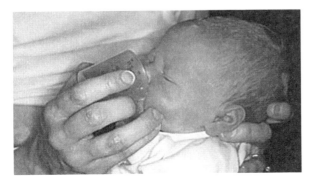

    a. Down syndrome
    b. Premature baby
    c. Direct breastfeeding is painful
    d. Giving medication to infant

5.3 **If you are working with a mother who is feeding her baby in this position, what should you say to her?**

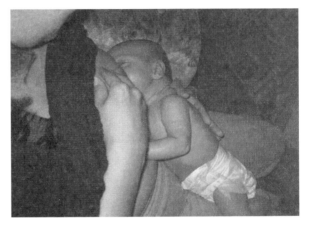

Courtesy of Catherine Watson Genna.

    a. Your semireclining position is triggering baby's instinctive behaviors for feeding.
    b. Move your right hand under your left breast to raise it slightly.
    c. Bring the baby's hips and legs in closer to your body.
    d. Your baby's eyes are closed, which means he is nearly finished with this feed.

5.4   **Based on what you can see in this photograph, what is the MOST LIKELY age of this baby?**

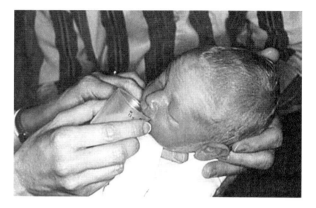

   a. 36 weeks' gestational age
   b. 38 weeks' gestational age
   c. 2 days postbirth
   d. 4 days postbirth

5.5   **What is the FIRST suggestion you would make to help this mother breastfeed more comfortably?**

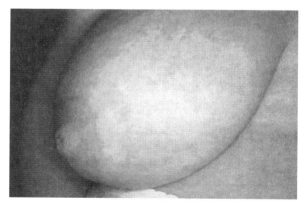

See color plate 28.

   a. Place a nipple shield over your nipple until the baby's suck improves.
   b. Wear a supportive bra 24 hours a day.
   c. Lean back with your baby on your bare chest and see if she will move to the breast.
   d. Use some lanolin on your nipple before feeds.

5.6   **This baby just came off the breast. What is this mother MOST LIKELY feeling?**

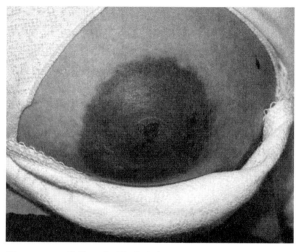

Courtesy of Carole Dobrich.

   a. Pinching nipple pain
   b. Aching breast pain
   c. Relaxation and sleepiness
   d. Relief that the baby fed well

5.7   **You are helping a frightened, overwhelmed mother on day 4 with her first baby. She has been calling everyone she knows to get advice on what to expect in the early days of breastfeeding, and she has heard confusing stories. You observe that she responds to her baby's cues and the baby nurses effectively for about 20 minutes before falling asleep and releasing her breast spontaneously. Your FIRST response should be:**

   a. Now that's what I call a textbook example of a great breastfeed!
   b. Does she usually take only one breast like she just did?
   c. Are you getting enough help at home?
   d. Your baby looks better today than when you were discharged.

5.8 **This baby has not been feeding well and needs a medically necessary supplement. Why is it being given in this manner?**

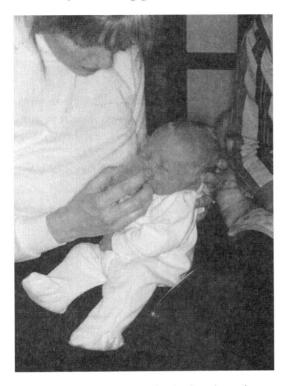

   a. Mother can't afford a bottle and teat
   b. Can pace to baby's ability
   c. Protects oral-motor functions for breastfeeding
   d. Can be easily cleaned

5.9 **The bulge on this mother's breast is MOST LIKELY:**

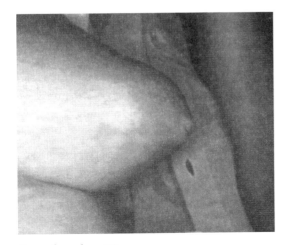

See color plate 29.

   a. a plugged duct.
   b. a galactocele.
   c. mastitis.
   d. an abscess.

5.10 **How would you document this baby's oral configuration?**

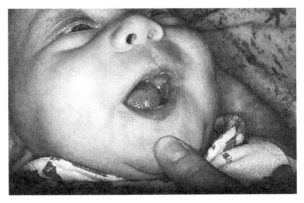

See color plate 30.

   a. Normal tongue position.
   b. Tongue is not moving normally.
   c. The tongue stays behind the inferior alveolar ridge.
   d. The baby has a poor tongue position.

5.11 **After trying to wean her baby to formula unsuccessfully, a mother of a 2-week-old baby requests help in restarting breast-feeding. She had trouble with latching in the early days, says her nipples are flat, and has been feeding pumped milk in a bottle with silicone teat. Your FIRST action should be:**

   a. Teach her suck-training techniques.
   b. Show her how to use a nipple-pulling device to extend her nipples.
   c. Have her place the bottle teat over her own nipple for a few feeds.
   d. Place the baby skin-to-skin on mother's body and support attempts at self-attachment

5.12   **The mother of a 5-day-old healthy term baby had reduction mammoplasty four years ago. Lactogenesis II occurred on day 3, but the mother's breasts have not felt full or shown any signs of engorgement. The baby has had one moderately heavy brown stool in the previous 24 hours. He has neither gained nor lost weight since day 3. What is your FIRST recommendation?**

a.   This baby's stool output and weight gain are sufficient and nothing needs to be done.

b.   This baby's stool output and weight gain are insufficient, but it is not yet necessary to supplement this baby. Nurse very frequently.

c.   This baby's stool output and weight gain are insufficient, and immediate supplementation of donated milk or formula is necessary.

d.   This baby's stool output and weight status are insufficient and supplementation is necessary. The mother should begin pumping and give her baby whatever she can pump.

5.13   **What would be the MOST APPROPRIATE use for this technique?**

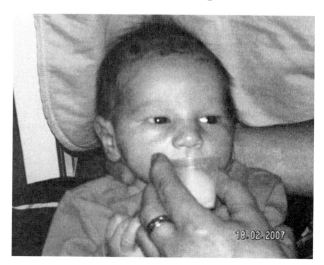

Courtesy of Carole Dobrich.

a.   Baby less than 24 hours old and not yet nursing

b.   Six-month-old refusing solid foods

c.   Baby has poor suck and mother's nipples are damaged

d.   Supplementing a 4-day-old baby who is 7% below birth weight

5.14   **A staff nurse called the lactation consultant (LC) to help assess an obese mother breastfeeding her baby on day 2. Which indicator would be the MOST REASSURING indicator of effective feeding?**

a.   Baby stays attached at least 10 minutes.

b.   Rooting and swallowing are observed.

c.   Baby's ear, shoulder, and hips are aligned.

d.   The mother reports gentle tugging on her breast.

5.15   **What is the MOST LIKELY reason this mother is experiencing pain in her left axilla?**

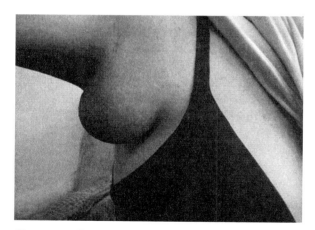

Courtesy of Maya Bolman/Ann Witt.

a.   Severe postpartum engorgement

b.   Lactogenesis II in axillary mammary tissue

c.   Allergic reaction to a new deodorant

d.   Overuse strain of the pectoral muscles

5.16 Lactoferrin in colostrum and mother's milk is important to the baby because it:

   a. binds iron in the baby's gut, thus withholding iron from pathogens.

   b. transports calcium to the infant.

   c. promotes the absorption of lactose.

   d. provides nutrients for *Lactobacillus bifidus* in the gut.

5.17 What structure in this baby's mouth is LIKELY preventing deep attachment at breast?

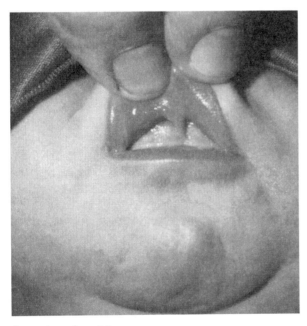

See color plate 31.

Courtesy of K. Jean Cotterman.

   a. Labial frenulum

   b. Lingual frenulum

   c. Recessed jaw

   d. Alveolar ridge

5.18 What is the MOST LIKELY explanation for the color of this milk, which was collected on day 5?

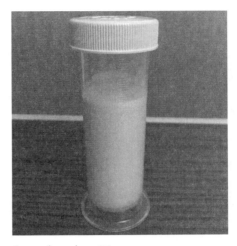

See color plate 32.

Courtesy of Laura Atkinson.

   a. The mother is taking prenatal vitamins containing beta-carotene.

   b. The milk contains pus from the mother's breast infection.

   c. Milk on day 5 has significant amounts of beta-carotene.

   d. The mother had carrots and sweet potatoes for dinner last night.

5.19 What are the dark dots around the outside (periphery) of the areola, on the skin?

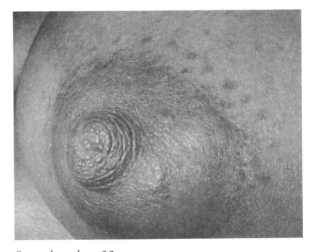

See color plate 33.

Courtesy of K. Jean Cotterman.

   a. Normal pigment variations

   b. Tattoos

   c. Pressure marks from an ill-fitting bra

   d. Scars from stitches after breast surgery

5.20 **What is the FIRST suggestion you would give this mother?**

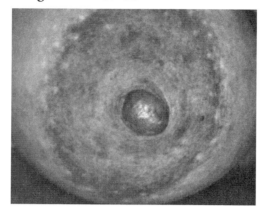

See color plate 34.

a. Use a nipple shield during feeds.
b. Have your baby's suck evaluated immediately.
c. Keep up the good work; everything looks great.
d. Bring your baby deeper onto your breast.

5.21 **A mother calls you complaining of breast pain. Her breasts are hot, hard, "knotty," and painful to the touch. She is 3 days postpartum. The FIRST suggestion you should give her is:**

a. Don't worry, your breasts will feel better in 24 hours.
b. Use a nipple shield during feedings.
c. Express or pump at least every 2 to 3 hours until the lumps are gone.
d. Restrict your fluid intake.

5.22 **What is the MOST LIKELY breastfeeding outcome for this baby?**

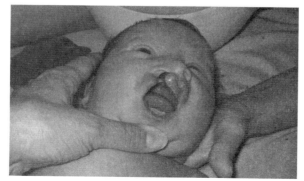

See color plate 35.

Courtesy of Catherine Watson Genna.

a. Exclusive breastfeeding without assistive devices for 6 months
b. 30% chance mother will need to support her milk production and supplement with expressed milk
c. 50% chance of failure-to-thrive on breastfeeding alone
d. Baby will need a fitted obturator and multiple surgeries to breastfeed

5.23 **A mother is concerned that her 1-week-old baby is passing one black, tarry stool per day. The baby nurses about every 3 hours for 15 to 20 minutes. Your FIRST recommendation is:**

a. Relax, the baby is still passing meconium stools.
b. Your baby needs to be examined by a physician today.
c. Stop drinking milk because your baby is reacting to the protein.
d. Begin supplementing, because the baby is not getting sufficient fluids.

5.24 **What, if anything, would you suggest to this mother regarding her baby's position and latch?**

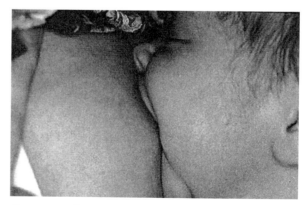

Courtesy of Greg Notestine.

a. Everything looks good.
b. Try uncurling his lower lip with your finger.
c. Tickle his feet so he wakes up during feeds.
d. Press down on your breast so his nostrils are clear.

5.25 **This mother's baby keeps bobbing on and off the breast and cannot quite latch on. The FIRST action she should take is to:**

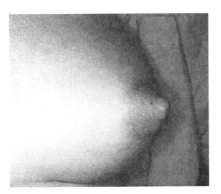

a. Place a nipple shield over her nipple.
b. Let her baby suck on her finger to calm him.
c. Express some milk to soften the breast.
d. Burp him first before trying again.

5.26 **This baby is 2 weeks old and still under his birth weight. The mother's nipples are cracked, scabbed, and painful. Feeds are 30 to 45 minutes long every 2 hours around the clock. The mother is exhausted. The FIRST recommendation you would make to his mother is:**

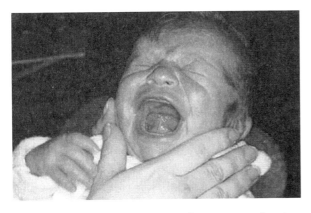

a. Have the baby's pediatrician or dentist evaluate his frenulum.
b. He's obviously upset; give him a pacifier to calm him before trying to breastfeed.
c. Are you willing to try feeding him some expressed milk in a cup?
d. Go to bed with him and try nursing lying down in a darkened room.

5.27 **The mother in this photograph is uncertain about how much milk she is making for her baby. Your FIRST action should be:**

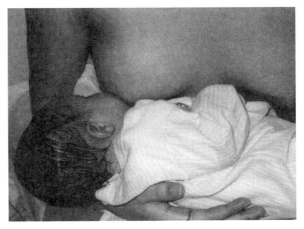

Courtesy of K. Jean Cotterman.

a. Reassure her that most mothers make plenty of milk.
b. Carefully observe a full nursing session.
c. Weigh the baby before and after the next feed, in the same clothes.
d. Suggest she pump her milk to see how much she's making.

5.28 **Which visual element of this baby's latch is MOST LIKELY to indicate a problem?**

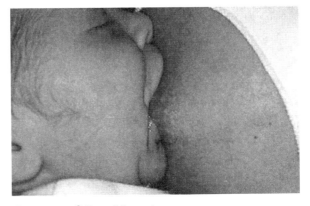

Courtesy of Greg Notestine.

a. Deep puckering at the nasolabial crease
b. Eyes are closed
c. Chin is driven into the breast
d. Nose is barely touching the breast

5.29 **A mother complains of a firm, tender area in her right breast that has persisted for 3 days, despite application of cool cabbage compresses, ice packs, and frequent milk expression using a hospital-grade electric breast pump. Your NEXT action should be:**

a. Suggest she continue this strategy for another 48 hours.

b. Switch to warm compresses before pumping.

c. Ask for a more thorough medical evaluation by a breast specialist.

d. Apply a breast binder and ask her to restrict fluids.

5.30 **The MOST APPROPRIATE guidance you can give this mother on feeding patterns is:**

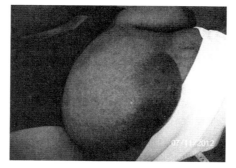

See color plate 36.
Courtesy of K. Jean Cotterman.

a. Your milk supply is very high, so use only one breast per feed.

b. Start on the fuller breast for about 10 minutes, then switch to the other.

c. Let the baby nurse on the first breast until he releases the breast on his own.

d. Switch sides several times during a feed to make sure both sides get stimulated.

5.31 **You are working with a baby who has a unilateral cleft of the hard palate. The MOST APPROPRIATE strategy to suggest is:**

a. Try nursing lying down to see if your breast will fill the cleft.

b. Gradually reduce your milk production while you switch to formula.

c. Hand-express after every attempted nursing session, and give the milk by cup.

d. If the baby can latch, try feeding in upright positions to avoid nasopharyngeal reflux.

5.32 **This mother is 4 days postbirth. What is the MOST LIKELY cause of the condition pictured?**

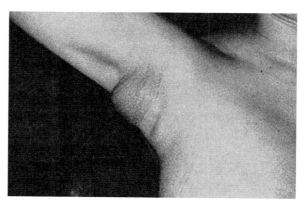

See color plate 37.

a. Plugged milk duct

b. Infected sweat gland in axilla

c. Mastitis in the tail of Spence

d. Milk stasis in accessory breast tissue

5.33 **A mother is concerned about low milk production 2 weeks after giving birth. Which of the following is MOST LIKELY to increase the rate of milk synthesis?**

a. Begin drinking ¼ cup of fenugreek tea 3 times a day.

b. Thoroughly drain the breasts every 2 to 3 hours by nursing, pumping, and/or expressing.

c. Put the baby to breast every 2 to 3 hours to stimulate the breasts even if the baby does not feed well.

d. Ask her physician to prescribe metoclopramide to increase prolactin.

5.34 **To properly use this device, the mother should:**

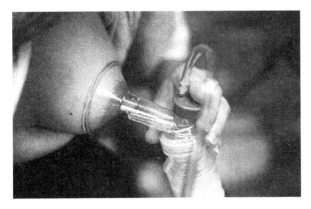

a. cycle the pressure rapidly in the beginning, then slower as milk flows.

b. hold the pressure steady for up to 5 minutes.

c. cycle the pressure about 80 to 100 times per minute.

d. use the pump vacuum to stretch the nipple forward into the flange.

5.35 **What is the MOST LIKELY condition pictured?**

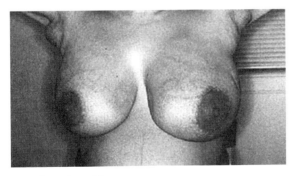

See color plate 38.

a. Abscess in the lower inner quadrant of the left breast

b. Bilateral primary engorgement

c. Large breasts with accessory breast tissue in both axilla

d. Bilateral mastitis extending to the axilla

5.36 **This 6-day-old baby has been nursing about every 4 hours during the day and once at night and has not regained birth weight. The mother has asked for help breastfeeding. At the time this picture was taken, he had been sleeping since his last feed ended 3 hours ago. What is your FIRST recommendation to the mother?**

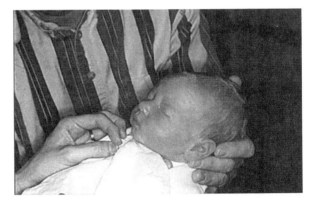

a. Try giving him some expressed breast-milk with a spoon right now.

b. Please undress him so we can check his weight.

c. Take him to his physician's office or an emergency clinic immediately.

d. Let's see what he does at breast, even while he's sleepy.

5.37 **At this postbirth stage, which statement is MOST ACCURATE?**

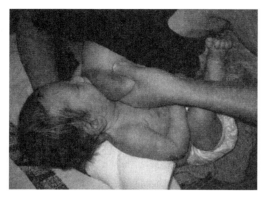

Courtesy of Carole Dobrich.

    a. Too many visitors can interfere with feeding.
    b. Mother is getting ready to go back to work.
    c. Baby does not consume all the milk that mother is making.
    d. Baby is sleeping 6 to 8 hours at night.

5.38 **This mother complains of sharp nipple pain. Which suggestion is MOST LIKELY to quickly relieve her discomfort?**

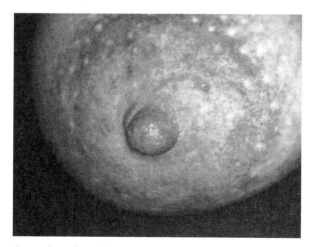

See color plate 39.

    a. Apply purified lanolin to the irritated area.
    b. Wear a silicone nipple shield during feeds.
    c. Wear breast shells between feeds.
    d. Bring the baby deeply onto the breast.

5.39 **What is the MOST LIKELY cause of the dark marks on this mother's areola?**

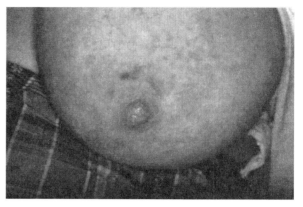

See color plate 40.

    a. Herpes lesions
    b. Tooth marks from toddler's biting
    c. Bruise from baby's off-center latch
    d. Improper use of breast pump

5.40 **A mother is concerned because her areola is over 4 inches (10 cm) in diameter, and drops of milk appear on the areola when her milk lets down. How will this affect her ability to breastfeed?**

    a. The areola is too large to fit completely inside the baby's mouth.
    b. The milk duct openings on the areola will make it difficult for her baby to latch.
    c. Very large areolas are associated with milk oversupply.
    d. Her breasts are normal, and she should easily be able to breastfeed.

5.41 **The MOST IMPORTANT reason to use this feeding position and device is to:**

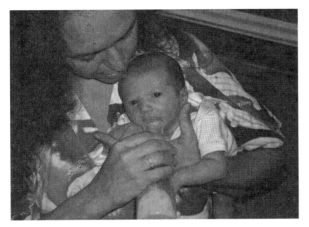

Courtesy of Catherine Watson Genna.

    a. simulate a breastfeeding position.
    b. prevent the tongue from falling back into the airway.
    c. prevent milk from being lost into the cleft.
    d. increase baby's muscle tone.

5.42 **5.42 This full-term baby is 36 hours old. The MOST LIKELY condition requiring this treatment is:**

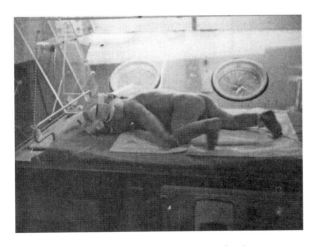

    a. exclusive, effective breastfeeding
    b. ABO incompatibility
    c. breastmilk jaundice
    d. hypoglycemia

5.43 **This mother complains of nipple pain while pumping. The MOST LIKELY cause is that:**

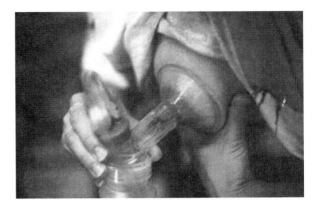

    a. she has a fungal infection on her nipples.
    b. the pump flange is not centered over her nipple.
    c. the pressure on the pump is too high.
    d. her lower hand is pulling the breast away from the pump.

5.44 **This baby has been feeding well for 4 days as pictured. What should you NEXT action be?**

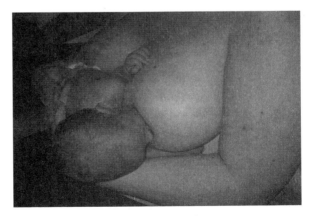

Courtesy of Catherine Watson Genna.

    a. Remind the mother to express or pump milk while this device is necessary.
    b. Begin cutting away the nipple shield so the baby does not become dependent on it.
    c. Sterilize the nipple shield by boiling it once a day.
    d. Tell the mother to lower the baby's hips to a more diagonal position.

5.45 This baby had trouble latching and staying on breast and was not gaining weight. The mother's nipples were very painful at every feed. Attempting a deeper latch and better positioning did not improve the situation. The practitioner shown is MOST LIKELY performing which of the following procedures?

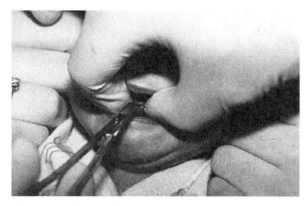

Courtesy of Greg Notestine.

   a. Frenectomy

   b. Frenotomy

   c. Tonsillectomy

   d. Myringotomy

5.46 A first-time mother and her 5-day-old infant called you for help. The baby is neither voiding nor stooling regularly and appears yellow. While the mother's breasts were engorged, all attempts at latching the baby onto the breast failed. She expressed 2 ounces of milk total (60 mL). What is the NEXT action she should take?

   a. Pour the milk into a bottle and feed it with a wide-base nipple (teat).

   b. Place the baby skin-to-skin on her chest and see if he will self-attach.

   c. Use a small open cup to pour the pumped milk into the baby's mouth.

   d. Drip the pumped milk into the baby's mouth with a small dropper.

5.47 What is this mother doing with the hand that is not holding the device?

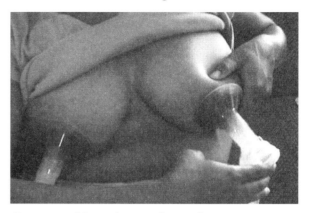

Courtesy of © Barbara Wilson-Clay.

   a. Tapping the breast to aid milk let-down

   b. Massaging milk toward the nipple to increase collected volume

   c. Pressing her breast more deeply into the flange

   d. Stroking the skin surface to increase milk synthesis

5.48 This mother says her breast feels very full and hard. Her 4-day-old baby cannot effectively latch because her breast is so full. What would your FIRST suggestion be?

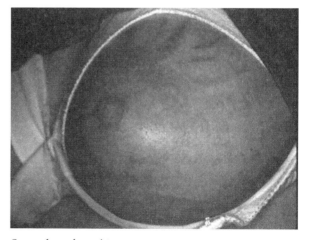

See color plate 41.

   a. Antifungal therapy

   b. Hand-express to soften the areola and nipple

   c. Fit mother with a breast binder

   d. Antibiotic therapy

5.49 **This mother is worried that her left breast is larger than her right. Your FIRST response should be:**

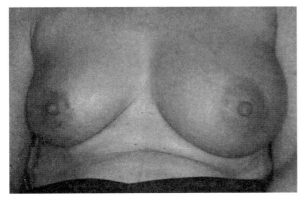

Courtesy of Carole Dobrich.

a. The left breast appears to have mastitis.
b. Different breast sizes are very common.
c. What size were your breasts before pregnancy?
d. The left will clearly make more milk than the right.

5.50 **A mother calls in a panic on day 3. She has been crying all morning, her breasts hurt, and her baby is having a hard time feeding. Your FIRST response to her should be:**

a. How many times did your baby stool today?
b. Things sure are overwhelming for you today!
c. Have you been pumping your breasts?
d. You'll be fine; lots of mothers have problems on day 3.

5.51 **A first-time mother and her 5-day-old infant called you for help. They live in a very remote area far from a health-care facility. The baby is 5 days old, neither voiding nor stooling regularly, and appears yellow. The mother's breasts are painfully engorged and all attempts at latching the baby onto the breast have failed. Your FIRST action should be:**

a. Take her name and contact information and refer her to a home-health-care provider.
b. Coach her on hand-expressing her milk over the phone.
c. Ask her if she has a breast pump or any formula at home.
d. Call the hospital where she gave birth and complain about lack of follow-up.

5.52 **At 14 days postbirth, a mother tells you that she has bright red vaginal bleeding and that her baby (birth weight 9 lb 2 oz) seems constantly hungry. The MOST LIKELY explanation for this is:**

a. large-for-gestational-age baby.
b. early return of menses.
c. uterine infection.
d. retained placental fragment.

5.53 **A mother sustained significant blood loss during birth requiring a blood transfusion. Four days later, her milk has not yet "come in." The MOST LIKELY reason for delay in onset of copious milk synthesis is:**

a. young age.
b. cesarean delivery.
c. first lactation cycle.
d. significant blood loss.

5.54 **You are helping a mother at her first postpartum visit on day 4. She has been limiting her baby's feeds to 10 minutes per breast because a hospital nurse told her "if he nurses longer than that, he's only using you as a pacifier and you'll get sore." Your FIRST statement to her should be:**

a. Let's see what he can do with nursing at breast at his own pace.
b. That advice was wrong; long feeds do not cause nipple pain.
c. The baby gets most of your milk in the first 10 minutes.
d. How are your breasts feeling today?

5.55 **On seeing this 14-day-old infant, the FIRST question you would ask the mother about her own health status is:**

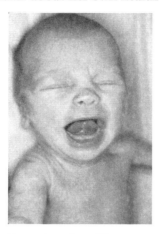

See color plate 42.

a. Are you getting enough rest?
b. Are you eating a well-balanced diet?
c. Do you have a fever?
d. What color and quantity is your vaginal discharge?

5.56 **A mother has begun breastfeeding successfully and is leaving the hospital with her 3-day-old baby today. Your BEST action is to:**

a. Call her in a week to see how things are going.
b. Give her information about local breast-feeding support groups.
c. Enroll her in a food supplement program in case she needs infant formula.
d. Make sure she has a written pamphlet on breastfeeding.

5.57 **A mother is trying to reduce milk production through pumping, and found that pumping for 15 minutes every 3 hours was producing excess milk. Which strategy would be MOST LIKELY to reduce total amount pumped per day?**

a. Pump at the highest comfortable pressure.
b. Use a large-diameter flange.
c. Pump only past one let-down (milk ejection reflex).
d. Pump more often so the breasts do not have time to fill.

5.58 **What is the FIRST THING you should say to the mother of this 5-day-old baby?**

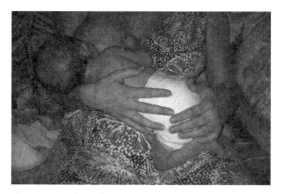

Courtesy of Catherine Watson Genna.

a. Can you see your baby's lips when you hold him like that?
b. How are your breasts feeling during and after each feed?
c. Would you like suggestions on feeding more discretely?
d. How is breastfeeding going for you and your baby today?

5.59 **Which strategy would be MOST EFFECTIVE for a mother who is producing far more milk than her healthy, term 2-week-old daughter needs?**

a. Breastfeed on cue (8 to 12 or more times a day) while milk production adjusts.
b. Drink 1 cup of sage tea 3 times a day to reduce milk production.
c. Wear a supportive bra and apply cold packs if overfull.
d. Offer only one breast per feed, and express the other breast.

5.60 **The mother of a 2-week-old baby asks for help drying up her milk, saying, "I don't know what to do anymore. I feel like the milk will just never dry up." Your FIRST response to her should be:**

a. You sound desperate! At 2 weeks, your breasts are still adjusting to making milk.
b. What did you expect when you decided to stop breastfeeding?
c. Have you tried using a breast binder?
d. Your milk will eventually dry up if you stop all that pumping.

5.61 A mother with epilepsy wants to breast-feed her third baby, after formula-feeding her first two. Which aspect of breastfeeding should you spend MOST TIME discussing with her?

a. Increased infant alertness

b. Looser and more frequent stools

c. More breast and nipple pain

d. More frequent infant spitting up

5.62 This mother is 4 days postpartum. Which of the following recommendations is MOST APPROPRIATE?

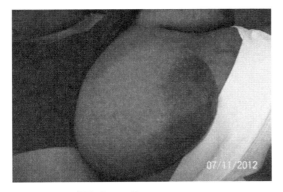

Courtesy of K. Jean Cotterman.

a. Apply cool cabbage compresses to the lump in your left armpit.

b. Feed your baby at least every 2 to 3 hours or more often if he cues.

c. Apply hot compresses to help milk flow in your left breast.

d. Use cool compresses after feeds if breasts feel full.

5.63 The mother of this baby complains of stinging, burning pain in her nipples. The strategy MOST LIKELY to resolve her pain is:

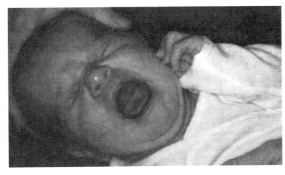

See color plate 43.

a. breastfeed for frequent short periods of time.

b. wear nipple shields during breastfeeding for 1 week.

c. treat mother and baby with antifungal medication.

d. boil all the baby's pacifiers.

5.64 A mother is 3 days postpartum and is worried that her milk is not flowing out, even though her breasts feel very full. She pumps 5 mL from one breast and 10 mL from the other. Your FIRST action should be to:

a. provide her with oxytocin nasal spray.

b. perform alternate breast massage.

c. apply cold packs to her breasts.

d. apply hot compresses to her breasts.

5.65 The MOST LIKELY result of this mother's dietary practices would be:

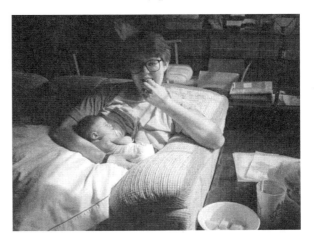

a. Her milk will contain more vitamin A.

b. Her milk supply will increase.

c. The baby's breath may smell like cantaloupe.

d. The baby will reject the cantaloupe-flavored milk.

5.66   **What is the FIRST thing you should say to this mother?**

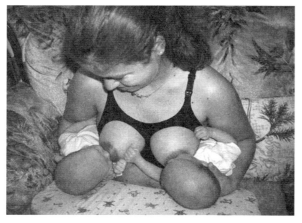

Courtesy of Catherine Watson Genna.

   a. Bring the baby on the right more deeply onto your breast.
   b. Shall I help restrain the baby's hands so he does not interfere with the other baby?
   c. How do you like breastfeeding both twins at once?
   d. Be sure to make eye contact with both babies during each feed.

5.67   **This mother has been using a piece of equipment to help resolve her breast-feeding problem. Which is the MOST LIKELY product that she used?**

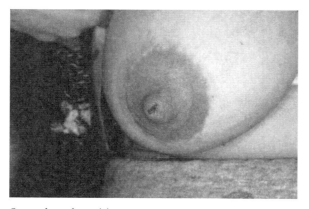

See color plate 44.

   a. Nipple shields
   b. Breast shells
   c. Bottle teat placed over her nipple
   d. Breast pump

5.68   **How would you document the appearance of this lactating mother's breast?**

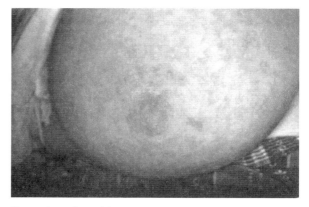

See color plate 45

   a. Unpigmented areola
   b. Poison ivy
   c. Normal breast
   d. Fungal infection

5.69   **A first-time mother at home calls you on day 5 for help with her painfully engorged breasts. What would have been the BEST way to prevent this situation?**

   a. She should have worn a supportive bra starting on the first day after delivery.
   b. The hospital could have provided her with cold compresses to reduce swelling.
   c. She should have been given a breast pump to relieve overproduction.
   d. The baby should have been put to breast in the first hour after birth and helped to feed effectively.

5.70 **Which statement in the mother's story is MOST LIKELY the cause of the condition of her nipple?**

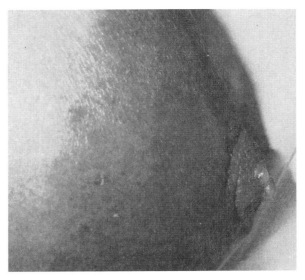

Courtesy of K. Jean Cotterman.

a. My nipples were tender, so I rubbed some expressed milk into the skin.

b. My baby can't stay latched very long; he latches then comes right off.

c. My breast pump has really strong suction when I first start using it.

d. During pregnancy, I was treated for several yeast infections

5.71 **What is the BEST suggestion you could make to this mother as she is expressing milk for her baby?**

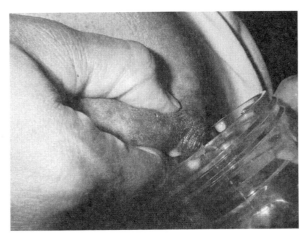

Courtesy of K. Jean Cotterman.

a. Move your hand back toward your chest wall.

b. Roll your fingers toward the nipple as you press inward.

c. That looks good; continue until the milk flow slows.

d. Massage your breast with the other hand while you express.

5.72 **A mother with delayed lactogenesis II was evaluated for hormone irregularities. Her levels of thyroid-stimulating hormone (TSH) and prolactin are normal; testosterone is 5 times higher than normal. Which of the following is the MOST LIKELY explanation for the delay in copious milk production?**

a. Hypothyroidism

b. Ovary theca lutein cyst

c. Anemia

d. Polycystic ovary syndrome

5.73 **What technique is MOST LIKELY being shown in this picture?**

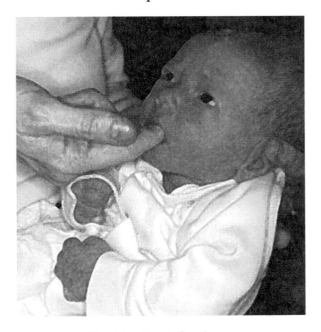

a. Checking for cleft palate

b. Comforting or calming

c. Digital oral assessment

d. Checking for short frenulum

5.74 **This mother is 4 days postpartum. Your FIRST action to assist her in breastfeeding should be:**

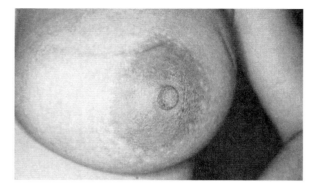

   a. Put your baby prone on your chest and let him self-attach.
   b. Use warm compresses to soften the areola.
   c. Use cool compresses to reduce edema.
   d. Express some milk to soften the breast.

5.75 **A LC operates a private breast pump rental depot from her home and is employed by a hospital maternity unit. If a mother must leave the hospital without her baby, the LC tells the mother about her own rental depot but not others in the community. This behavior is:**
   a. legal and ethical.
   b. illegal and unethical.
   c. a conflict of interest.
   d. a valuable service to patients.

5.76 **This mother is only able to express a few drops of milk, and her mother is telling her to supplement her 8-day-old baby. Your FIRST action would be to:**

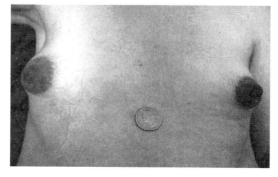

Courtesy of Catherine Watson Genna.

   a. help her position her baby deeply onto her breast.
   b. instruct her in use of a tube-feeding device to be used during feeds.
   c. contact her physician for a prescription galactagogue.
   d. explore her options for supplementing her baby.

5.77 **You are helping a mother exclusively breastfeed her 2-month-old child. Assuming the mother is responsive to her baby's cues, what is the MOST LIKELY feeding pattern to expect for this infant over the first 6 months?**
   a. Feeding from both breasts every session including at night
   b. Feeding from one breast each time he feeds
   c. Feeding from one or both breasts in no particular pattern
   d. Clusters of two or three feeds close together, then long stretches between

5.78 **What is the MOST LIKELY explanation for the condition pictured?**

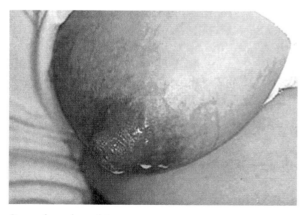

See color plate 46.

   a. Milk residue after pumping
   b. Nipple candidiasis
   c. Herpes lesions
   d. Lanolin

5.79 **A healthy, thriving 10-day-old baby is diagnosed with a bilirubin level of 120 mg/dL (17 mmol/L). The FIRST suggestion for his care should be to:**
   a. replace most of the breastfeeds with artificial baby milk.
   b. institute phototherapy except during feedings.
   c. continue to ensure 10 to 12 effective breastfeedings every day.
   d. spend several sessions undressed in a sunny window.

5.80 **Which visual aspect of this baby's latch is the FIRST INDICATION of potential problems in breastfeeding?**

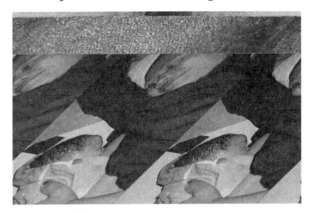

Courtesy of Greg Notestine.

   a. Angle of the lips/mouth is about 90 degrees
   b. Puckering along the nasolabial crease
   c. Chin barely touches the breast
   d. Areola is nearly completely in baby's mouth

5.81 **An 8-day-old infant has been at breast constantly since birth. His mother complains of nipple pain and states that her baby makes a clicking sound and loses his grasp of her nipple frequently during the feed. You have corrected her latch-on technique. Your NEXT action should be to:**

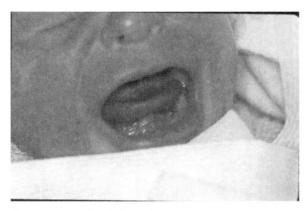

Courtesy of Greg Notestine.

   a. provide her with a sterile nipple shield.
   b. instruct her to use several different breastfeeding positions.
   c. instruct her in suck training to correct the baby's sucking.
   d. refer her to a health professional qualified to evaluate for tongue-tie.

5.82 **The MOST COMMON cause of inadequate milk supply is:**
   a. impaired let-down reflex.
   b. restricted maternal fluid intake.
   c. inadequate or infrequent milk removal.
   d. inadequate maternal diet.

5.83 **A healthy, full-term newborn is found to have a total bilirubin level of 14.2 mg/dL (245 µmol/L) on the 4th day of life. The BEST recommendation is to:**
   a. breastfeed the baby at least 10 times a day.
   b. feed artificial baby milk after breastfeedings.
   c. feed artificial baby milk for 24 hours; maintain supply through pumping.
   d. tell the mother that this level of bilirubin is rarely a problem.

5.84 **How is the baby pictured responding to this technique?**

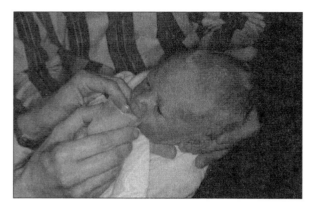

a. Stressed
b. Shut down
c. Relaxed
d. Agitated

5.85 **The FIRST action you would suggest to assist this baby is to:**

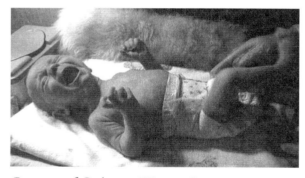

Courtesy of Catherine Watson Genna.

a. attempt direct breastfeeding, correcting positioning as needed.
b. send the baby to an oral surgeon for a frenotomy.
c. cup-feed 2 ounces of expressed mother's milk.
d. have mother place the baby skin-to-skin for 30 minutes.

5.86 **This baby is having difficulty latching on and breastfeeding. The MOST LIKELY reason is:**

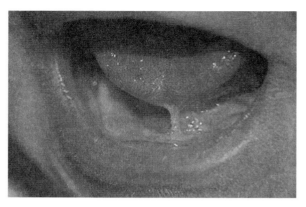

Courtesy of Greg Notestine.

a. the baby is crying too hard to latch well.
b. the lingual frenulum is restricting tongue movement.
c. the lips are too tense.
d. the baby's mouth is not open wide enough.

5.87 **This baby's mother is concerned about a clicking, smacking sound that occurs during nursing. Her nipples are mildly tender. Your FIRST action would be to:**

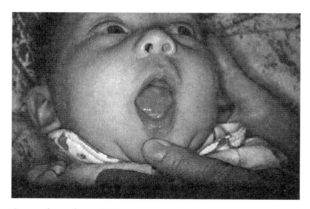

See color plate 47.

a. refer her for evaluation of the baby's tongue musculature.
b. ensure good alignment and deep latch at breast.
c. perform a digital examination to assess tongue movement.
d. reassure her that some nipple tenderness is normal in early lactation.

5.88 **What is the MOST LIKELY cause of the lumps on this woman's areola?**

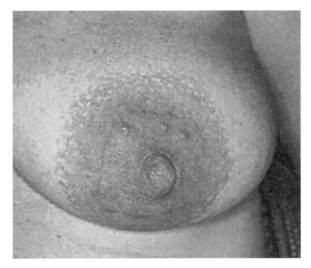

See color plate 48

   a. Irritation from wet bra pads
   b. Infected Montgomery glands
   c. Poison ivy
   d. Normal anatomy

5.89 **A 38-week neonate with a birth weight of 3573 g (7 lb 12 oz) is referred to you with a discharge weight of 3171 g (6 lb 12 oz) at 72 hours postdelivery. The FIRST thing you should do is:**

   a. weigh the infant to see if the hospital's scale was correct.
   b. tell the mother that the weight loss is within normal range.
   c. take a thorough history of the dyad's breastfeeding practices.
   d. suggest she discuss any interventions with her baby's doctor.

5.90 **A mother is concerned that tandem nursing may be harmful to her new baby or older breastfeeding child. Your FIRST recommendation would be to:**

   a. wean the older child.
   b. reassure that tandem breastfeeding is not harmful to either child.
   c. reduce the time the older child is at the breast.
   d. feed the new baby first, before breastfeeding the older child.

5.91 **This mother says she is enjoying breastfeeding. Your FIRST response should be:**

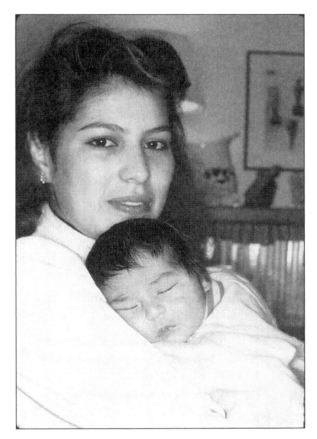

   a. Your baby looks a bit jaundiced; has he seen the doctor?
   b. How many times has your baby nursed in the past 24 hours?
   c. How many wet diapers have you changed so far today?
   d. Wonderful! You were ambivalent, and now you look so confident. How are things going?

5.92 **This mother's baby was having trouble latching on and breastfeeding. The MOST LIKELY maternal reason for the baby's difficulty is:**

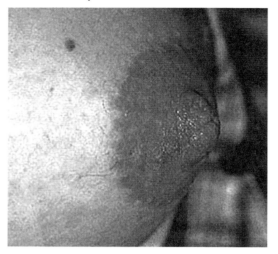

See color plate 49.

Courtesy of Greg Notestine.

   a. her nipple is somewhat short and flat.

   b. her breast is engorged, preventing deep latch.

   c. her nipple is very small, and the baby couldn't feel it.

   d. her nipple is very large, and the baby was choking on it.

5.93 **Which of the following breastfeeding-related behaviors is this baby MOST LIKELY to exhibit?**

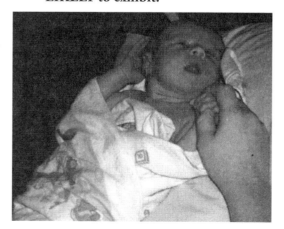

   a. Gazes up and smiles at mother

   b. Hands relax as baby obtains milk

   c. Reaches for mother's face

   d. Cues to feed by crying

5.94 **This picture was taken immediately after a baby ended a feeding. Which statement MOST LIKELY describes the preceding feed?**

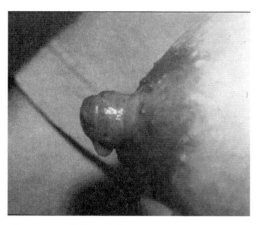

Courtesy of Greg Notestine.

   a. Comfortable, with good milk transfer

   b. Comfortable, but with poor milk transfer

   c. Painful, but with good milk transfer

   d. Painful, with poor milk transfer

5.95 **This mother is having difficulty getting her baby to take the breast. What is the FIRST thing you would do?**

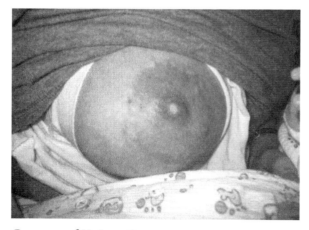

Courtesy of K. Jean Cotterman.

   a. Attempt deeper attachment at breast.

   b. Put a nipple shield over her nipple.

   c. Cup-feed the baby before trying again.

   d. Try nursing lying down instead of sitting up.

5.96 **This mother's baby is 8 days old. The MOST LIKELY cause of the condition pictured is:**

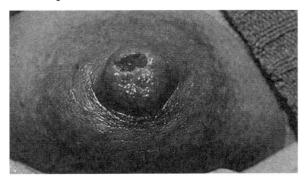

See color plate 50.

Courtesy of Greg Notestine.

    a. normal breastfeeding.
    b. baby is tongue-tied.
    c. baby is not latching deeply.
    d. baby is biting during feeds.

5.97 **What is the MOST LIKELY reason this baby cannot make a good seal on the mother's breast?**

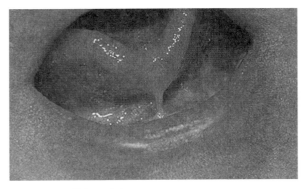

Courtesy of Greg Notestine.

    a. The tongue is trough-shaped.
    b. The tongue is too thick.
    c. The baby has a small mouth opening.
    d. The lingual frenulum is short and tight.

5.98 **A mother contacts you with a tender, hot, swollen breast with a wedge-shaped red area. She says she is running a fever, and wonders if she has the flu. Her baby is nursing 6 or 7 times a day and uses a pacifier to stretch out the time between feeds, especially at night. What is the MOST IMPORTANT suggestion you could make to resolve this situation?**

    a. Contact your physician to request a prescribed antibiotic.
    b. Rest in bed with the baby for the next 10 days.
    c. Empty your breast much more often by nursing or hand-expressing.
    d. Bind your breasts with a non-stretchy cloth to reduce swelling.

5.99 **The condition pictured appeared suddenly 3 days postbirth. The FIRST suggestion you would give to this mother is:**

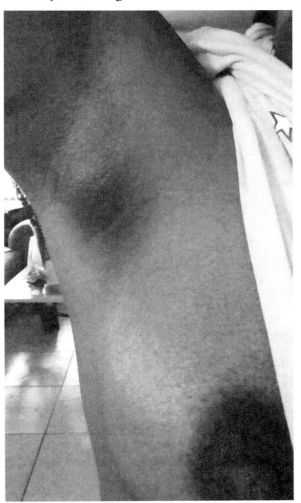

See color plate 51.

    a. try massaging the plug of milk toward your nipple.
    b. see whether the lump changes size after you nurse your baby.
    c. put hot compresses on the swollen area.
    d. make an appointment with a breast surgeon for a biopsy.

5.100 **After being bottle-fed for several weeks, this baby's mother is transitioning to direct breastfeeding. What is the NEXT action she should take?**

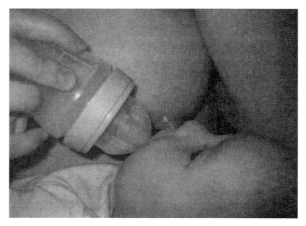

Courtesy of Catherine Watson Genna.

    a. Moisten the nipple shield with more expressed milk.

    b. Quickly move the baby from the bottle to the breast.

    c. Change to a standard-shaped bottle nipple and keep trying.

    d. Stop trying direct breastfeeding; the baby is doing well on the bottle.

5.101 **The MOST LIKELY explanation for what this mother is doing is:**

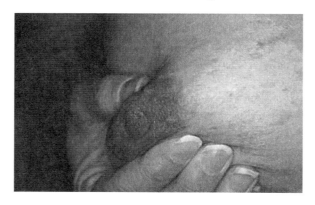

    a. doing a pinch test for retraction.

    b. doing nipple rolling technique.

    c. measuring the size of her areola.

    d. hand-expressing her milk.

5.102 **A 5-day-old baby has yellow-tinged skin and is not feeding well. After the baby's primary care provider has ruled out any pathology, the MOST IMPORTANT action would be to:**

    a. give 1 oz (30 mL) of infant formula after each breastfeed for the next 24 hours.

    b. place the unwrapped baby near a window with direct sunlight to reduce the level of bilirubin.

    c. give the baby 1 oz (30 mL) of glucose water after feeds to flush out the bilirubin.

    d. keep the mother and baby together and assure the baby has at least 8 to 12 effective feeds each day.

5.103 **Breast shells would be MOST HELPFUL for this mother to:**

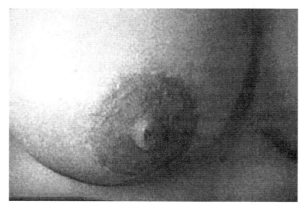

See color plate 52.

    a. evert her nipples.

    b. protect the damaged skin from clothing.

    c. protect the nipple tip from the baby's palate.

    d. reduce areolar edema.

5.104 **A mother trying to rapidly dry up her milk develops mastitis when her baby is 10 days old. Which is the MOST LIKELY predisposing factor?**

    a. Flat nipples that retain bacteria in skin folds

    b. Bacterial contamination of her absorbent bra pads

    c. Recurring milk stasis

    d. Inadequate cleaning of breast pump parts

5.105 **Once lactogenesis II has occurred, mothers usually get the most milk during pumping if they:**
   a. pump at its preset minimum suction level throughout pumping session.
   b. raise suction level to the pump's maximum level when milk ejection reflex occurs.
   c. raise suction level to mother's own maximum comfortable level when milk ejection reflex occurs.
   d. gradually increase suction level little by little throughout the pumping session.

5.106 **What is the FIRST thing you would do to help this mother's baby attach to the breast?**

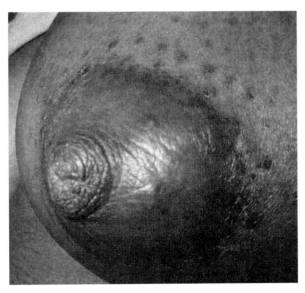

Courtesy of K. Jean Cotterman.

   a. Help her express a bit of milk to get the flow started.
   b. Gently press the areola back toward the chest to reduce edema.
   c. Massage and stroke the breast to stimulate let-down.
   d. Help her semirecline with the baby lying prone on her bare chest.

5.107 **A mother with a 5-day-old infant repeatedly requests "rules" for how many times a day she should feed her baby. This behavior is typical of which stage of maternal role acquisition?**
   a. Anticipatory
   b. Formal
   c. Informal
   d. Personal

5.108 **This mother's baby is 4 days old. She is MOST LIKELY using this equipment to:**

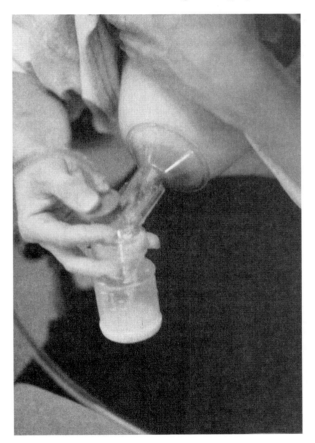

   a. remove excess milk.
   b. stimulate the breast to make milk.
   c. correct inverted nipples.
   d. prevent mastitis.

5.109 **The MOST APPROPRIATE action for the LC to take with this mother–baby pair is to:**

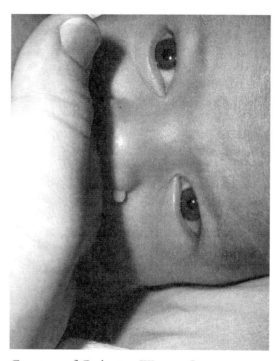

Courtesy of Catherine Watson Genna.

a. instruct mother to stop compressing the breast, as she is causing milk to flow too forcefully.

b. help mother use an upright position to reduce nasal regurgitation.

c. teach mother to use a special slow-flow teat to prevent aspiration.

d. show mother how to use a bulb syringe to aspirate baby's nose after feeds.

Answers for 3–14 Days Questions

5.1 **The answer is c.** The "orange peel" or "peau d'orange" texture of the breast pictured is most likely early postpartum edema. The most important strategy is to reduce edema and support frequent milk removal. Choice b, hand-expression, may be useful if the edema is not blocking milk release. Choice a would be advised if this condition is seen at other times during lactation or in a nonlactating breast, as it is an indication of inflammatory carcinoma. Choice d is not necessary and not appropriate. (Difficulty: 4; Discipline: Techniques; Taxonomy: Collaboration)

5.2 **The answer is c.** When a baby cannot breastfeed directly, an open cup is the safest and recommended first choice for feeding device by BFHI Step 5. Although an open cup could be used for all the choices listed, in this case the baby's appearance is that of a term, normal baby. (Difficulty: 4; Discipline: Clinical Skills; Taxonomy: Plan)

5.3 **The answer is a.** A semireclining position often triggers baby's instinctive feeding behaviors. Suzanne Colson's research on "biological nurturing" suggests that the mother's upright position is not ideal for either mother or baby. (Difficulty: 4; Discipline: Clinical Skills; Taxonomy: Goals)

5.4 **The answer is d.** This baby is 4 days old. The milk in the cup is slightly yellow, suggesting transitional milk. The baby's skin is slightly yellow, suggesting mild jaundice, which would be considered pathological if the baby were younger than 3 to 4 days. (Difficulty: 4; Discipline: Development; Taxonomy: Assessment)

5.5 **The answer is c.** The FIRST suggestion to prevent nipple damage and assure a good latch is to allow the baby to attempt self-attachment. Lanolin or a nipple shield is not appropriate for this mother. Wearing a bra is irrelevant. (Difficulty: 2; Discipline: Techniques; Taxonomy: Plan)

5.6 **The answer is a.** The flattened nipple is most likely causing a pinching nipple pain. This type of postfeed distortion is an indication that the baby did not feed well. (Difficulty: 4; Discipline: Pathology; Taxonomy: Evaluate)

5.7 **The answer is a.** Supporting the mother with a positive, enthusiastic statement about her skills or ability is very confirming, especially for uncertain mothers. The other questions address clinical progress and might be appropriate after praising and re-inforcing the mother's breastfeeding-related behavior. (Difficulty: 5; Discipline: Clinical Skills; Taxonomy: Goals)

5.8 **The answer is c.** BFHI Step 9: Give no artificial teats or pacifiers (also called dummies or soothers) to breastfeeding infants. Choices b and d are also true. (Difficulty: 4; Discipline: Clinical Skills; Taxonomy: Collaboration)

5.9 **The answer is b.** The bulge is a galactocele. Plugged ducts are rarely visible on the breast surface. Inflammation is characteristic of both mastitis and abscess and would appear as a reddened area on the breast. (Difficulty: 5; Discipline: Pathology; Taxonomy: Knowledge)

5.10 **The answer is c.** This is the most accurate description of this baby's tongue. Unseen in the photograph is the baby's very short, tight lingual frenulum. (Difficulty: 4; Discipline: Clinical Skills; Taxonomy: Document)

5.11 **The answer is d.** Placing the baby skin-to-skin on mother's chest often leads to infant self-attachment by triggering the infant's instincts. After 2 weeks, any early minor suck problems should have resolved. Babies with normal suck can latch onto many different nipple configurations, and the pumping would likely have improved her nipple elasticity. (Difficulty: 5; Discipline: Techniques; Taxonomy: Plan)

5.12 **The answer is c.** Immediate supplementation is warranted for this baby because his diaper output and weight gain are insufficient. Choices a and b are wrong because stool output and weight gain are insufficient, and immediate supplementation is necessary. Choice d is wrong because there is no breast fullness. (Difficulty: 3; Discipline: Pathology; Taxonomy: Evaluate)

5.13 **The answer is c.** Cup-feeding is one appropriate technique for improving a baby's suboptimum suck, providing food, allowing nipples to heal, and behavior modification. (Difficulty: 4; Discipline: Clinical Skills; Taxonomy: Plan)

5.14 **The answer is b.** Rooting and observed swallowing are reliable indicators that the baby is effectively breastfeeding during the first 4 days. Length of feeds can vary and still be effective. Alignment can vary. The mother's sensation is not a reliable indicator of a good feed. The mother's obesity is irrelevant. (Difficulty: 3; Discipline: Techniques; Taxonomy: Assessment)

5.15 **The answer is b.** This mother has axillary mammary tissue that has no outlet, and the photograph was taken 4 days postbirth. Lactogenesis II is causing milk secretion in the axillary mammary tissue. (Difficulty: 3; Discipline: Pathology; Taxonomy: Evaluate)

5.16 **The answer is a.** Lactoferrin is a potent iron-transport agent. More is present in milk than needed by the baby; thus, it is able to bind and rob pathogens of iron needed for proliferation. Lactoferrin also promotes the absorption of iron and indirectly helps establish intestinal flora, by keeping the pathogenic population in check. Lactoferrin is not known to be related to calcium metabolism. (Difficulty: 4; Discipline: Development; Taxonomy: Knowledge)

5.17 **The answer is a.** This baby has a short, thick labial frenulum, sometimes called a lip tie, which inhibits the upper lip from flanging outward and thus prevents a deep attachment at breast. The lingual (lower) frenulum does not show in this image. The jaw is normal, and the alveolar ridge does not show. (Difficulty: 4; Discipline: Pathology; Taxonomy: Assessment)

5.18 **The answer is c.** Milk collected on day 5 is composed of colostrum plus increasing levels of lactose; the yellow color is from the beta-carotene in colostrum. Milk collected during mastitis does not contain pus, and there is no indication that the mother has a breast infection. Yellow-color milk can be caused by foods or drugs the mother has consumed. (Difficulty: 4; Discipline: Development; Taxonomy: Knowledge)

5.19 **The answer is a.** The dark dots around the periphery of the areola are normal pigment variations. This is a normal breast. (Difficulty: 4; Discipline: Development; Taxonomy: Assessment)

5.20 **The answer is d.** The compression stripe from 1:00 to 7:00 indicates a shallow latch. The first intervention should be correcting the positioning and latch during feeds. (Difficulty: 5; Discipline: Techniques; Taxonomy: Plan)

5.21 **The answer is c.** The mother is experiencing milk stasis and inflammation, a common event on day 3. Removal of milk to support ongoing lactogenesis is the top priority. (Difficulty: 3; Discipline: Techniques; Taxonomy: Plan)

5.22 The answer is b. Many babies with a unilateral cleft lip can breastfeed and grow normally without assistive devices. However, about one-third will not grow adequately on direct breastfeeding alone. Mother may need to pump or express to maintain milk production, and supplement the pumped milk with a cup. Human milk is especially important for babies with facial anomalies. (Difficulty: 4; Discipline: Pathology; Taxonomy: Collaboration)

5.23 The answer is b. Passing black, tarry stools after day 4 is abnormal. The baby needs a thorough medical evaluation to rule out gastrointestinal bleeding. By day 7, the baby should be passing three or five or more profuse loose yellow stools every day. (Difficulty: 4; Discipline: Pathology; Taxonomy: Plan)

5.24 The answer is b. The baby's lower lip is curled in and needs to be turned (flanged) outward. Tickling the baby's feet is ineffective, and there is no need to press down on the breast to clear his nostrils. (Difficulty: 4; Discipline: Techniques; Taxonomy: Plan)

5.25 The answer is c. This mother's breasts are full and taut with milk, which inhibits her baby from a good deep latch. She should express or pump some milk to soften her breasts before trying to feed him again. (Difficulty: 3; Discipline: Techniques; Taxonomy: Plan)

5.26 The answer is c. This baby's most immediate need is for calories. His skin is slightly yellow, suggesting some amount of jaundice. That fact, combined with 2 weeks of poor feeding at breast, indicates inadequate milk transfer. The baby needs calories immediately while other approaches to remedy this situation are explored. (Difficulty: 5; Discipline: Pathology; Taxonomy: Plan)

5.27 The answer is b. Careful observation of a feed will reveal effective or ineffective milk transfer, mother's ability to read her baby's cues, and more. The first response could be patronizing and does not address the mother's concerns. Weighing after observing a full feed may be a reasonable next strategy. Pumping to "see how much" is inappropriate and inaccurate. (Difficulty: 4; Discipline: Clinical Skills; Taxonomy: Assessment)

5.28 The answer is a. Deep puckering suggests poor tongue position or motion. In this case, the baby was tongue-tied. Feeding with the eyes closed is a lesser indicator of a problem. The chin and nose are well-positioned. (Difficulty: 3; Discipline: Techniques; Taxonomy: Assessment)

5.29 The answer is c. When standard, appropriate treatment for breast engorgement does not quickly resolve the problem, a thorough medical evaluation is warranted to confirm or rule out serious pathology. (Difficulty: 3; Discipline: Pathology; Taxonomy: Collaboration)

5.30 The answer is c. Allowing the baby to set the pace of feeds is most appropriate. This mother has very large breasts, and the baby may even want to feed more than one time from one breast before switching sides. (Difficulty: 4; Discipline: Techniques; Taxonomy: Plan)

5.31 The answer is d. Some babies with a cleft of the hard palate can breastfeed effectively, and an upright position may be easiest for both mother and baby. There is no known advantage to nursing lying down; a soft breast may fill the cleft regardless of position. Choice c may be necessary if the baby does not nurse well directly. Choice b is inappropriate. (Difficulty: 4; Discipline: Techniques; Taxonomy: Plan)

5.32 The answer is d. The swelling is accessory breast tissue that is producing milk in the immediate postbirth period. (Difficulty: 5; Discipline: Development; Taxonomy: Evaluate)

5.33 **The answer is b.** Thorough removal milk will increase the RATE of milk synthesis. Stimulation without removal is not effective because milk stasis slows the rate of milk synthesis. Galactagogues are not well researched. Metoclopramide will increase prolactin but needs to be combined with adequate milk removal. (Difficulty: 5; Discipline: Physiology; Taxonomy: Plan)

5.34 **The answer is a.** The pumping pattern should closely mimic the baby's feeding pattern of rapid cycling until the milk lets down, then about 40 to 60 cycles of alternating vacuum and release per minute during milk flow. (Difficulty: 3; Discipline: Clinical Skills; Taxonomy: Plan)

5.35 **The answer is c.** This woman's large breasts are normal; she has accessory mammary tissue in both axilla. This photograph was taken on day 4 postbirth. (Difficulty: 5; Discipline: Development; Taxonomy: Assessment)

5.36 **The answer is d.** Attempting direct breastfeeding is always the first strategy in a breastfeeding consult. The baby is slightly yellow (jaundiced) and sleepy, so the other choices are appropriate. Emergency action is not warranted for this baby, as there are no obvious indications of a life-threatening condition. (Difficulty: 4; Discipline: Techniques; Taxonomy: Plan)

5.37 **The answer is c.** Most mothers produce more milk than their baby needs, especially in the early 2 weeks. Milk production gradually adjusts to baby's needs over the first 6 weeks or so. Babies typically consume about two-thirds of the milk available in the breast. (Difficulty: 4; Discipline: Development; Taxonomy: Goals)

5.38 **The answer is d.** Improved positioning at breast is most likely to result in immediately more comfortable feeding. The other suggestions may be considered only if improved positioning and latch is ineffective. (Difficulty: 3; Discipline: Clinical Skills; Taxonomy: Plan)

5.39 **The answer is c.** The dark marks are bruises from her baby's off-center latch. The photograph was taken on day 3. (Difficulty: 4; Discipline: Pathology; Taxonomy: Assessment)

5.40 **The answer is d.** This mother's breasts are entirely normal. Dripping milk is from duct openings and is unlikely to have any effect on the baby's latch. Areolar size is unrelated to milk supply and ability to breastfeed. (Difficulty: 3; Discipline: Development; Taxonomy: Evaluate)

5.41 **The answer is b.** This baby's cleft is complete, and his tongue is small and posteriorly placed and drops easily into his airway. He has great difficulty feeding by any method. The Haberman feeder puts pressure on the tongue and positions it more anteriorly in the baby's mouth. (Difficulty: 4; Discipline: Techniques; Taxonomy: Plan)

5.42 **The answer is b.** ABO incompatibility is a cause of early-onset jaundice. "Breastmilk jaundice" becomes apparent or continues to rise after the 3rd day, and bilirubin levels may peak at any time from the 7th to the 10th day, or even as late as the 15th day. Effective, exclusive breastfeeding does not result in high-enough levels of bilirubin to warrant treatment with light therapy. Hypoglycemia is not treated in this manner. (Difficulty: 4; Discipline: Pathology; Taxonomy: History)

5.43 **The answer is b.** The most likely cause of her nipple pain is off-center placement of the nipple in the pump flange. At one time, this was thought to increase milk yield. Off-center positioning or a too-narrow-diameter flange can cause friction and pain and inhibit milk flow. (Difficulty: 4; Discipline: Clinical Skills; Taxonomy: History)

5.44 **The answer is a.** When a nipple shield is being used correctly as pictured, the mother often needs to express or pump milk to support milk production. Cutting back the nipple shield can leave sharp edges and is therefore not recommended. The shield needs to be cleaned; boiling is usually not needed. The baby's position is fine as is. (Difficulty: 3; Discipline: Clinical Skills; Taxonomy: Evaluate)

5.45 **The answer is b.** The practitioner is performing a frenotomy, an incision of the baby's lingual frenulum that was short and tight. Frenectomy is removal of tissue, not a simple incision. Tonsillectomy (removal of the tonsils) would have no relationship to the breastfeeding problem, and myringotomy is ear surgery. (Difficulty: 3; Discipline: Pathology; Taxonomy: Collaboration)

5.46 **The answer is b.** Direct breastfeeding is preferred over using a device to feed the baby, so an attempt at self-latching would be the next best strategy. If the attempt is unsuccessful, feeding the pumped milk with open cup is the next best option, allowing the baby to lap or sip the milk. A dropper may work but can be tedious for all. A bottle with teat is the least desirable of these options. (Difficulty: 4; Discipline: Techniques; Taxonomy: Plan)

5.47 **The answer is b.** Massaging the breast toward the nipple during pumping or feeding may help move milk from the alveoli toward the nipple. (Difficulty: 4; Discipline: Techniques; Taxonomy: Assessment)

5.48 **The answer is b. Hand-expressing prior to or in addition to pumping will help release milk. There are no signs of infection.** Breast binders have not been found to be safe or effective for inflammatory conditions of the lactating breast. (Difficulty: 6; Discipline: Techniques; Taxonomy: Plan)

5.49 **The answer is b.** Uneven breast size is very common. Total milk production is not related to breast size. The most appropriate first response is providing factual information to the mother. (Difficulty: 4; Discipline: Development; Taxonomy: Goals)

5.50 **The answer is b.** Beginning your interaction with an empathetic response such as b helps validate the mother's emotions, helps her integrate her experience, and moves her into problem solving. (Difficulty: 4; Discipline: Psychology; Taxonomy: Goals)

5.51 **The answer is b.** Teaching hand-expression by phone is the fastest and usually the easiest way to solve two urgent issues: her breast engorgement and obtaining milk to feed her baby. (Difficulty: 2; Discipline: Techniques; Taxonomy: Assessment)

5.52 **The answer is d.** Bright red lochia at 14 days with signs of low milk supply suggest that retained placental fragments are suppressing the onset of lactogenesis II. (Difficulty: 3; Discipline: Pathology; Taxonomy: History)

5.53 **The answer is d.** Severe blood loss can cause pituitary shock (Sheehan syndrome), which blocks prolactin responses needed for lactogenesis II. (Difficulty: 5; Discipline: Pathology; Taxonomy: History)

5.54 **The answer is a.** Feeding the baby is the FIRST action to take, and feeding on cue for length and frequency is the first issue to address. Choice b is incorrect because feed length and nipple pain are not correlated. Although choice c is somewhat correct, that response does not take the baby's ability to feed into consideration. Addressing her breast comfort would be one of the next issues to address. (Difficulty: 4; Discipline: Clinical Skills; Taxonomy: Goals)

5.55 **The answer is d.** The baby is thin and crying, and clearly not thriving. This mother still had bright red vaginal bleeding and a very low milk supply. This situation strongly suggests a retained placenta, which suppresses the onset of lactogenesis II. (Difficulty: 4; Discipline: Pathology; Taxonomy: History)

5.56 **The answer is b.** Step 10 of the Baby-Friendly Hospital Initiative addresses the importance of referring new mothers to peer support groups and other community-based breastfeeding support programs. The other actions are less likely to result in her continuing to breastfeed successfully. (Difficulty: 5; Discipline: Clinical Skills; Taxonomy: Goals)

5.57 **The answer is c.** Milk is released in a bolus-type pattern during milk ejections. Limiting total pumping time to only one let-down would result in less total milk collected. The other three options would increase the rate of production and/or amount collected. (Difficulty: 3; Discipline: Clinical Skills; Taxonomy: Plan)

5.58 **The answer is d.** Asking an open-ended question about what is going right are the FIRST comments you should make. Once you have positive rapport with a mother, then addressing any concerns that she has would be next. (Difficulty: 4; Discipline: Psychology; Taxonomy: Goals)

5.59 **The answer is a.** Lactating breasts will calibrate and adjust to the baby's needs by around six weeks. There is no indication of discomfort, so remedies for engorgement are inappropriate. Herbal products to reduce production are poorly researched; suppression of production so early in lactation is inappropriate. Patterns of breast usage are unrelated to total milk volume produced. (Difficulty: 3; Discipline: Techniques; Taxonomy: Plan)

5.60 **The answer is a.** Your FIRST response should be a validation of her concern and a factual statement related to her situation. Blaming her for stopping is inappropriate; breast binders do not hasten weaning and may increase pain; and sudden cessation of pumping may result in more breast pathology. (Difficulty: 2; Discipline: Clinical Skills; Taxonomy: Goals)

5.61 **The answer is a.** Breastfed infants are more alert and responsive compared to formula-fed babies due to the increased interaction with mother, composition of milk, and sucking at breast instead of a bottle. Formula-fed babies may sleep longer than breastfed babies, putting them at higher risk for SIDS. The stool composition may surprise her; breast and nipple pain should not occur. Breastfed babies are less likely to spit up than formula-fed babies. (Difficulty: 4; Discipline: Clinical Skills; Taxonomy: Goals)

5.62 **The answer is b.** This woman's chief complaint is the accessory breast tissue in her armpit; her breasts are neither overfull nor swollen, and the baby is nursing well. Choices a and d might be helpful. There is no research supporting the use of HOT compresses to relieve milk stasis or edema. (Difficulty: 4; Discipline: Development; Taxonomy: Plan)

5.63 **The answer is c.** The baby's mouth is infected with thrush (*Candida*), which is a fungus. Mother and baby need to be treated simultaneously with an antifungal agent. The LC should be in close contact with the primary care providers in this situation. (Difficulty: 5; Discipline: Pathology; Taxonomy: Goals)

5.64 **The answer is c.** Cold packs will reduce edema, the most likely cause of impeded milk flow in early postpartum. There is no research supporting the use of hot compresses to improve milk flow. (Difficulty: 3; Discipline: Techniques; Taxonomy: Plan)

5.65 **The answer is c.** Mothers' milk contains traces of flavors present in the mother's food choices, which helps the baby learn and enjoy family food preferences. Shortly after this picture was taken, the baby's breath smelled faintly of cantaloupe. (Difficulty: 3; Discipline: Development; Taxonomy: History)

5.66 **The answer is c.** Supporting what the mother is doing is the FIRST thing to do or say in nearly every situation. This mother and her babies are completely normal and thriving. The NEXT step might be to ensure that she is in contact with other mothers who are breastfeeding twins or triplets. (Difficulty: 3; Discipline: Clinical Skills; Taxonomy: Goals)

5.67 **The answer is b.** The indentation visible on the areolar skin was caused by a breast shell placed over her nipple to allow air drying of the wound. (Difficulty: 4; Discipline: Clinical Skills; Taxonomy: History)

5.68 **The answer is a.** This mother's breast has no visible areola. She experienced no breast changes during pregnancy, and this breast did not produce any milk postbirth. Sometimes one unusual anatomical finding, such as the lack of pigmented areola, indicates other unusual or pathological conditions. (Difficulty: 3; Discipline: Pathology; Taxonomy: Document)

5.69 **The answer is d.** Immediate breastfeeding in the first hour followed by at least 8–12 effective feeds per day is the most effective strategy to ensure normal lactogenesis and prevention of engorgement after birth. A supportive bra may be comfortable but not relevant to engorgement. If edema does occur, cool compresses may be comforting and helpful. Pumps are appropriate only if the baby is not feeding well and mother cannot hand-express for comfort. (Difficulty: 3; Discipline: Techniques; Taxonomy: Assessment)

5.70 **The answer is c.** The blisters at the nipple tip are likely from excess pressure of the breast pump. None of the other choices are likely to result in blisters on the nipple tip. (Difficulty: 5; Discipline: Pathology; Taxonomy: History)

5.71 **The answer is c.** Supporting and encouraging what she is doing are the most appropriate suggestions. Moving her hand back toward the chest wall may not improve anything. Rolling her fingers toward the nipple as she presses inward may help. Massage is not needed for this mother, as there is no indication that expression of milk is inadequate; besides, she's using the other hand to hold the collection container. (Difficulty: 4; Discipline: Clinical Skills; Taxonomy: Goals)

5.72 **The answer is b.** Ovary theca lutein cysts secrete large amounts of testosterone, which explains the markedly increased levels of that hormone. TSH and prolactin are within normal levels. Testosterone range of normal is 15 to 70 ng/dL. All of these conditions may be related to delayed onset of lactogenesis II. (Difficulty: 4; Discipline: Pathology; Taxonomy: Evaluate)

5.73 **The answer is c.** The mother is doing a digital oral assessment to feel her own baby's palate. This also explains why she is not wearing gloves. (Difficulty: 4; Discipline: Techniques; Taxonomy: Assessment)

5.74 **The answer is a.** Babies can find the breast by themselves if they are placed on the mother's chest and supported in their movements. This mother's breast is large, but there is no evidence of milk stasis, edema, or excessive fullness. (Difficulty: 3; Discipline: Techniques; Taxonomy: Plan)

5.75 **The answer is c.** Referring to one's self is a conflict of interest. (Difficulty: 4; Discipline: Clinical Skills; Taxonomy: Collaboration)

5.76 **The answer is d.** This mother's breasts are severely underdeveloped (hypoplastic) with very little visible glandular tissue and veining. At 8 days, she should be producing substantial quantities of milk. The first action is to ensure the infant's nutrition (choice d) while you and she explore other strategies for supporting her lactation. The metal disk is a U.S. 25-cent coin for size comparison. (Difficulty: 5; Discipline: Pathology; Taxonomy: Collaboration)

5.77 **The answer is c.** The most common 24-hour feeding pattern observed (57%) in a cohort of normal exclusively breastfed babies in Australia is feeding from one or both breasts in no particular pattern. The other patterns were also observed, although less frequently. Also, 30% of babies studied never took both breasts; 13% always took both breasts, and some babies tended to cluster their feeds more than others. (Difficulty: 4; Discipline: Development; Taxonomy: Assessment)

5.78 **The answer is a.** The white substance is milk residue. The mother had just finished pumping her milk. (Difficulty: 4; Discipline: Clinical Skills; Taxonomy: History)

5.79 **The answer is c.** Prolonged elevated bilirubin in a healthy, thriving baby at the level listed is not considered pathological. Continued appropriate breastfeeding practices are the BEST suggestions. (Difficulty: 3; Discipline: Pathology; Taxonomy: Plan)

5.80 **The answer is a.** In appropriate latch, the angle of the lips is between 120 and 160 degrees; therefore, the narrow angle is a key visual indicator of shallow latch. In this picture, the puckering at the nasolabial crease and chin failing to touch the breast are also indications of a poor latch. The amount of areola in the mouth is the least important indicator of a problem latch. The baby in this picture was tongue-tied. (Difficulty: 4; Discipline: Techniques; Taxonomy: Evaluate)

5.81 **The answer is d.** This baby is tongue-tied. Frenotomy (incision of the lingual frenulum) is an appropriate and effective treatment, especially when ordinary lactation techniques have not been helpful. The next action for the LC is to put the mother in contact with a professional who is qualified to evaluate and treat this anatomic condition of the infant. (Difficulty: 5; Discipline: Clinical Skills; Taxonomy: Collaboration)

5.82 **The answer is c.** Persistent milk stasis is the chief cause of suppressed lactation (inadequate milk supply). Frequent, thorough removal of milk is necessary to sustain lactation. The other factors listed are old myths and not central to maintaining milk synthesis. (Difficulty: 5; Discipline: Pathology; Taxonomy: Knowledge)

5.83 **The answer is a.** It is always appropriate to make sure the baby is feeding well as the FIRST strategy. While that level of bilirubin is rarely a problem for a healthy, full-term newborn, the LC should always make sure the baby is effectively feeding as a top priority. (Difficulty: 3; Discipline: Techniques; Taxonomy: Goals)

5.84 **The answer is c.** This 7-day-old baby is relaxed and feeding well from the cup, which is being used correctly. (Difficulty: 2; Discipline: Clinical Skills; Taxonomy: Assessment)

5.85 **The answer is a.** This baby's most urgent need is for food. Direct breastfeeding is almost always the first strategy. In this child's case, breastfeeding has not been going well, as evidenced by his failure to thrive. Providing mother's own expressed milk would be the next strategy, combined with skin-to-skin care for comfort. (Difficulty: 5; Discipline: Techniques; Taxonomy: Plan)

5.86 **The answer is b.** The baby's short, tight frenulum is restricting proper tongue movement needed for latch and feeding. (Difficulty: 4; Discipline: Development; Taxonomy: Assessment)

5.87 **The answer is b.** Ensuring good alignment and deep latch is the FIRST action to take. After that, choice c would be the next step to take. Nipple tenderness is not normal during any stage of lactation, and referral for evaluation of the tongue musculature would be rarely needed. (Difficulty: 4; Discipline: Techniques; Taxonomy: Plan)

5.88 **The answer is d.** This is a normal breast. The slight pink color of the nipple and areola is normal for this woman. (Difficulty: 5; Discipline: Development; Taxonomy: Evaluate)

5.89 **The answer is c.** Assessing the dyad's current feeding patterns is the first step. After that, the other strategies may be appropriate. (Difficulty: 4; Discipline: Clinical Skills; Taxonomy: History)

5.90 **The answer is b.** There is no evidence that continuing to breastfeed both children is harmful to either child or the mother. (Difficulty: 3; Discipline: Physiology; Taxonomy: Goals)

5.91 **The answer is d.** Reinforcing the mother is the first strategy to support her decision and build confidence. After rapport is established, attending to the baby's possible jaundice and breastfeeding management questions is appropriate. (Difficulty: 4; Discipline: Psychology; Taxonomy: Goals)

5.92 **The answer is a.** This nipple is somewhat short and flat. Most babies would have no problem with this nipple. The breast is not engorged, and the nipple is in the normal range of sizes. (Difficulty: 3; Discipline: Pathology; Taxonomy: Assessment)

5.93 **The answer is b.** In the early weeks, babies often feed with closed fists that open and relax as the baby becomes satiated at breast. (Difficulty: 4; Discipline: Development; Taxonomy: Evaluate)

5.94 **The answer is a.** The nipple is normal shape and the breast is not full postfeed. Both of these suggest maternal comfort with effective milk transfer. If milk transfer was poor, there should be breast fullness postfeed. If the mother experienced pain, there is usually nipple distortion visible postfeed. (Difficulty: 3; Discipline: Techniques; Taxonomy: Evaluate)

5.95 **The answer is a.** Attempting a deeper latch is the first and usually most effective intervention. If that does not eliminate the pain and result in better feeding, further investigation is needed. (Difficulty: 4; Discipline: Techniques; Taxonomy: Plan)

5.96 **The answer is b.** This nipple wound was caused by a baby with tongue-tie (short and/ or tight lingual frenulum). Normal breastfeeding does not cause this kind of wound; shallow latch is unlikely to cause this much damage in just 8 days, and an 8-day-old is unlikely to be biting during feeds. (Difficulty: 3; Discipline: Pathology; Taxonomy: Evaluate)

5.97 **The answer is d.** The baby's lingual frenulum is short and tight, attached at the tongue tip and on the bottom (alveolar) gum ridge. This prevents the tongue from creating a good seal at breast. (Difficulty: 4; Discipline: Development; Taxonomy: Evaluate)

5.98 **The answer is c.** Frequent, thorough breast emptying to reduce milk stasis is the most important action in this situation. She should also rest in bed safely with her baby. If the fever does not resolve very quickly or gets worse, her physician should be involved immediately. Binding the breasts is inappropriate and can be harmful. (Difficulty: 4; Discipline: Pathology; Taxonomy: Goals)

5.99 **The answer is b.** Feeding the baby and noticing any changes related to milk flow is the FIRST action to take. If the swelling decreases after nursing, it is likely that the accessory breast tissue in the axilla has an outlet. There is no indication that this lump is painful for the mother. (Difficulty: 4; Discipline: Development; Taxonomy: Plan)

5.100 **The answer is b.** This photograph shows the "bait and switch" technique in which the baby takes some milk from the bottle then is quickly moved onto the breast with nipple shield in place, moistened with expressed milk. If the baby refuses the breast, the baby is given more milk from the bottle and the process repeated. This technique is described in "Supporting Sucking Skills in Breastfeeding Infants," Chapter 5. (Difficulty: 3; Discipline: Techniques; Taxonomy: Plan)

5.101 **The answer is d.** This mother is hand-expressing her milk. The retracted nipple is not causing a problem. Note that her fingers are approximately at the edge of the areola. (Difficulty: 4; Discipline: Techniques; Taxonomy: Evaluate)

5.102 **The answer is d.** Frequent effective breast-feeds are the best way to reduce bilirubin levels. If the baby is not feeding well, mother should hand-express and cup-feed her milk until the baby feeds better. Giving formula exposes the baby to a foreign protein. Direct sunlight may help, if the baby is getting sufficient milk. Bilirubin is not water-soluble, so choice c is incorrect. (Difficulty: 4; Discipline: Pathology; Taxonomy: Collaboration)

5.103 **The answer is b.** Breast shells with wide backs will protect the injured skin from the rubbing of her bra or clothing. (Difficulty: 3; Discipline: Clinical Skills; Taxonomy: Plan)

5.104 **The answer is c.** Milk stasis is the most likely predisposing factor in developing mastitis. Once milk stasis occurs, commonly occurring bacteria can multiply. (Difficulty: 4; Discipline: Pathology; Taxonomy: History)

5.105 **The answer is c.** Volume of milk collected during a pumping session is related to level of negative pressure (suction) in the pump flange unless the level is painful for the mother or the flange compresses the milk ducts. The current best practice is to pump at the maximum comfortable pressure. (Difficulty: 5; Discipline: Techniques; Taxonomy: Plan)

5.106 **The answer is d.** Facilitating the baby's self-attachment is the best approach and nearly always is quickly successful. The other actions are older approaches that have not been shown to be consistently effective. There is nothing shown in this photograph that would suggest a problem with self-attachment. (Difficulty: 5; Discipline: Techniques; Taxonomy: Plan)

5.107 **The answer is b.** During the formal stage, mothers seek consistent, concrete "rules" to govern their actions. (Difficulty: 4; Discipline: Psychology; Taxonomy: Knowledge)

5.108 **The answer is a.** On day 4, many mothers make more milk than their infants can consume. Use of a pump to remove excess milk can help prevent milk stasis and help the baby latch on and feed more effectively. (Difficulty: 5; Discipline: Techniques; Taxonomy: Goals)

5.109 **The answer is b.** Upright positions will help this baby to feed. This baby had velopharyngeal insufficiency, and milk dripped out of whichever nostril was lower during the feeding. (Difficulty: 4; Discipline: Techniques; Taxonomy: Goals)

CHAPTER 6

15–28 Days Questions

6.1 To comfortably breastfeed, this mother may want to use:

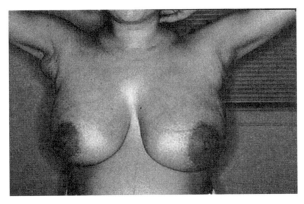

See color plate 53.

   a. a breast pump to remove excessive milk before feeding.
   b. ice packs to reduce swelling.
   c. a nipple shield to help her baby latch on.
   d. a well-fitting bra to support her large breasts.

6.2 What is the MOST LIKELY reason this grandmother would engage in the behavior shown?

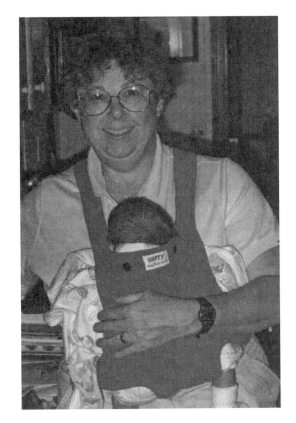

   a. Competition with the baby's mother
   b. Soothe the baby while mother finishes a nap
   c. Baby has a medical condition that requires upright posture
   d. Genuine affection for her grandchild

6.3 **A mother complains that her baby "cries constantly." She has been feeding her baby on a strict schedule found in a popular "parenting" book. Your BEST response to her is:**

a. It is acceptable to limit your baby's feeds to 10 minutes per breast.

b. You can give a pacifier to help your baby extend the time between feeds.

c. Babies do best when there are no restrictions on length or frequency of breastfeeds.

d. Giving water between feeds will get your baby onto a more regular feeding schedule.

6.4 **This baby feeds for 30 to 45 minutes at each breast, each feeding, in the exact position shown in this picture. The MOST LIKELY cause of this behavior is:**

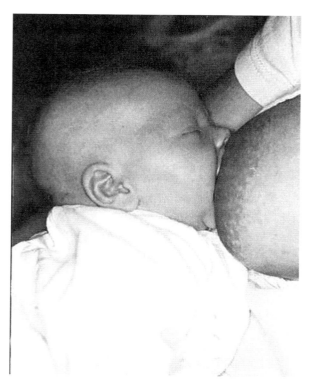

a. normal behavior.

b. disorganized sucking.

c. mother has low milk supply.

d. delayed clearing of labor drugs.

6.5 **This mother reports that her 3-week-old baby seems hungry after feeds and has not yet regained her birth weight. The MOST LIKELY reason for this situation is:**

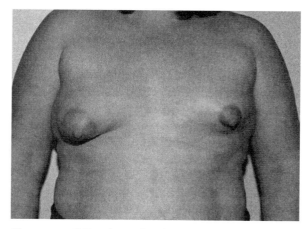

Courtesy of Carole Dobrich.

a. too many hours of pacifier use.

b. scheduled feeds.

c. insufficient glandular tissue.

d. shallow latch at breast.

6.6 **The asymmetry of this woman's breasts is MOST LIKELY due to:**

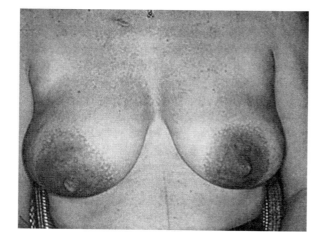

a. normal development.

b. low milk supply in the smaller breast.

c. insufficient glandular tissue in the smaller breast.

d. hypermastia in the larger breast.

6.7 This mother's nipple pain has persisted for over two weeks. Which of the following is the MOST LIKELY cause?

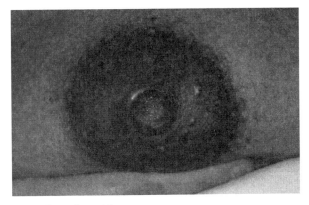

See color plate 54.
Courtesy of Carole Dobrich.

   a. Fragile nipple skin in red-headed mother
   b. Baby has small mouth
   c. Tongue thrust movements
   d. Cleft of the soft palate

6.8 This baby prefers this head position and has significant difficulty nursing in other positions. What is the MOST LIKELY cause of this preference?

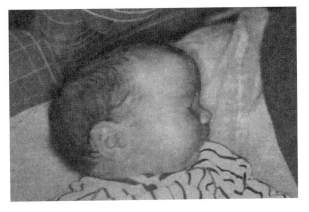

   a. Interesting objects on one side of his crib
   b. Mother feeds only on one breast
   c. Torticollis
   d. Ankyloglossia

6.9 The grandmother of a 4-week-old exclusively breastfed baby who has five or six profuse yellow loose stools every day is worried, and asks for an explanation. The MOST LIKELY cause for stools of this kind is:

   a. diarrhea.
   b. infection with an intestinal parasite.
   c. mother recently ate bright yellow squash.
   d. normal stools.

6.10 This baby has been bottle-fed with expressed mother's milk for 4 weeks, and the mother has asked for your help transitioning to direct breastfeeding. What should be your NEXT suggestion?

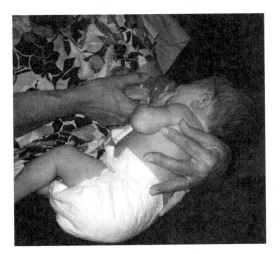

Courtesy of Catherine Watson Genna.

   a. Tilt the bottle more upright so air does not mix with milk.
   b. Remove the bottle after the baby swallows three times, then resume.
   c. Jiggle the bottle so the milk flows faster.
   d. Position the baby in a more upright posture.

6.11   **What is the AVERAGE volume of milk consumed per 24 hours by a breastfed baby of this age?**

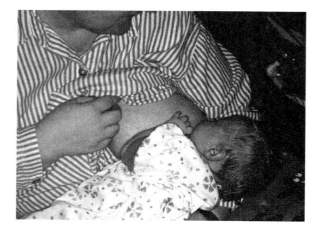

    a. 550 to 600 mL (18 to 20 oz)
    b. 650 to 700 mL (21.5 to 23 oz)
    c. 750 to 800 mL (25 to 26.5 oz)
    d. 850 to 900 mL (28 to 30 oz)

6.12   **This baby attaches to the breast, feeds steadily and comfortably for about 17 minutes, then releases the breast. Which of the following actions is MOST APPROPRIATE for mother?**

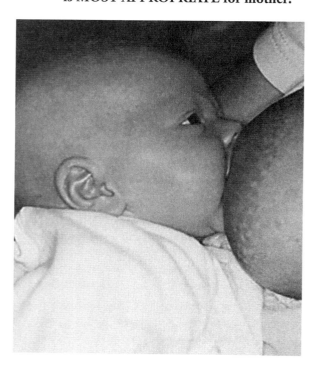

    a. Use your other hand to support your breast during feeds.
    b. Bring your arm closer to your baby's neck.
    c. Continue doing what you are doing.
    d. Pull your baby's legs closer to you.

6.13   **This exclusively breastfed baby is gaining well and otherwise healthy. For the condition pictured, your BEST recommendation to the mother is to:**

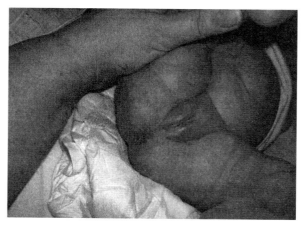

See color plate 55.
Courtesy of Erika Nehlsen.

    a. try eliminating dairy products from your diet for a week to rule out an allergic response.
    b. give the baby water in between breastfeeds because her urine is too concentrated.
    c. start supplementing with soy formula because your milk supply is inadequate.
    d. ask the baby's pediatrician to prescribe an antifungal ointment for the baby's skin.

6.14 **What neurodevelopmental state is this baby in?**

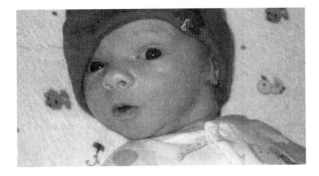

   a. Drowsy
   b. Quiet alert
   c. Active alert
   d. Rapid eye movement (REM) sleep

6.15 **What is your BEST recommendation for the condition pictured?**

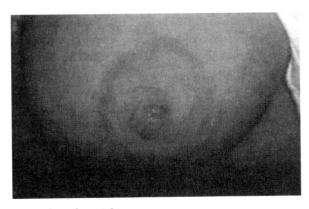

See color plate 56.

   a. Rub cocoa butter into the sore area.
   b. Rinse with hydrogen peroxide several times a day.
   c. Use a dressing designed for moist-wound healing on the wound.
   d. Apply vitamin E oil to the nipple tip.

6.16 **The baby in this picture has the same genetic disease as her mother: arthrogryposis. The MOST LIKELY difficulty this mother will have with breastfeeding is related to:**

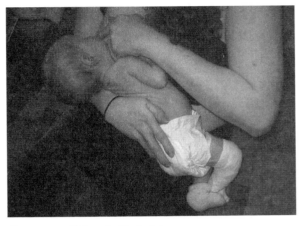

Courtesy of Carole Dobrich.

   a. latching her infant to her breast due to the baby's low tone.
   b. positioning and latching her infant due to mother's hand deformity.
   c. low milk production.
   d. holding the baby due to the leg cast.

6.17 **What is the MOST LIKELY evidence-based sleep pattern for a mother in the early weeks postpartum?**
   a. Awake during the daylight hours, then 8 hours of uninterrupted sleep
   b. Sleeps longer when her baby is in the same room in a crib
   c. Sleeps longer and deeper when her baby is formula-fed by someone else
   d. Sleeps longer and has better quality sleep when bedsharing with her nursing baby

6.18 **Which is the MOST LIKELY cause of the condition pictured?**

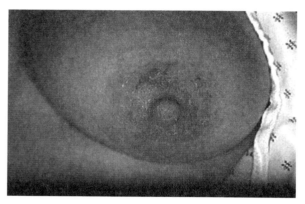

See color plate 57.

   a. Baby is teething

   b. Allergic response to laundry soap used to wash bra

   c. Suction too high on breast pump

   d. Baby has a bacterial infection of the mouth

6.19 **A mother and baby are MOST LIKELY to prefer the underarm (vertical) position for which of the following reasons?**

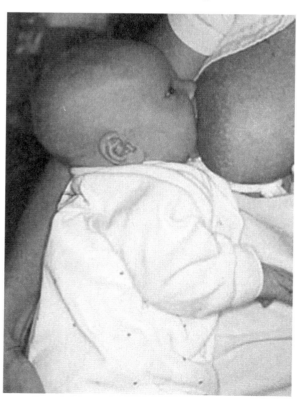

   a. Infant has greater head stability

   b. Coping with a strong let-down reflex

   c. Less chance of plugged milk ducts

   d. Reduces infant colic

6.20 **A breastfeeding mother fractured her pelvis and right leg in a car accident. She is in traction and taking pain medications. Her exclusively breastfed 3-month-old baby has never taken a bottle. The MOST HLEPFUL action to support this family is to:**

   a. get her an electric breast pump so she does not become engorged.

   b. encourage her husband to teach the baby to take milk from a spoon or cup.

   c. help her position the baby for nursing in a way that does not disturb her injuries.

   d. obtain a prescription for birth control pills to dry up her milk.

6.21 **Within the first minute or two of beginning a breastfeed, a 2-week-old infant gulps, coughs, and chokes, then releases the breast. This incident MOST LIKELY describes:**

   a. infant with decreased oral tone.

   b. poor coordination of sucking, swallowing, and breathing.

   c. strong milk ejection reflex.

   d. gastroesophageal reflux.

6.22 **If an exclusively breastfed baby has eczema and blood in his stools, your FIRST action should be to:**

   a. make sure the baby is truly exclusively breastfed.

   b. refer the baby to his primary care provider for evaluation.

   c. suggest the mother modify her nursing pattern to increase hindmilk.

   d. recommend the mother stop all consumption of dairy products.

6.23 Which milk component causes the stools of exclusively breastfed babies to have a mild, yeast-like odor?

    a. Glycopeptides

    b. Candida albicans

    c. Phospholipids

    d. Bifidus factor

6.24 This baby has been at breast about 20 minutes. What is your BEST recommendation to this mother?

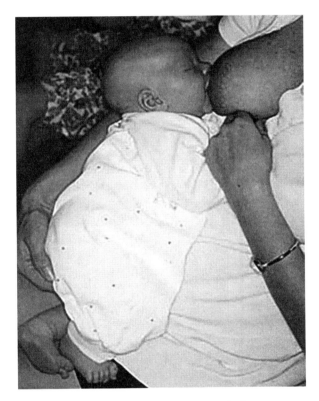

    a. Insert your finger to break the suction, then remove him.

    b. Pull his buttocks in closer to you for a better latch.

    c. Watch his sucking slow down as he prepares to self-detach.

    d. Tickle his feet to wake him so he can finish the feed.

6.25 A mother is inducing lactation for her adopted baby. After 4 weeks of effort, she reports pumping both breasts simultaneously about 4 times a day with a consumer-grade electric breast pump, getting about 1 oz per breast each time. Which strategy would be MOST LIKELY to increase her milk production?

    a. Change to pumping sequentially (not simultaneously).

    b. Use a hospital-grade (multiuser) pump instead of a consumer (single-user) pump.

    c. Increase the number of pumping sessions per day to at least eight.

    d. Use a larger-diameter flange on the collection containers.

6.26 Which is the MOST EFFECTIVE strategy for increasing milk supply?

    a. Take fenugreek tea or capsules.

    b. Drink more fluids.

    c. Eat more nutritious food.

    d. Express milk frequently and thoroughly.

6.27 Which of the following is the MOST LIKELY cause of the condition pictured?

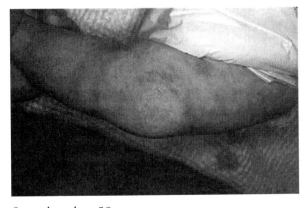

See color plate 58.

    a. Cold temperature in the room

    b. Supplements of cow's milk–based formula

    c. Supplements of rice cereal

    d. Baby recently had a tetanus immunization

6.28 This baby is being breastfed with a silicone nipple shield, jaw support, and a straddle position at breast. The underlying condition that is being helped by these strategies is MOST LIKELY:

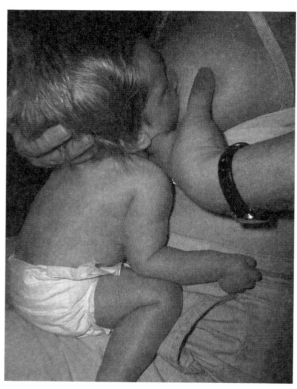

Courtesy of Catherine Watson Genna.

    a. hypertonia.
    b. hypotonia.
    c. ataxia.
    d. hypoglycemia.

6.29 Which behavioral state is illustrated by the infant in this picture?

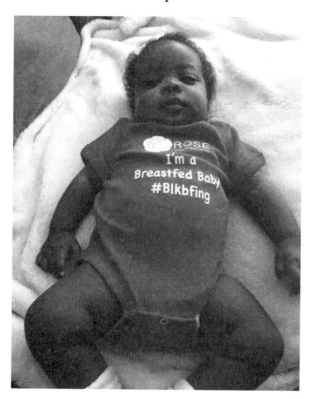

    a. Active alert
    b. Quiet alert
    c. Light sleep
    d. Drowsy

6.30 **What is the MOST LIKELY cause of the condition pictured?**

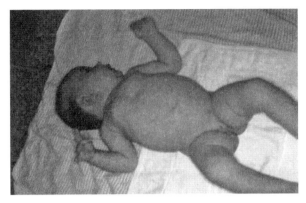

See color plate 59.

a. Acidic urine from human milk feedings
b. Yeast infection (*Candida*)
c. Allergic reaction to cow milk protein passing through mother's milk
d. Sensitivity to chemicals in disposable diapers

6.31 **This mother says her nipples started itching and stinging a few days ago. The MOST LIKELY cause of her symptoms is:**

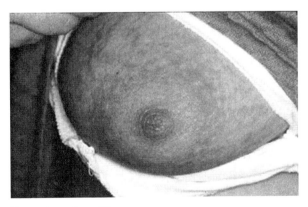

See color plate 60.

a. dry skin.
b. eczema.
c. nipple thrush.
d. positional soreness.

6.32 **A mother of a 2-week-old baby states that her baby's suck feels weak compared with her first baby's suck. This second baby, she states, "always seems hungry," and has also lost weight since birth. Which statement undermines the mother's confidence?**

a. The baby had a low birth weight.
b. The baby is lazy.
c. There is poor intraoral tone.
d. There is shallow attachment at breast.

6.33 **You have just observed this mother feeding her baby. She describes nipple pain all throughout the feed. At the next feed, which should be your FIRST suggestion?**

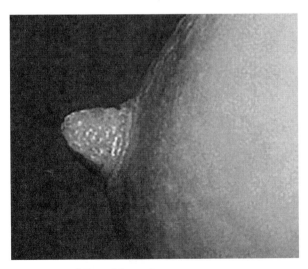

Courtesy of Greg Notestine.

a. Bring the baby onto the breast more deeply.
b. Wait till the baby's mouth is very widely open before latching
c. Everything looks good; do what you've been doing all along.
d. Make sure the baby's lips are turned outward (flanged).

6.34 **Which suggestion MOST SUPPORTS continued exclusive breastfeeding for the mother of a 3-week-old baby who complains that her baby won't sleep alone?**

   a. Give your baby some formula so he will sleep more soundly.
   b. Baby-proof your bed, then lie with your baby's face near your breast. You'll both fall asleep easily.
   c. Nurse your baby to sleep, then slowly ease him into his own crib near where you sleep.
   d. If you let him cry for a short time, he'll learn to put himself to sleep.

6.35 **This mother is uncomfortable in this situation. Your BEST response to her is:**

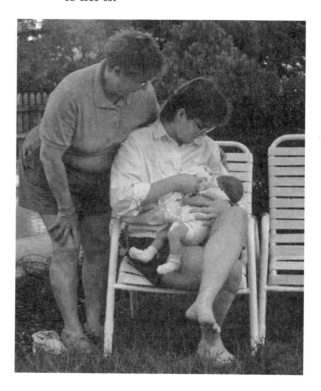

   a. You'll get used to it; many mothers breastfeed in public.
   b. You could always try the ladies' room.
   c. It won't hurt to give the baby a bottle when you're out shopping.
   d. It can be embarrassing the first few time you breastfeed away from home.

6.36 **This baby is having trouble feeding. Which suggestion is MOST LIKELY to improve the situation?**

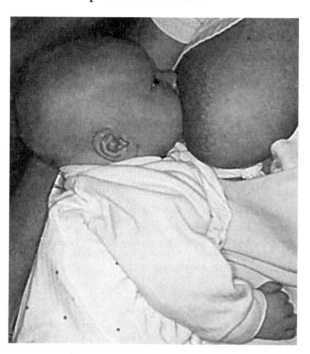

   a. Mother should support her breast with her left hand.
   b. Pull baby's hips and legs in closer to mom's body.
   c. Place a pillow under baby's body.
   d. Change to a horizontal position.

6.37 **This picture was taken 3 hours after the baby fed on this breast. The condition pictured is MOST LIKELY:**

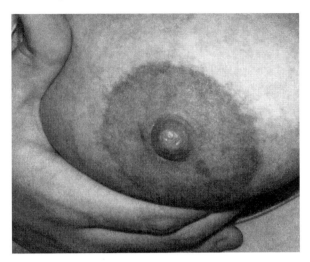

See color plate 61.

Courtesy of K. Jean Cotterman.

a. infectious mastitis in the upper, outer quadrant.

b. galactocele on the lateral side (toward the mother's arm).

c. moderate postfeed breast fullness.

d. edema caused by milk stasis.

6.38 **Which is the MOST LIKELY cause of severely low milk volume at 3 weeks postpartum in a mother with a normal newborn?**

a. Breast surgery

b. Retained placental fragments

c. Breastfeeding mismanagement

d. Environmental estrogenic compounds

6.39 **A mother comes to you for help with breastfeeding her 3-week-old baby, stating, "He just doesn't seem to be able to get it right." When you observe the baby breastfeeding, you note that the baby has a highly erratic suck–swallow pattern and that he never develops a good rhythmic suckling action. Which of the following is MOST LIKELY to explain his sucking behavior?**

a. Some babies do not establish effective suckling patterns for 4 to 6 weeks after birth.

b. The baby's head is still quite molded.

c. The baby was born at 37½ weeks' gestation.

d. The baby has cerebral palsy.

6.40 **A breastfeeding mother complains of a lump in her breast. Which characteristic is MOST LIKELY to be dangerous and require medical evaluation?**

a. The lump feels like a soft fluid-filled sac.

b. The skin over the lump is red and warm.

c. Mother began running a low-grade fever at the same time the lump appeared.

d. The lump does not change size before and after the baby feeds.

6.41 **The behavior exhibited by this baby often occurs about 2 hours after the last breastfeed. What is your BEST recommendation to the mother?**

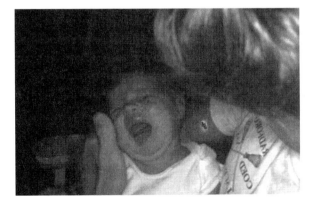

a. Offer her a pacifier to satisfy her need to suck.

b. Breastfeed her again, now.

c. Let her cry a bit so her feedings get spaced out.

d. Give her some water to tide her over until the next feed.

6.42 **What is the MOST LIKELY reason that you would recommend this feeding technique and equipment?**

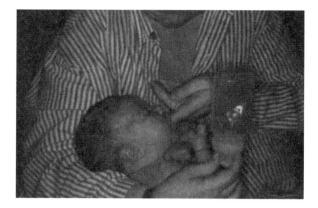

a. Baby has cleft palate.
b. Baby has a weak suck.
c. Baby is clamping down on mom's nipple.
d. Baby is failing to thrive.

6.43 **This mother asks for advice on family planning. She wishes to continue breastfeeding yet does not want to become pregnant again. Your BEST response to her is to:**

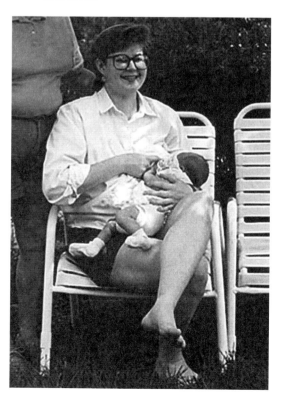

a. Begin taking a progestin-only oral contraceptive.
b. Use a condom every time you have intercourse.
c. An intrauterine device is your best option.
d. Breastfeed exclusively around the clock without supplements or pacifiers.

6.44 **A 3-week-old exclusively breastfed baby with a strong family history of allergy has a severe reaction the first time he is fed with a cow's milk–based formula. The MOST LIKELY explanation for this is that the:**

a. baby was sensitized by intact cow's milk protein that passed into mother's milk.
b. baby was given a bottle of formula in the hospital nursery.
c. mother consumed large amounts of dairy products during pregnancy.
d. allergic reaction was more likely due to the latex in the bottle nipple than the cow's milk.

6.45 **This baby's mother complains of persistent sore nipples. Of the following, which is the first question you should ask?**

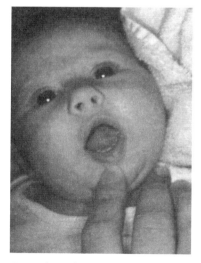

See color plate 62.

a. How did you prepare your nipples during pregnancy?
b. May I watch you breastfeed right now?
c. Are you feeling a stinging, burning sensation?
d. How long do you intend to breastfeed?

6.46 **Which of these behaviors is MOST COMMON for a baby of this age?**

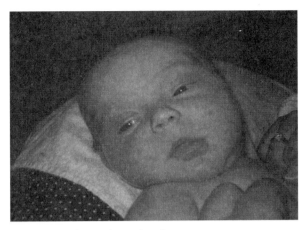

Courtesy of Carole Dobrich.

  a. Hands frequently open
  b. Eye focal distance is about 8 to 12 inches
  c. Reaches for object
  d. Differentiated cries and sounds

6.47 **This mother has a 2-week-old baby who has difficulty attaching to her smaller breast, has been fussy after feeds, and has not regained birth weight. She claims that she does not have enough milk. The MOST LIKELY cause of this situation is that the:**

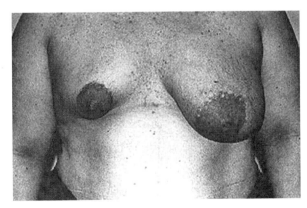

Courtesy of Kay Hoover.

  a. mother is not feeding her baby frequently enough.
  b. smaller breast has insufficient glandular tissue.
  c. baby is attached incorrectly to the breast.
  d. baby is sensitive to an allergen in his mother's milk.

6.48 **What is the FIRST action that an adopting mother should take to start transitioning her baby to nursing at breast?**
  a. Try feeding the formula using a tube-feeding device at breast.
  b. Hold the baby in a nursing position near the breast during feeds.
  c. Replace the standard nipple (teat) with a slow-flow design.
  d. Wait until the baby is very hungry before attempting at breast.

6.49 **What is a normal duration of sleep for a 3-week-old exclusively breastfed infant?**
  a. Three to 4 hours between feeds, around the clock
  b. About 1 hour, with some longer and shorter periods
  c. Irregularly during the day and 5 to 6 hours at night
  d. Two-hour naps during the day, plus a longer stretch at night

6.50 **When evaluating this mother and her 3-week-old baby, which would you suspect is the major reason for the condition pictured?**

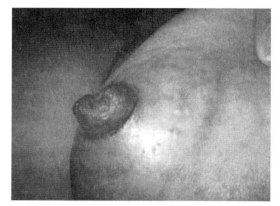

Courtesy of K. Jean Cotterman.

   a. Shallow latch

   b. Baby's mouth is small

   c. Nursing lying down

   d. Tight lingual frenulum

6.51 **A baby gained 19 oz in the past 5 days but is fussy and gassy much of the day. His mother feeds him on both breasts at each feed. Your BEST suggestion to her is:**

   a. cut down your own fluid intake, because you have too much milk.

   b. let him finish nursing on the first breast before you offer the other one.

   c. stop drinking cow's milk for the next 2 weeks.

   d. try giving him some lactose-free supplement three times a day.

6.52 **What is the mother of this baby MOST LIKELY to be feeling?**

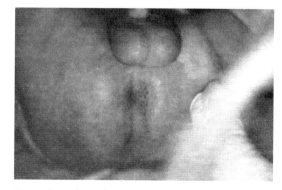

See color plate 63.

   a. Stinging, burning nipple pain

   b. Deep aching pain in her breast

   c. Comfortable breasts and nipples

   d. Sharp pain after and between feedings

6.53 **This mother–infant dyad needs to be carefully assessed for:**

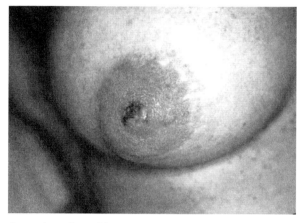

See color plate 64.

   a. duration of feeds.

   b. thrush.

   c. nipple shield use.

   d. latch-on technique.

6.54 **A breastfeeding mother of a 3-week-old baby needs oral surgery for an abscessed tooth. Her dentist is concerned that the anti-inflammatory drug he plans to prescribe may appear in her milk and cause problems for her baby. Which of the following statements is TRUE?**

   a. Anti-inflammatory drugs cause severe bleeding in breastfed babies.

   b. Most drugs appear in high concentrations in milk.

   c. Breastfeeding will retard healing of her surgical incision.

   d. Anti-inflammatory drugs are generally compatible with breastfeeding.

6.55 **Which of the following is MOST LIKELY to be found in the mouth of this mother's baby?**

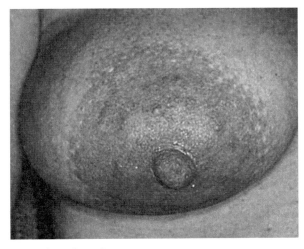

See color plate 65.

    a. Dried milk on the tongue
    b. Normal tongue
    c. Oral thrush (*Candida*)
    d. Strep throat

6.56 **Which of the following sensations is this mother MOST LIKELY to be experiencing?**

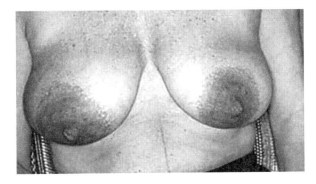

    a. Comfort during and between feeds
    b. Systemic fever and chills
    c. Deep, aching breast pain
    d. Burning, stabbing pain of both nipples/ areolas

6.57 **A mother is concerned because her 3-week-old exclusively breastfed baby suddenly became very fussy in the evenings. Her breastfeeding pattern did not change, and the baby is otherwise healthy. Which recently added item in her diet is MOST LIKELY to be related to her baby's reaction?**

    a. lemonade
    b. herbal tea
    c. green vegetables
    d. vitamin supplements

6.58 **The MOST LIKELY reason for this infant's low weight gain is**

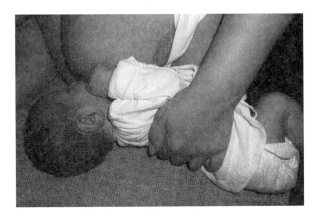

Courtesy of Catherine Watson Genna.

    a. Hyperextended neck which prevents comfortable swallowing
    b. Hypertonia as demonstrated by the baby's position
    c. Breast hypoplasia and insufficient glandular tissue
    d. Damage to the milk ducts and sensory tissue under the scarred area of the breast

6.59 **What visual cue(s) do you see in this photograph that would increase your concern about the effectiveness of this baby's feeding ability?**

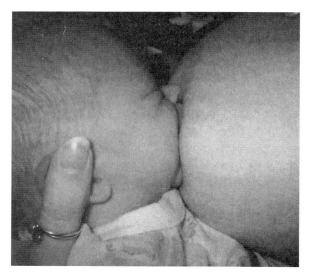

Courtesy of K. Jean Cotterman.

    a. Mother's finger is covering the baby's ear
    b. Baby's eyes are closed
    c. Baby's nose is too close to the breast
    d. Mother's breast is not supported

6.60 **The mother of this baby is having difficulty keeping the baby latched on. Based on what you see, what should be your NEXT course of action?**

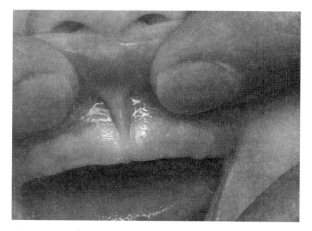

Courtesy of Greg Notestine.

    a. Refer her to a credentialed provider to evaluate the thick, tight labial frenulum.
    b. Suggest she pull the baby onto her breast deeper at the start of feeds.
    c. Teach her how to use a silicone nipple shield for improved milk transfer.
    d. Weigh the baby before and after a feed to assess milk transfer.

6.61 **Any breastfeeding difficulties experienced by this infant are MOST LIKELY related to:**

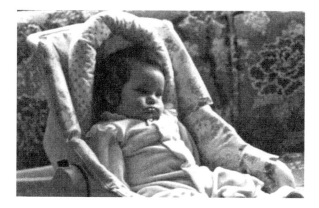

    a. Fetal Alcohol Syndrome
    b. Congenital hypothyroidism
    c. Down Syndrome
    d. Pierre Robin Syndrome

6.62 **A mother is concerned about her baby's feeding pattern. The baby nurses 10–30 minutes on one breast then self-detaches. Your BEST response to her is:**

    a. This is a normal, common pattern.
    b. Babies get all they need in the first 10 minutes.
    c. Your baby has a sucking problem.
    d. Your let-down reflex is too slow.

6.63 **A mother reports her 16-day-old baby is suddenly quite fussy and wants to breastfeed very frequently. Your FIRST response should be:**

a. Suggest several galactogogues that may help to raise milk supply.

b. Reassure the mother that the baby is going through a growth spurt and all is well.

c. Tell her to pump for 10 minutes after every feeding.

d. Ask the mother to describe how breastfeeding was going before baby got fussy.

6.64 **A 3-week-old, exclusively breastfed baby nurses every 1.5 to 2 hours in the late afternoon and evenings. She is gaining over 1 ounce (28 g) per day and has 5–6 profuse, yellow stools and 8+ wet diapers per day. The MOST LIKELY explanation for this frequent nursing pattern is:**

a. normal behavior for this age

b. low milk supply

c. baby is becoming too dependent

d. baby is ready for solid foods.

6.65 **This 4-week-old exclusively breastfed baby was 6 lbs, 3 oz (2.8 kg) at birth. The MOST LIKELY reason for her appearance at this age is:**

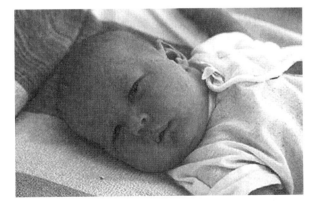

a. Her mother's milk is too high in fat

b. She is taking steroid drugs for a medical condition

c. Mother feeds her on cue, 24 hours a day, without a pacifier

d. Mother's milk is too high in lactose

6.66 **A baby now 4 weeks old was adopted when she was 3 days old and has been formula-fed from birth. Her adoptive mother's goal is to have her baby nurse at breast. The FIRST action the adoptive mother should take toward this goal is to:**

a. feed Mindy using an open cup instead of a bottle

b. get donor human milk from a milk bank to replace the formula

c. change to a slow-flow nipple to mimic at-breast-feeding

d. put the baby to breast for non-nutritive sucking

6.67 **A mother is planning to induce lactation for her 4-week-old adopted baby. She has never been pregnant. The simplest strategy for inducing lactation at this point in time is to:**

a. put the baby to breast very frequently and for as long as the baby will nurse.

b. put the baby to breast using a tube-feeding device.

c. take prescribed pharmaceutical hormone supplements.

d. use a multi-user breast pump several times a day.

Answers for 15–28 Days Questions

6.1 **The answer is d.** Mothers with large breasts may enjoy the support of a well-fitting bra. Bra wearing has no therapeutic value other than maternal comfort, and no portion of the bra should press on or compress breast tissue. There is no pathology shown in this picture. Her baby is nursing well on day 4 postbirth. (Difficulty: 4; Discipline: Clinical Skills; Taxonomy: Goals)

6.2 **The answer is b.** Other loving adults can support the breastfeeding mother in ways other than breastfeeding. Choices c and d are reasonable choices. This picture shows the author carrying her perfectly normal, wonderful, gorgeous, and brilliant grand-daughter at about 4 weeks of age. Competition with the baby's own mother is highly unlikely. (Difficulty: 4; Discipline: Psychology; Taxonomy: Collaboration)

6.3 **The answer is c.** Babies feed for varying lengths and at varying intervals according to their hunger, emotional needs, growth and developmental stages, and other physiological factors. Placing restrictions on length or frequency or offering substitutes disrupts the breastfeeding relationship and interferes with fulfillment of infant needs. (Difficulty: 2; Discipline: Clinical Skills; Taxonomy: Plan)

6.4 **The answer is b.** A common sign of disorganized sucking is the baby feeds for extended periods with its eyes closed. Also, 30 to 45 minutes per breast is not normal behavior for this healthy 3-week-old. Mother's milk supply cannot be ascertained by infant feeding behavior, and the effect of most labor drugs would have diminished by now. (Difficulty: 5; Discipline: Pathology; Taxonomy: Evaluate)

6.5 **The answer is c.** The mother's breasts have not developed sufficient glandular tissue to support lactation for her baby. (Difficulty: 3; Discipline: Pathology; Taxonomy: History)

6.6 **The answer is a.** Differences in breast size during lactation are normal and common. (Difficulty: 2; Discipline: Development; Taxonomy: Assessment)

6.7 **The answer is d.** This mother's baby was thrusting her tongue forward to compensate for the mother's abundant supply of milk and strong milk ejection reflex. The picture was taken at 2 1/2 weeks postbirth. Choices a and b are possible but unlikely. A cleft palate is unlikely to cause the horizontal crack in this mother's nipples. (Difficulty: 4; Discipline: Pathology; Taxonomy: Evaluate)

6.8 **The answer is c.** Torticollis is the most likely reason that this baby prefers to turn his head right. Torticollis is an abnormal condition of the neck muscles, especially the sterno-cleidomastoid. (Difficulty: 3; Discipline: Pathology; Taxonomy: Evaluate)

6.9 **The answer is d.** Stools of exclusively breast-fed babies in the first month are exactly as described. (Difficulty: 3; Discipline: Development; Taxonomy: Assessment)

6.10 **The answer is d.** Using a more upright posture removes gravity as an aid to feeding, which is more like breastfeeding. Air mixing with milk from bottle position or type of nipple can trigger a need to burp. Pacing by bottle removal should coordinate with baby's behavior, not a set number of swallows. Flow rate should match baby's tolerance, so jiggling may be detrimental. (Difficulty: 4; Discipline: Techniques; Taxonomy: Goals)

6.11 **The answer is c.** The average 2- to 4-week-old baby's milk consumption is approximately 750 to 800 mL [25 to 26.5 oz] per day. The amount can vary widely among normal babies. (Difficulty: 5; Discipline: Development; Taxonomy: Assessment)

6.12 **The answer is c.** This baby is adequately attached and positioned for feeding, and the pattern is normal in length and comfortable for both mother and baby. While choices a, b, and d would be appropriate if the feeding pattern was uncomfortable or ineffective, suggesting too many technique changes could undermine the mother's confidence in breastfeeding. (Difficulty: 2; Discipline: Techniques; Taxonomy: Goals)

6.13 **The answer is a.** The baby is entirely healthy and thriving except for an allergic diaper rash caused by dairy in her mother's diet. The other options are inappropriate and incorrect. There are no signs of fungal infection on the baby in this picture. (Difficulty: 3; Discipline: Pathology; Taxonomy: Plan)

6.14 **The answer is b.** This baby is in the quiet alert state. (Difficulty: 4; Discipline: Development; Taxonomy: Assessment)

6.15 **The answer is c.** Dressings designed for moist-wound healing are appropriate treatments for nipple wounds. The source of the damage needs to be identified and corrected. The other suggestions are inappropriate. (Difficulty: 2; Discipline: Pharmacology; Taxonomy: Plan)

6.16 **The answer is b.** The mother's condition prevents her hand from grasping, so positioning must be done with her full arm. The other choices are not an issue in this condition. (Difficulty: 4; Discipline: Techniques; Taxonomy: History)

6.17 **The answer is d.** Research studies report that a breastfeeding mother who shares a safe bed with her baby has the best nocturnal sleep of every group of new parents tested. All postpartum women tend to have fragmented sleep regardless of how they feed their babies. (Difficulty: 4; Discipline: Development; Taxonomy: Assessment)

6.18 **The answer is d.** This is a bacterial infection of the nipple skin. The baby had just begun treatment for a staph infection on his mouth that was acquired at day care. (Difficulty: 4; Discipline: Pathology; Taxonomy: Evaluate)

6.19 **The answer is a.** The vertical position is helpful when the baby has a head injury or needs help maintaining good alignment. Let-down reflex is not affected by baby's position; the "colic hold" is holding the baby prone on the mother's forearm. Plugged milk ducts are rarely found in the upper quadrant. (Difficulty: 2; Discipline: Techniques; Taxonomy: Plan)

6.20 **The answer is c.** The only limiting factor to breastfeeding is the mother's injuries. Compatible pain medications are available. She and her baby still need each other while she recovers. (Difficulty: 4; Discipline: Clinical Skills; Taxonomy: Plan)

6.21 **The answer is b.** By 2 weeks, most term infants should be able to handle mother's milk-ejection reflex. If the baby cannot coordinate sucking and swallowing with breathing, he may choke and gasp for breath as the milk releases. Occasionally, a normal baby may still have difficulty handling a mother's strong milk-ejection reflex. (Difficulty: 3; Discipline: Pathology)

6.22 **The answer is a.** First, confirm that the baby is taking no other substances including vitamins, medications, and herbs and is not using a pacifier. Any intake of other foods including infant formula, fluids, herbs, or medications can confuse the clinical picture. Once that has been done, eliminating all dairy products in all forms from the mother's diet is the next most appropriate action. The baby's primary care provider should always be notified of the lactation care plan. Modifying nursing to increase hindmilk is ineffective if the cause is something in the mother's diet. (Difficulty: 4; Discipline: Pathology; Taxonomy: Assessment)

6.23 **The answer is d.** Bifidus factor supports gut colonization with *Lactobacillus bifidus*, a friendly bacterium that protects the gut mucosa from pathogens. Bifidus factor is not found in the milk of other animals. (Difficulty: 3; Discipline: Development; Taxonomy: Assessment)

6.24 **The answer is c.** This baby is nearing the end of the feed on this breast and should be allowed to self-detach at his own pace. He is correctly positioned for effective nursing. (Difficulty: 4; Discipline: Clinical Skills; Taxonomy: Goals)

6.25 **The answer is c.** Adding additional sessions is the most likely strategy to increase production. Sequential pumping is less effective than simultaneous pumping for most women because simultaneous pumping takes advantage of the let-down reflex in both breasts. Any pump with sufficient pressures and appropriate rhythms would be effective, not whether the pump is designed for multiple or single users. A larger-diameter flange might be helpful if the flange diameter is inhibiting movement of the breast/nipple in the flange. (Difficulty: 4; Discipline: Techniques; Taxonomy: Goals)

6.26 **The answer is d.** The most important regulatory mechanism for milk synthesis is frequent and thorough milk removal. (Difficulty: 4; Discipline: Techniques; Taxonomy: Plan)

6.27 **The answer is b.** This was diagnosed as eczema, an allergic reaction that began soon after this baby was given supplements of cow's milk–based formula. Rice cereal is a less common allergen. It is unlikely that cold temperature or a tetanus immunization triggered this response. (Difficulty: 3; Discipline: Pathology; Taxonomy: History)

6.28 **The answer is b.** This baby's hypotonia (low muscle tone) is caused by Prader-Willi syndrome. The nipple shield (barely visible), jaw support, and upright straddle position are all techniques that can assist a baby with low tone to maximize milk obtained directly at breast. (Difficulty: 2; Discipline: Pathology; Taxonomy: History)

6.29 **The answer is b.** In the quiet alert state, the baby's eyes are open, arms extended and relaxed, and hands loosely open. The baby's expression is calm and relaxed. (Difficulty: 4; Discipline: Development; Taxonomy: Goals)

6.30 **The answer is c.** The reddened skin is found only on the genitalia and anal opening, suggesting an allergic response. Yeast infections are characterized by blisters or papules. Acidic urine does not result from human milk feedings, and chemical sensitivities would likely appear under the entire diaper area. This baby was in fact allergic to dairy products ingested by her mother. (Difficulty: 3; Discipline: Pathology; Taxonomy: Evaluate)

6.31 **The answer is c.** Nipple thrush often has few visible signs—identification is based on clinical symptoms of itching, stinging, and/or burning. The slightly pink color of her nipples, combined with the sensations reported, is highly suggestive of nipple thrush (*Candida*). (Difficulty: 5; Discipline: Pathology; Taxonomy: Evaluate)

6.32 **The answer is b.** Babies are not lazy. Labeling babies in this manner prevents looking for, finding, and resolving the cause of the problem. All of the other choices are possible causes of poor milk transfer and low weight gain in a newborn. (Difficulty: 5; Discipline: Psychology; Taxonomy: Goals)

6.33 **The answer is a.** Deep attachment is usually the first and most important strategy for preventing nipple pain. The peaked shape of the nipple does not "look good"; it suggests a shallow latch and/or poor sucking technique, both of which need attention and correction. Choices b and d are reasonable and appropriate suggestions. (Difficulty: 4; Discipline: Techniques; Taxonomy: Plan)

6.34 **The answer is b.** Breastfeeding mothers instinctively sleep with their baby in a unique, protective posture. Exclusively breastfeeding mothers who sleep with their babies on a safe surface get the most sleep of all postpartum parents. Formula may suppress arousal, is a significant risk factor for many reasons, and interferes with exclusive breastfeeding. Crying is stressful for babies, with significant long-term negative consequences. (Difficulty: 4; Discipline: Psychology; Taxonomy: Goals)

6.35 **The answer is d.** Identifying with the mother's feelings rather than offering solutions allows her to think about her options. (Difficulty: 2; Discipline: Psychology; Taxonomy: Goals)

6.36 **The answer is b.** The baby's head is too extended relative to his trunk, so pulling the legs closer to mother will better align hip and shoulders. Supporting the breast will not correct the infant's position. The horizontal position and use of a pillow are not likely to help. (Difficulty: 2; Discipline: Techniques; Taxonomy: Plan)

6.37 **The answer is c.** This is an entirely normal breast with moderate fullness. There are no visual indications of mastitis, galactocele, or edema. (Difficulty: 5; Discipline: Development; Taxonomy: Assessment)

6.38 **The answer is b.** Retained placenta is the most likely maternal factor in severely low milk production. Choices a and c are common maternal factors to investigate in low milk volume at 3 weeks postpartum. (Difficulty: 4; Discipline: Pathology; Taxonomy: History)

6.39 **The answer is b.** Persistent cranial molding can interfere with nervous system functioning in the early weeks, which can interfere with the suck–swallow pattern. Birth-related cranial molding should resolve within the first few weeks. (Difficulty: 3; Discipline: Pathology; Taxonomy: Evaluate)

6.40 **The answer is d.** Lumps that do not change size related to milk flow are considered ominous. The mother should be evaluated by a physician immediately. The other characteristics are fairly common during lactation. (Difficulty: 2; Discipline: Pathology; Taxonomy: Collaboration)

6.41 **The answer is b.** Babies should be breastfed when they show signs of hunger. Crying, as shown in the picture, is a LATE hunger cue. The other options do not meet the baby's need for frequent feedings. (Difficulty: 3; Discipline: Clinical Skills; Taxonomy: Goals)

6.42 **The answer is c.** Finger-feeding is a therapeutic method that may help a baby get back to direct breastfeeding after early difficulties. (Difficulty: 3; Discipline: Clinical Skills; Taxonomy: Plan)

6.43 **The answer is d.** The Lactation Amenorrhea Method (LAM) offers the highest (at least 98%) protection against unplanned pregnancy and is the most compatible method with continued breastfeeding. (Difficulty: 5; Discipline: Physiology; Taxonomy: Goals)

6.44 **The answer is c.** Prenatal sensitization to bovine protein does occur, especially in genetically susceptible children. Choices a and b are also sources of sensitization. (Difficulty: 4; Discipline: Development; Taxonomy: History)

6.45 **The answer is b.** Observing a breastfeed is the first step in identifying the cause of painful nipples. (Difficulty: 3; Discipline: Clinical Skills; Taxonomy: Assessment)

6.46 **The answer is b.** A newborn's eye focal distance is about 8 to 12 inches, or the approximate distance between the baby's eyes and the mother's eyes during nursing. Choices a and d are correct. The 2- to 4-week-old is not yet capable of reaching for objects. (Difficulty: 4; Discipline: Development; Taxonomy: Assessment)

6.47 **The answer is b.** The smaller breast has characteristics of insufficient glandular tissue. (Difficulty: 4; Discipline: Pathology; Taxonomy: History)

6.48 **The answer is b.** The first goal is to encourage the baby to view the breast as the source of food, so holding the baby in nursing position with the baby's cheek touching the mother's bare breast is the best first strategy. Tube-feeding devices may be an option after the baby can latch and attempt to feed at breast, if the mother's milk production is low. Replacing the standard nipple with a slow-flow is still not breastfeeding. Hungry babies are in no mood to change feeding methods easily, so attempting to directly breastfeed when the baby is not excessively hungry is more effective. (Difficulty: 4; Discipline: Techniques; Taxonomy: Goals)

6.49 **The answer is b.** Newborn sleep patterns are irregular, and short periods of sleep are typical. Babies do not sleep for long stretches for several months. By 3 months, some have begun to consolidate short sleep stretches into longer ones occasionally. (Difficulty: 4; Discipline: Development; Taxonomy: Assessment)

6.50 **The answer is d.** This mother's baby had a short, tight lingual frenulum that was pushing her nipple tip up against the rugae on his hard palate, causing the damage on the top surface of her nipple. Choice a might have been reasonable had the baby's mouth anatomy been normal. Choice b is unlikely, and choice c is not a typical cause of nipple damage. (Difficulty: 4; Discipline: Pathology; Taxonomy: Assessment)

6.51 **The answer is b.** The baby should be allowed to feed in his own preferred pattern, which may be one breast per feed or even several feeds on one breast before switching to the other. Getting too little fat-rich hindmilk is one possible factor in rapid weight gain with fussy, gassy behavior. (Difficulty: 4; Discipline: Pathology; Taxonomy: Plan)

6.52 **The answer is a.** This baby's diaper-area rash was caused by *Candida* (thrush) infection, which was also present in his mouth and on mother's nipples. Mother was experiencing itching, stinging, burning nipple pain consistent with thrush infection of the nipples. (Difficulty: 4; Discipline: Pathology; Taxonomy: Evaluate)

6.53 **The answer is d.** The location of the abrasions suggests that the baby is nursing on the nipple tips instead of taking a large, deep grasp of the nipple–areola complex. (Difficulty: 5; Discipline: Techniques; Taxonomy: Assessment)

6.54 **The answer is d.** Anti-inflammatory drugs are generally compatible with breastfeeding. The other statements are false. (Difficulty: 3; Discipline: Pharmacology; Taxonomy: Knowledge)

6.55 **The answer is c.** The shiny, reddened color of this mother's nipple and areola is typical of thrush (*Candida*) infection. Her baby's mouth is likely to show white plaques that do not rub off and are typical of oral thrush/fungal (*Candida*) infections. (Difficulty: 4; Discipline: Pathology; Taxonomy: Assessment)

6.56 **The answer is d.** The reddened areola and nipple area indicate the probable presence of nipple thrush (*Candida*) infection, which is commonly accompanied by burning, stinging, or itching. Fever & chills and deep, aching breast pain are more likely to be caused by a bacterial breast infection. A few mothers will feel no discomfort even with this amount of nipple thrush. (Difficulty: 3; Discipline: Pathology; Taxonomy: Assessment)

6.57 **The answer is b.** Herbal teas may contain substances that exert a pharmacological effect on the baby. (Difficulty: 4; Discipline: Pharmacology; Taxonomy: Knowledge)

6.58 **The answer is d.** This mother had breast reduction surgery with significant tissue removal many years ago. The scars on the lateral surface of her breast, near her arm, are the only visible clues of this underlying condition. The baby is in an effective (and perhaps awkward) position for feeding, and shows no signs of hypertonia. (Difficulty: 4; Discipline: Pathology; Taxonomy: History)

6.59 **The answer is b.** The baby's eyes are closed even though he or she is still deeply attached to the breast. This baby was tongue-tied and struggling to stay at breast. None of the other choices are relevant. (Difficulty: 2; Discipline: Clinical Skills; Taxonomy: Evaluate)

6.60 **The answer is a.** Referral to a credentialed provider to evaluate lip-tie (tight and/or thick labial frenulum) and possibly release the tissue is the next best course of action. The baby's upper lip needs to curl outward for effective deep latch. Choice b might be an interim strategy. Choice c is unlikely to help. Choice d is an appropriate part of evaluation, but won't fix the baby's latch-on problem. (Difficulty: 4; Discipline: Clinical Skills; Taxonomy: Collaboration)

6.61 **The answer is c.** This baby has Down Syndrome (Trisomy 21). However, not all babies with Down Syndrome have problems with breastfeeding. (Difficulty:3; Discipline: Pathology; Taxonomy: Evaluate)

6.62 **The answer is a.** Research and experience shows that a range of 7–30 minutes per breastis normal and common. About 30% of babies always feed from only one breast (always unpaired feeds). (Difficulty: 3; Discipline: Development; Taxonomy: Goals)

6.63 **The answer is d.** Although some babies seem to go through benign "growth spurts" in the early weeks, ongoing unrecognized problems need to be first ruled out. The LC should always take a history before offering suggestions. (Difficulty: 3; Discipline: Development; Taxonomy: Assessment)

6.64 **The answer is a.** This is a normal pattern. (Difficulty: 2; Discipline: Development; Taxonomy: Evaluate)

6.65 **The answer is c.** This 4-week-old baby has gained weight appropriately and is entirely normal. (Difficulty: 3; Discipline: Development; Taxonomy: Assessment)

6.66 **The answer is a.** Changing from a teat/nipple to an open cup is the BEST of the strategies and the first one to try. Donor milk is an independent issue and not central to establish breastfeeding in an adoptive situation. There is no evidence that a slow-flow nipple would help transitioning to the breast. Non-nutritive sucking at breast could help, but wouldn't be the first or most promising strategy to try. (Difficulty: 4; Discipline: Techniques; Taxonomy: Goals)

6.67 **The answer is a.** The simplest method of inducing lactation is frequent sucking at breast while supplementing as needed using an open cup with donor milk or formula. The other methods are known to be effective, but are generally more complicated. (Difficulty: 5; Discipline: Physiology; Taxonomy: Plan)

CHAPTER 7

1–3 Months Questions

7.1 The breastfeeding equipment shown in this photograph is MOST LIKELY being used for:

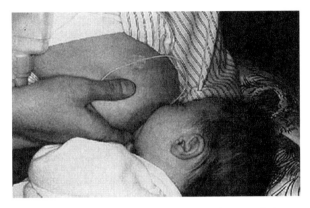

   a. provision of sufficient calories while increasing the milk supply.

   b. training the baby at the breast to suck correctly and effectively.

   c. ensuring adequate caloric intake because this baby is too small to obtain enough nourishment.

   d. aiding this baby to attach correctly to the breast and continue sucking.

7.2 According to studies of breastfed babies in an industrialized society, which of the following feeding patterns MOST CLOSELY approximates that of an exclusively breastfed 3-month-old baby?

   a. 4 to 6 feeds per day, total 60 minutes or more

   b. 6 to 8 feeds per day, total 100 minutes or more

   c. 8 to 10 feeds per day, total 120 minutes or more

   d. 10 to 12 feeds per day, total 140 minutes or more

7.3 A woman requests information on allowing her children to take this action together. Your BEST response is:

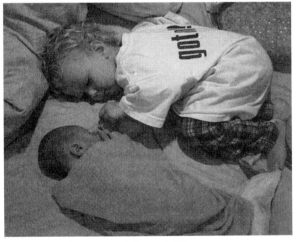

Courtesy of Virginia (Ginny) Kooyman.

   a. The children look very cute when they are asleep.

   b. The infant is at some danger from overlying, so make sure they sleep where you can see them.

   c. Children should learn to sleep in their own beds; both children should be in cribs.

   d. Siblings sleeping together is common around the world. There is no risk to this practice.

7.4 **What factor below is MOST RELATED to the age of the child pictured?**

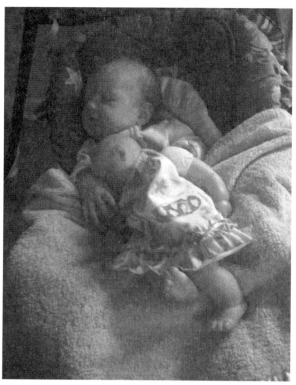

Courtesy of Virginia (Ginny) Kooyman.

    a. Will no longer take a pacifier
    b. Highest risk of SIDS
    c. Ability to roll over
    d. Highest risk of otitis media

7.5 **When comparing the 2006 WHO Growth Standards to the pre-2006 growth charts used for many years, which statement BEST describes the growth of exclusively breastfed babies in the first 6 months?**
    a. Breastfed babies gain more weight.
    b. Breastfed babies are longer in length.
    c. There is no difference in weight gain.
    d. Breastfed babies are leaner per height.

7.6 **This baby's weight gain and development are normal. What is the FIRST question you would ask the mother?**

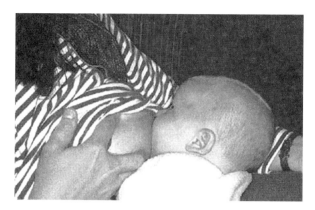

    a. Do you use this position at all feeds?
    b. Is your baby sleeping through the night yet?
    c. How is breastfeeding going for you?
    d. Have your menstrual periods returned?

7.7 **This mother's nipple pain began after several months of comfortable breastfeeding. The MOST IMPORTANT action you would take to help relieve this mother's discomfort is to:**

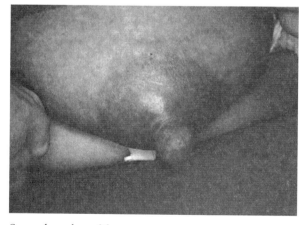

See color plate 66.

    a. teach her how to keep her baby from squirming during feeds.
    b. assist her baby to take more of the breast during latch-on.
    c. provide a silicone nipple shield to reduce abrasion on the nipple skin.
    d. help her get treatment for a probable nipple thrush infection.

7.8 The mother of a 5-month-old baby is practicing the lactational amenorrhea method (LAM) of family planning. Which behavior is not related to the effectiveness of the method?

    a. Intercourse more than twice a week

    b. Relief bottle every other day

    c. Baby sleeping through the night

    d. Return of menstruation

7.9 This baby's mother complains of clicking and smacking during breastfeeds. The MOST LIKELY explanation is that:

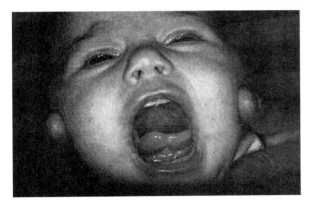

    a. high-domed palate prevents deep latch.

    b. tongue-tie prevents deep attachment.

    c. tongue shape causes intermittent loss of seal.

    d. buccal fat pads are interfering with tongue movement.

7.10 The condition on this mother's nipple appeared a few weeks after she a suspicious lump was surgically removed from her breast. Her baby has no signs of oral thrush or other infections. The lactation consultant's (LC) MOST IMPORTANT role in this situation is to:

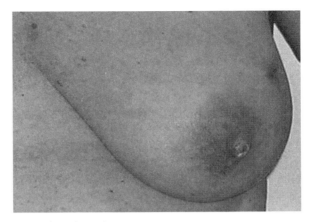

See color plate 67.

Courtesy of Catherine Watson Genna.

    a. advise her on which nipple creams have been shown to be effective.

    b. take a thorough history including photographing the affected area.

    c. suggest she clean the affected area with an antibacterial soap daily.

    d. show her how to hand-express milk from that breast.

7.11 Which method of family planning would MOST INTERFERE with breastfeeding?

    a. Tubal ligation

    b. Progestin-only oral contraceptives

    c. Intrauterine devices

    d. Natural family planning (periodic abstinence)

7.12 A thriving, exclusively breastfed 3-month-old baby suddenly begins nursing much more frequently, around the clock. Her mother calls you, worried that something has happened to her milk. Your BEST response to her is:

    a. Has the baby been exposed to illness lately?

    b. Babies usually nurse more frequently beginning at 3 months of age.

    c. This is probably a growth spurt; her usual pattern will probably resume soon.

    d. Your milk is higher in casein now, making her fussier.

7.13 **Which of the following events is MOST LIKELY to be associated with a baby of this age?**

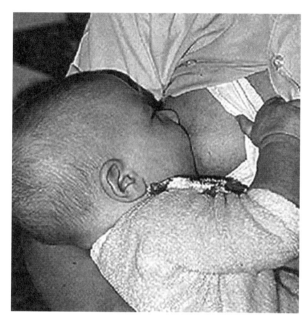

a. Breastfeeds 6 to 8 times per 24 hours
b. May sleep for 2 to 3 hours once a day
c. Grasps his toes during nursing
d. Recognizes other adults and smiles

7.14 **A mother asks about a book she has read that recommends letting a baby "cry it out" to teach him to sleep all night by 3 months of age. The authors claim that responding immediately to baby's cries will teach the baby to be manipulative. Based on Erickson and Piaget's work regarding the development of trust, your BEST response to her is:**

a. Three month-old babies are learning trust. Not responding to him teaches him that he can't trust you.
b. The book is correct. Babies can learn to self-soothe at that age.
c. Babies learn to manipulate parents at an early age. You can learn to differentiate his cries of real distress.
d. By 3 months, his ability to trust you is already developed, and crying it out won't hurt him.

7.15 **What is the MOST LIKELY cause of gastroesophageal reflux disease (GERD) in a 1-month-old term baby who is otherwise healthy?**

a. Overanxious mother
b. Cow's milk protein allergy
c. Lactose intolerance
d. Overactive letdown in the mother

7.16 **Which of the following feeding patterns would be MOST LIKELY in a 2-month-old exclusively breastfed baby?**

a. Clustering feeds in the late morning
b. No feeding for 6 to 8 hours at night
c. Feeds about every 3 to 4 hours during the day and one or two at night
d. 8 to 12 or more feeds spaced throughout the 24-hour day

7.17 **This mother of a 3-month-old began feeling pinpoint pain on her nipple tip 2 days ago. The pain is MOST LIKELY due to:**

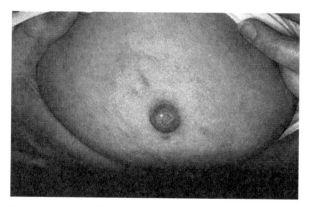

See color plate 68.

a. mastitis
b. a plugged nipple pore.
c. a bacterial infection.
d. a friction blister.

7.18 **A mother of a fussy, gassy baby has been drinking 10 glasses of cow's milk per day on her doctor's recommendation. Your FIRST action would be to:**

a. encourage her to follow her doctor's dietary advice.

b. take a thorough history including allergy and food sensitivity in the family.

c. tell her that 6 to 8 glasses of any liquid is adequate during lactation.

d. tell her that consumption of dairy products is not related to her baby's symptoms.

7.19 **A mother expresses fear that her milk supply is faltering. Her baby is nursing effectively on cue at least 12 times per 24 hours, and she is feeling tired and chilly. Which is the MOST LIKELY cause of these signs?**

a. Low serum prolactin levels

b. Low thyroid hormone level

c. Anemia

d. Chronic fatigue syndrome

7.20 **A breastfeeding mother 6 weeks post-birth tells you "None of your suggestions have worked, and I'm at the end of my rope. I'm a complete failure as a mom!" Which is the MOST LIKELY condition affecting the mother?**

a. Bipolar disorder

b. Anxiety disorder

c. Postpartum depression

d. Asperger's syndrome

7.21 **Which of the following is the highest risk factor for SIDS?**

a. bedsharing (co-sleeping)

b. Maternal smoking during pregnancy

c. Formula feeding

d. Alcohol use in pregnancy

7.22 **Which situation puts the infant at LOWEST risk of smothering?**

a. Baby alone, placed supine on a soft adult mattress

b. Adult sleeping with baby on a sofa (couch)

c. Nursing mother sleeping with her baby on a firm adult mattress

d. Swaddled infant alone, supine, in a crib

7.23 **When this condition is seen in a breastfeeding infant, which is the MOST APPROPRIATE recommendation?**

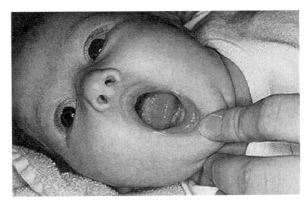

See color plate 69.

a. Simultaneous treatment of the baby and mother's breast should begin.

b. Unless the mother has signs of infection, treat only the baby's mouth with an antifungal medication.

c. Check mother's nipples for signs or symptoms of infection.

d. Boil all pacifiers and burp cloths.

7.24 **Both children in this photograph are nursing. What are the MOST LIKELY implications for the younger baby while his older sister continues to nurse?**

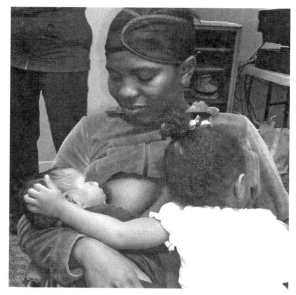

Courtesy of Melissa Courts.

   a. The older child will take too much of the infant's milk.
   b. The younger child will be distracted by the older one.
   c. The older child will be jealous of the younger's frequent nursing
   d. Both children will receive adequate milk at breast.

7.25 **What is the FIRST action you would take to assist this mother?**

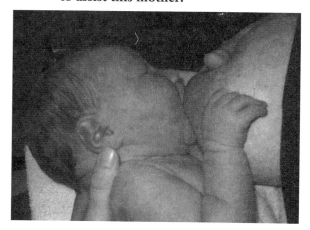

Courtesy of Carole Dobrich.

   a. Correct positioning and latch-on technique
   b. Apply an antibacterial ointment
   c. Apply an antifungal preparation
   d. Provide her with a silicone nipple shield

7.26 **The rash on this baby's face appeared when he began receiving supplements of cow's milk–based artificial baby milk. What is the MOST LIKELY cause of the rash?**

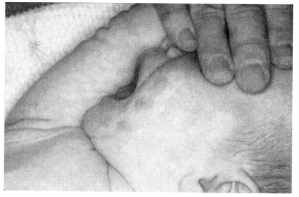

See color plate 70.

   a. Normal infant acne
   b. Reaction to nonhuman protein in the artificial baby milk
   c. Presence of bovine antigen in mother's milk
   d. Allergic reaction to latex in bottle teat

7.27 **Which method of family planning is MOST LIKELY to interfere with breastfeeding?**
   a. Progestin-containing medications
   b. Estrogen-containing medications
   c. Cervical cap or diaphragm
   d. Natural family planning (periodic abstinence)

7.28 A mother tells you that the pediatrician has recommended that she give artificial baby milk after each breastfeeding to her slow-gaining 9-week-old infant. What should be your FIRST response?

    a. Explore the mother's breastfeeding patterns.

    b. Refer her to a different pediatrician.

    c. Refer her to a breastfeeding support group.

    d. Give information on how to provide complementary feeding without compromising breastfeeding.

7.29 The MOST LIKELY consequence of this behavior is:

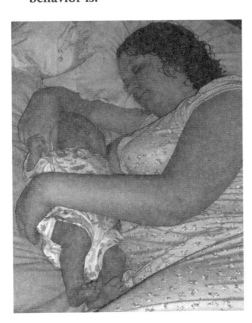

    a. baby receives up to 30% of calories at night.

    b. increased risk of baby smothering.

    c. higher likelihood of longer and exclusive breastfeeding.

    d. reduced risk of pregnancy.

7.30 What could you do to DECREASE this baby's risk of SIDS?

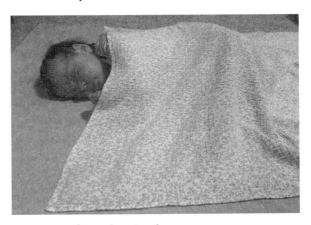

Courtesy of Heather Spada.

    a. Use a sleep sack instead of the blanket.

    b. Put the baby in a crib.

    c. Give the baby a pacifier.

    d. Roll the baby onto her back.

7.31 What is the MOST LIKELY reason that the mother is using the equipment pictured?

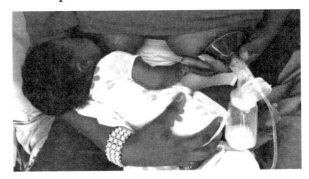

Courtesy of Kimarie Bugg.

    a. Her baby is premature and has a weak suck.

    b. Her milk production is low because of her cultural background.

    c. She plans to return to paid employment soon.

    d. The baby's father insists on feeding the baby.

7.32 **The normal and safest nighttime sleep and breastfeeding pattern for the 3-month-old exclusively breastfed baby is that:**

a. mother and baby share a bed and feed several times at night.

b. baby sleeps in another room away from parents.

c. baby is put to bed at a regular time and allowed to self-comfort to go to sleep.

d. baby is nursed to sleep, then put down with a pacifier in a crib.

7.33 **A mother of 10-week-old twins calls. She says that all she does all day is feed babies and she can't take it anymore. She asks how she can introduce some artificial baby milk or infant cereal without weaning her babies from the breast. The FIRST thing you should do is:**

a. suggest she feed her infants simultaneously in order to save time.

b. tell her that offering other foods will decrease milk production.

c. ask if she has any help with household chores.

d. actively listen, and praise her for breastfeeding two babies.

7.34 **This mother had surgery to drain a breast abscess 3 days ago, and you are visiting her in her home for the second time since the surgery. What is your MOST IMPORTANT action at this point?**

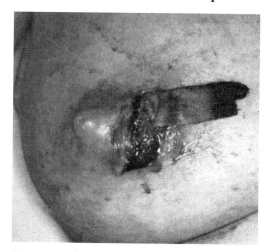

See color plate 71.

a. Advise her to stop breastfeeding on this breast.

b. Assist her to express milk from this breast every few hours.

c. Encourage her to rest and continue breastfeeding on the other breast.

d. Support her taking any prescribed antibiotics.

7.35 **During breastfeeding, this baby's mother has noticed loud clicking and smacking. The MOST LIKELY reason for the clicking is:**

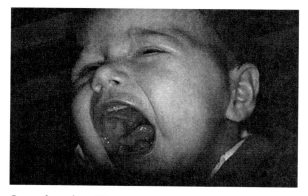

See color plate 72.

a. prominent buccal fat pads compromising tongue motion.

b. oddly shaped tongue tip, causing loss of seal during sucking.

c. short, tight labial frenulum preventing deep attachment at breast.

d. tight muscles around the mouth causing overuse of lips to create seal.

7.36 **A 3-month-old exclusively breastfed baby is suddenly hospitalized for treatment of a cardiac abnormality. The mother is told she must stop breastfeeding because the baby's intake and output need to be carefully measured. Of the following options, which is MOST SUPPORTIVE of her desire to continue breastfeeding?**

a. Mother expresses her milk and gives it by an alternative feeding device.

b. Weigh the baby before and after feeds.

c. Weigh the mother before and after feeds.

d. Carefully count the baby's swallows and record duration of breastfeeding.

7.37 **What is the MOST LIKELY reason that the mother and baby are using this feeding position?**

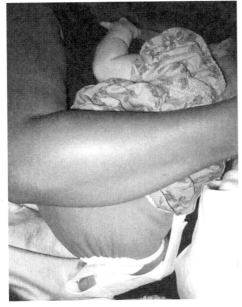

Courtesy of Catherine Watson Genna

a. Mother has an overactive let-down reflex.
b. Baby cannot tolerate pressure on either hip.
c. Baby can't handle mother's overabundant milk production
d. Mother is recovering from cesarean surgery.

7.38 **What is the MOST LIKELY cause of the condition shown? The condition has persisted for 2 months.**

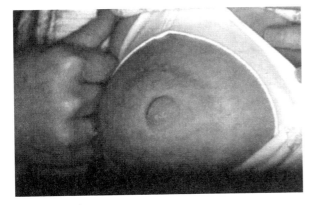

See color plate 73.

a. Paget's disease
b. Plugged nipple pore
c. Persistent wound from baby's tongue thrust
d. Nipple thrush (*Candida*)

7.39 **This activity is appropriate or necessary during which of the following maternal conditions?**

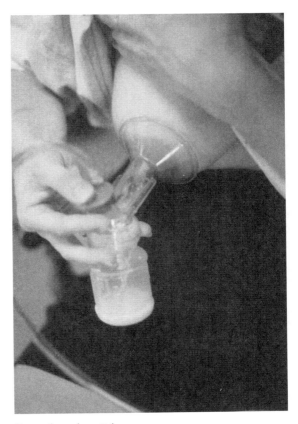

See color plate 74.

a. Chickenpox
b. Infectious mastitis
c. Breast abscess near the nipple
d. Toxoplasmosis

7.40 **Which of the following statements about this practice is MOST ACCURATE?**

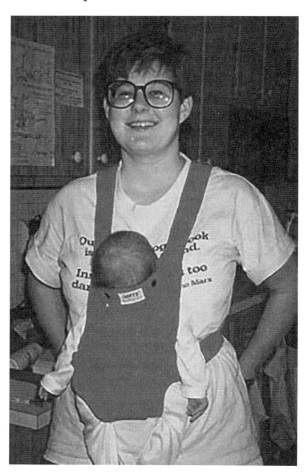

a. Helps the baby maintain body temperature
b. Promotes psychomotor development
c. Increases risk of hip dysplasia
d. Prolongs dependency on the mother

7.41 **This mother had persistent deep breast pain and low-grade fever for 2 weeks. What is the MOST LIKELY reason for the treatment pictured?**

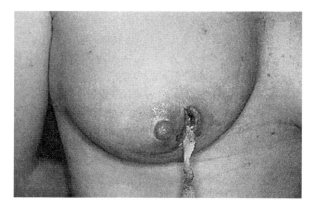

a. Infectious mastitis
b. Breast abscess
c. Intraductal papilloma
d. Mammary duct ectasia

7.42 **Why do the breastfed baby's stools become firmer over time, even before the addition of solid foods?**

a. Casein increases in proportion to whey over time.
b. There is less liquid in proportion to minerals in the milk over time.
c. Breastmilk supplies inadequate fluids over time, necessitating adding other drinks.
d. The baby perspires more, using more of the liquid in milk for metabolism.

7.43 Which of the following is MOST ASSO-CIATED with this sleep position?

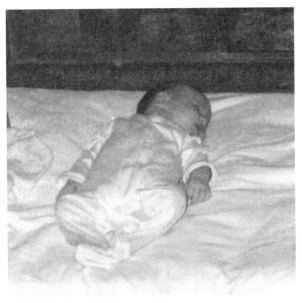

    a. Increased time in deep sleep
    b. Less risk of sudden infant death syndrome
    c. Less chance of aspiration of milk
    d. Decreased number of awakenings at night

7.44 The husband of a breastfeeding woman is eager for his wife to be as amorous as she was before his son was born 3 months ago. He asks you for some suggestions that will help her feel more eager for his lovemaking. Your BEST response is:
    a. You'll just have to learn to live with it. When the baby weans, your relationship will get better.
    b. Try helping her with the baby, house-work, and cooking. She would probably consider that as great "foreplay."
    c. It would be more appropriate for me to talk directly with your wife about this subject.
    d. You may want to use some lubricant, time your lovemaking around the baby's sleep and nursing pattern, and take your time to help her get into the mood.

7.45 The mother of a 3-month-old hospital-ized for sudden failure to thrive asks for your help in resuming breastfeeding. The baby is allegedly allergic to breast-milk, cow's milk, and soy. In addition to increasing her milk production by pumping, the next MOST IMPORTANT strategy for helping her is:
    a. Teach the mother why and how to elim-inate all bovine and soy protein from her own diet.
    b. Tell her to stop drinking whole cow's milk for a week.
    c. Provide her with a dietary supplement of calcium to replace cow's milk
    d. Send a letter to her baby's care providers disputing the baby's allergy to breastmilk.

7.46 The MOST LIKELY and important out-come from this practice is:

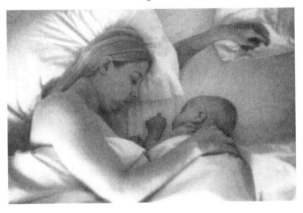

    a. baby is breastfed exclusively and longer.
    b. increased risk of suffocation for the infant.
    c. fragmented sleep for the mother.
    d. delayed return of fertility for mother.

7.47 A 3-month-old baby was hospitalized for sudden failure to thrive when his mother began giving supplements of formula. He was diagnosed with an allergy to breastmilk, cow's milk protein, and soy, and is being fed a bovine-based elemental formula. The mother wants to resume breastfeeding. Which is the MOST LIKELY cause of the baby's sudden growth problem?

a. Alpha-lactalbumin in the mother's milk

b. Beta-lactoglobulin in cow's milk formula

c. Absence of lactose in soy formula

d. Nipple confusion from bottle supplements

7.48 Which breastfeeding behavior is MOST LIKELY practiced by women using the Lactational Amenorrhea Method (LAM) of family planning?

a. Baby sleeps 6 or more hours alone at night.

b. Mother feeds baby every 2 to 3 hours during the day.

c. Baby breastfeeds on cue 8 or more times in 24 hours.

d. Mother gives water between feeds in hot weather.

7.49 At a well-baby clinic affiliated with a Baby-Friendly Hospital, the mother of an exclusively breastfed 6-week-old baby asks whether she should introduce a pacifier to her baby. Your BEST response is:

a. Breastfeeding is well-established, so introducing a pacifier will help protect against SIDS.

b. Pacifiers will help your baby learn to self-soothe and fall asleep alone.

c. Pacifiers are never recommended for breastfed babies.

d. Pacifiers increase your baby's risk of ear infections (otitis media).

7.50 A mother has been feeding her baby on a rigid schedule for several months on the advice of friends. Her child is now underweight, appears anxious, and cries frequently. She strongly desires to continue breastfeeding. Your BEST recommendation is to

a. Increase the amount of solid food he is getting.

b. Pump your milk between feeds to keep up your supply.

c. Add artificial milk to his feeds so he can stay on this schedule.

d. Feed the baby whenever he is hungry, at least 8 or more times a day.

7.51 A mother of a 10-week-old adopted baby consults you inquiring about induced lactation. The FIRST thing you would tell her is:

a. Adoptive breastfeeding is possible.

b. The baby is the deciding factor.

c. How to provide supplementary feeds.

d. She won't have a full milk supply.

7.52 You are working with a breastfeeding mothers whose 4-week-old baby is barely above birth weight. She tells you that she can't sleep, has not showered in 3 days, and feels hopeless that breastfeeding will ever be easy for her. After observing her breastfeeding appropriately, the NEXT action you should take is to:

a. give her information about local breastfeeding support groups.

b. identify family members who can care for the baby while she sleeps and bathes.

c. explore the possibility of postpartum depression with her and her primary care provider.

d. tell her that many new mothers feel overwhelmed at 4 weeks and that her feelings will pass.

7.53 **A mother complains that her baby is not fitting the feeding schedule recommended by a book she has read. Your BEST response to her is:**
   a. It's acceptable to limit your baby's feeds to 10 minutes per side.
   b. You can give a pacifier to help your baby space out his feeds.
   c. Breastfeed "on cue," or when your baby signals hunger is always best.
   d. Giving water between feeds will get him onto a better pattern.

7.54 **A mother contracts rubella while breastfeeding her 2-month-old baby. Which of the following actions is MOST APPROPRIATE?**
   a. Mother should continue breastfeeding.
   b. Mother should immediately stop breastfeeding.
   c. Baby should be isolated from mother.
   d. Mother and baby should immediately receive rubella vaccine.

7.55 **This condition has persisted for 2½ months. What is the MOST HELPFUL action you could take for this mother?**

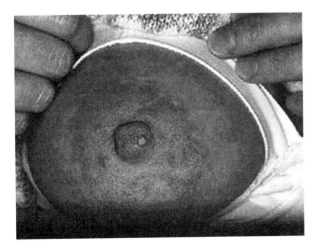

   a. Thoroughly examine the baby's nursing technique at breast.
   b. Refer her to a dermatologist for further evaluation.
   c. Provide her with moist-wound healing preparations.
   d. Recommend she pump or express and feed the baby with a device.

7.56 **This condition is MOST LIKELY associated with which of the following?**

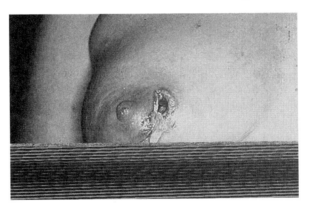

   a. Delayed or inadequate treatment of mastitis
   b. Ductal yeast infection
   c. Transmission of oral bacteria from the baby's mouth
   d. Bruising or trauma to the breast

7.57 **Which of the following findings is MOST LIKELY to be related to this mother's breastfeeding problem?**

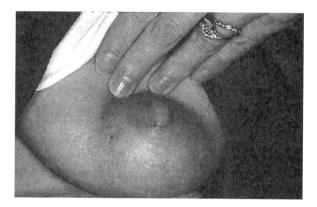

a. The mother's partner has an oral yeast infection.
b. The baby recently had strep throat.
c. Her baby is 7 months old and teething.
d. The mother has many allergies, including atopic dermatitis.

7.58 **The mother of this infant is MOST LIKELY to complain of:**

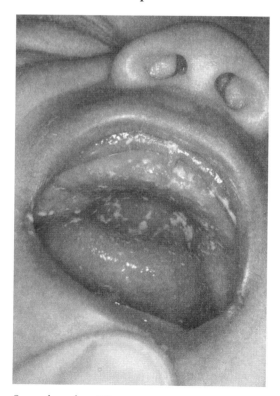

See color plate 75.

a. difficulty getting baby to latch on.
b. stinging, burning nipples.
c. vaginal discharge.
d. plugged ducts.

7.59 **In which of these sleep environments is the baby at HIGHEST risk for SIDS?**

a. Unattended, away from adult noises and contact
b. Sleeping on the same surface as an adult
c. Lying supine in a firm, flat, clean crib
d. Sleeping next to a drunk or drugged adult

7.60 **A dark-skinned 3-month-old exclusively breastfed baby lives in a location with limited sunlight many months of the year. Which recommendation to the mother is MOST APPROPRIATE?**

a. Give the child multivitamin supplements containing at least 200 IU of vitamin D daily.
b. Expose the baby's face and hands to direct sunlight at least 30 minutes per week.
c. Supplement the mother's diet with 2000 to 4000 IU of vitamin D per day.
d. Encourage the mother to feed child two servings of dark green or orange vegetables daily.

7.61 **Which is the MOST LIKELY outcome from "sleep training" regimens that allow a baby to "cry it out" to "teach them to sleep alone?**

a. Parents get a full night's uninterrupted sleep within 3 days.
b. Baby relaxes into a restful sleep when put to bed alone.
c. Baby's nighttime cortisol levels remain elevated even when the baby appears to be asleep.
d. Mother's daytime milk production adjusts to fewer nursings at night.

Answers for 1–3 Months Questions

7.1 **The answer is a.** Feeding tube devices were designed to provide food at breast for an adopted baby so that the baby's sucking will help stimulate the mother's breast to make milk. There is no research evidence that feeding tube devices accomplish any of the other outcomes. (Difficulty: 4; Discipline: Techniques; Taxonomy: Goals)

7.2 **The answer is d.** Experience and research show that 8 to 12 feeds totaling 140 to 160 minutes or more are most typical in industrialized cultures. Under 100 minutes at breast per day may indicate a problem. Many normal babies nurse for many more minutes per day. (Difficulty: 4; Discipline: Development; Taxonomy: Assessment)

7.3 **The answer is b.** Although siblings sleeping together is a practice found in many cultures, new research on sudden unexpected deaths in infancy (SUDI) suggests that infants under 6 months are at increased risk of suffocation from bed partners who are relatively unaware of the infant's presence, such as young siblings. Babies should sleep in close proximity to an attentive adult. (Difficulty: 4; Discipline: Psychology; Taxonomy: Goals)

7.4 **The answer is b.** The highest risk for SIDS is 2 to 4 months of age; the baby pictured is 3 months old. (Difficulty: 5; Discipline: Development; Taxonomy: Evaluate)

7.5 **The answer is d.** Breastfed babies initially gain more weight and by 6 months have begun to be leaner per height. By 12 months, there is a significant difference; the breastfed babies are even more lean per height than artificially fed babies. (Difficulty: 3; Discipline: Development; Taxonomy: Evaluate)

7.6 **The answer is c.** It is always appropriate to begin a counseling session with an open-ended, general, supportive question. Option b is inappropriate at 2 months, the age of the baby pictured. Choice a would be a reasonable question, especially if nipple soreness is a problem. Choice d might be asked on a routine screening form. (Difficulty: 4; Discipline: Psychology; Taxonomy: Assessment)

7.7 **The answer is d.** The crack at the base of the nipple and the shiny, reddish skin are common signs of nipple thrush (*Candida* infection). The other suggestions may provide some relief until the nipple thrush is dealt with. (Difficulty: 5; Discipline: Pathology; Taxonomy: Collaboration)

7.8 **The answer is a.** Frequency of sexual intercourse is unrelated to the LAM method (Difficulty: 2; Discipline: Physiology; Taxonomy: Goals)

7.9 **The answer is c.** This baby's tongue shape is unusual. This baby's other oral anatomic structures are normal. (Difficulty: 3; Discipline: Development; Taxonomy: Evaluate)

7.10 **The answer is b.** Taking a thorough history is always the first step in evaluating an unusual breast condition. This is Paget's disease, a form of cancer, often associated with other cancers in the breast. Choice a is inappropriate. Choice c is benign and irrelevant. Choice d may be useful. She needs to be evaluated by a physician specializing in breast conditions immediately. (Difficulty: 3; Discipline: Pathology; Taxonomy: History)

7.11 **The answer is b.** Use of progestin-containing contraceptives can diminish milk supply if given prior to 8 weeks postbirth. (Difficulty: 4; Discipline: Physiology; Taxonomy: Evaluate)

7.12 **The answer is c.** Growth occurs in spurts that may parallel changes in breastfeeding frequency, which may occur around 3 months of age. (Difficulty: 4; Discipline: Development; Taxonomy: Goals)

7.13 **The answer is b.** A 1- to 3-month-old exclusively breastfed babies may consolidate 2-hour-long sleep stretches occasionally. Longer sleep stretches are rare before at least 6 to 9 months. Babies of this age usually breastfeed at least 8 to 12 times per day in irregular patterns. The other behaviors typically occur at older ages. (Difficulty: 4; Discipline: Development; Taxonomy: History)

7.14 **The answer is a.** Forcing a baby to "cry it out" destroys the baby's growing sense of trust. Once broken, trust is difficult to repair. Babies' trust develops by consistently and promptly responding to his needs. Over time, his needs diminish and the baby can tolerate delays in mother's response. (Difficulty: 2; Discipline: Psychology; Taxonomy: Goals)

7.15 **The answer is b.** Cow's milk protein allergy is responsible for approximately 50% of reflux in otherwise healthy babies. (Difficulty: 5; Discipline: Pathology; Taxonomy: History)

7.16 **The answer is d.** The 1- to 3-month-old's feeds are usually spaced throughout the day and night. Clustering is more likely in the late afternoon or early evening. Choices b and c are unusual patterns for a thriving, exclusively breastfed 2-month-old. (Difficulty: 4; Discipline: Development; Taxonomy: Assessment)

7.17 **The answer is b.** This is a plugged nipple pore, also known as a "bleb" or "white spot." These are thought to be due to plugs of milk that solidify at the opening of a milk duct on the nipple skin. (Difficulty: 3; Discipline: Pathology; Taxonomy: Evaluate)

7.18 **The answer is b.** Taking a thorough history is top priority when solving a breastfeeding problem. The baby may be having an allergic reaction to the large amount of milk consumed by the mother. (Difficulty: 3; Discipline: Pathology; Taxonomy: Document)

7.19 **The answer is b.** Low thyroid hormone levels can cause suppressed milk synthesis, fatigue, and chilliness. The mother should have a full medical evaluation. (Difficulty: 5; Discipline: Pathology; Taxonomy: Knowledge)

7.20 **The answer is c.** Unresolved stress from the birth can trigger or exacerbate postpartum depression. She needs to see her primary care provider immediately for thorough evaluation, diagnosis, and treatment. Meanwhile, maintain contact with the mother and her primary care provider. (Difficulty: 4; Discipline: Clinical Skills; Taxonomy: Goals)

7.21 **The answer is b.** Maternal smoking during pregnancy is the highest risk factor of the factors listed. Any smoking in the household is also a high risk. Formula feeding is the second-highest of the listed risk factors for SIDS. Alcohol use during pregnancy is a less frequent risk factor for SIDS. Bedsharing is not a risk factor for SIDS but can be a risk for smothering under specific conditions, including if the bed partner is using alcohol or is on a sofa or couch. (Difficulty: 4; Discipline: Psychology; Taxonomy: Assessment)

7.22 **The answer is c.** A sober, nonsmoking breastfeeding mother on a safe surface poses no known risk to her baby of smothering. Babies alone on soft mattresses are at risk of rolling prone and smothering or becoming entrapped. Sofas are a high-risk situation for anyone sleeping with a baby, especially if the baby is on the inside (next to the back cushions). A swaddled baby alone in a crib is at increased risk of SIDS and smothering. (Difficulty: 4; Discipline: Psychology; Taxonomy: Evaluate)

7.23 **The answer is a.** The LC should collaborate with the primary care providers to assure adequate and immediate treatment of the dyad. Choices b, c, and d are appropriate after assurance of treatment has been confirmed. Mother-baby cross infection is likely when the baby has an oral infection. Assume that the mother's nipples are also infected with the same organism, as well as other infant body parts and any/all sucking objects. (Difficulty: 5; Discipline: Clinical Skills; Taxonomy: Plan)

7.24 **The answer is d.** Both children are obviously thriving in this photograph. The infant is thriving and exclusively breastfed. His sister is eating a wide variety of family foods and nurses sporadically. Tandem nursing is not a threat to either child's nutritional or emotional well-being. (Difficulty: 4; Discipline: Development; Taxonomy: Goals)

7.25 **The answer is a.** Correcting positioning is nearly always the first and most important intervention. This mother's nipple was abraded from positional soreness, which was completely relieved when her technique was corrected. (Difficulty: 4; Discipline: Techniques; Taxonomy: Plan)

7.26 **The answer is b.** Facial rashes are a common allergic reaction to cow's milk proteins. Direct exposure from artificial baby milk is the most likely trigger. (Difficulty: 4; Discipline: Pathology; Taxonomy: History)

7.27 **The answer is b.** Use of estrogen-containing contraceptives will nearly always diminish milk supply. Progestin-containing drugs may also lower milk supply in some women, especially if given prior to 8 weeks postbirth. The other methods do not use hormones and are compatible with breastfeeding. (Difficulty: 3; Discipline: Physiology; Taxonomy: History)

7.28 **The answer is a.** The first step in a consultation is always to explore the situation thoroughly. The LC is expected to communicate relevant information to the primary care provider(s). Referring her to another physician as the first strategy in helping her is inappropriate, although if she asks for the names of other providers, the LC should follow appropriate referral guidelines and provide these names. (Difficulty: 4; Discipline: Clinical Skills; Taxonomy: Assessment)

7.29 **The answer is c.** Breastfeeding dyads who safely bedshare have been shown to breastfeed longer and more exclusively. There is no research evidence of increased risk to the baby sleeping with a sober, nonsmoking breastfeeding mother on a safe surface. Choices a and d are also likely. (Difficulty: 4; Discipline: Psychology; Taxonomy: Goals)

7.30 **The answer is d.** Side-sleeping is a higher risk than supine sleeping for most babies, especially if the baby is sleeping alone. This firm, flat mattress on the floor is not a risk, nor is the proximity of the unused fireplace. The child is sleeping in proximity to her mother, who is out of the picture shown working in the same room. Pacifier use to "prevent SIDS" is not fully supported by research, and often interferes with breastfeeding. (Difficulty: 4; Discipline: Psychology; Taxonomy: Knowledge)

7.31 **The answer is c.** She is pumping her milk in anticipation of returning to paid employment soon, and lives in a country with limited maternity protection laws. The baby is about 6 weeks old and is thriving with exclusive breastfeeding. There is no indication that the baby is premature, has a week suck, or her milk production is low. Nothing about this photograph is relevant to the father's role or desires. (Difficulty: 4; Discipline: Clinical Skills; Taxonomy: Goals)

7.32 **The answer is a.** This is the biological norm and most common nighttime arrangement worldwide. Separate sleeping is associated with higher risk of SIDS. Self-comforting is distressful for many babies. Pacifiers can compromise breastfeeding. (Difficulty: 3; Discipline: Psychology; Taxonomy: Knowledge)

7.33 **The answer is d.** Active listening is the first action because the mother is obviously emotionally upset. Understanding, addressing, and exploring feelings are key to counseling the breastfeeding mother. (Difficulty: 4; Discipline: Psychology; Taxonomy: Goals)

7.34 **The answer is b.** Expressing milk every few hours will reduce the risk of milk stasis, and milk components will assist in wound healing. Choice a is rarely appropriate. Choices c and d are appropriate. (Difficulty: 4; Discipline: Clinical Skills; Taxonomy: Plan)

7.35 **The answer is b.** This baby's tongue is an unusual shape and could not maintain a seal around the breast. Her labial (upper) frenulum is normal. The tight oral muscles may or may not be related to the clicking and smacking. The buccal pads are exceptionally prominent and were unrelated to the noisy feeding behavior. (Difficulty: 5; Discipline: Pathology; Taxonomy: Assessment)

7.36 **The answer is b.** Prefeed and postfeed weight checks on a sensitive scale is the most accurate and least disruptive of the options listed. Expressing is disruptive. Weighing the mother and counting swallows are less accurate. (Difficulty: 4; Discipline: Techniques; Taxonomy: Goals)

7.37 **The answer is b.** The baby pictured is being treated for bilateral hip dysplasia with a harness that maintains the hip-leg position. The baby cannot tolerate pressure on either hip. The mother is holding her baby across her chest while lying flat, which is comfortable and effective for feeding. There is no indication of overactive milk ejection or production, and the baby is 2 months old. (Difficulty: 3; Discipline: Clinical Skills; Taxonomy: Goals)

7.38 **The answer is c.** The lesion is an unhealed wound caused by the baby's poor suck due to a short frenulum that was uncorrected for 2½ months. A plugged pore is likely to have resolved more quickly. Thrush usually causes the skin to be inflamed. Paget's disease is a type of nipple cancer and the least likely cause of the small wound shown. (Difficulty: 5; Discipline: Pathology; Taxonomy: Evaluate)

7.39 **The answer is c.** Expressing or pumping milk may be helpful if a breast abscess is so close to the nipple that the baby cannot effectively feed. The other conditions are compatible with continued breastfeeding. (Difficulty: 3; Discipline: Techniques; Taxonomy: Plan)

7.40 **The answer is b.** Continuous/frequent carrying with unrestricted breastfeeding fosters all aspects of infant mental and physical development. (Difficulty: 4; Discipline: Development; Taxonomy: History)

7.41 **The answer is b.** This surgery (incision and drainage) was performed to treat a breast abscess. The location of the incision may have long-term consequences to lactation in this breast. (Difficulty: 3; Discipline: Pathology; Taxonomy: History)

7.42 **The answer is a.** The whey-casein ratio changes from 90:10 in the newborn period to closer to 60:40 around 6 months. (Difficulty: 3; Discipline: Development; Taxonomy: Knowledge)

7.43 **The answer is b.** Supine sleeping is strongly associated with lower risk of SIDS. This position also makes breastfeeding at night easier. (Difficulty: 3; Discipline: Pathology; Taxonomy: Knowledge)

7.44 **The answer is d.** Libido varies widely among breastfeeding women. Men/fathers should be helped to find new ways to please the mother that are compatible with the biology and psychology of the breastfeeding period. (Difficulty: 3; Discipline: Clinical Skills; Taxonomy: Goals)

7.45 **The answer is a.** Assuming the baby is truly allergic, eliminating cow's milk protein and soy from the mother's diet is the most important strategy. Cow's milk protein takes more than 1 week to be eliminated. LCs do not provide dietary supplements as part of their role. Although directly disputing a medical diagnosis is unethical, providing accurate information on allergen transfer into mother's milk to the mother and her providers is appropriate. (Difficulty: 4; Discipline: Pathology; Taxonomy: Goals)

7.46 **The answer is a.** Safe bedsharing support exclusive breastfeeding, according to several studies. Nursing mothers who bedshare get more sleep. There is no documented risk to the infant unless the mother and environment has certain risk factors. Nearly all new mothers have fragmented sleep. Exclusive breastfeeding does help delay the return of fertility. (Difficulty: 5; Discipline: Psychology; Taxonomy: Goals)

7.47 **The answer is b.** Beta-lactoglobulin in cow's milk protein is a common allergen, and most likely to have caused this child's allergic reaction and failure to thrive. Soy is the second most common allergen. Babies are never allergic to mother's own milk or any of its natural components but may react to foreign proteins that pass into milk. Nipple confusion is unlikely to begin at 3 months. (Difficulty: 2; Discipline: Pathology; Taxonomy: Evaluate)

7.48 **The answer is c.** Women who choose LAM practice closer to optimal breastfeeding behaviors. Feeding on cue day and night is the most optimal of the above behaviors. Sleeping alone and giving water are likely to weaken the effect of LAM on fertility. Feeding on a schedule (every 2 to 3 hours) is less appropriate and suboptimal. (Difficulty: 3; Discipline: Physiology; Taxonomy: Knowledge)

7.49 **The answer is d.** Pacifier use increases the risk of otitis media, especially for babies who are in day care settings. A is questionable, because pacifiers fall out of babies' mouths very soon after they fall asleep, and the explanation for any statistically protective factor for SIDS is unknown. Choice b is inappropriate because babies learn to soothe by being soothed by nursing. There are some valid therapeutic uses for pacifiers in some breastfed babies. (Difficulty: 5; Discipline: Clinical Skills; Taxonomy: Goals)

7.50 **The answer is d.** Scheduled feeds are inappropriate and can result in underfeeding and failure to thrive. Feeding on cue is appropriate regardless of the baby's age. (Difficulty: 3; Discipline: Psychology; Taxonomy: Goals)

7.51 **The answer is a.** The first statement to the mother should be a positive statement. Afterward, a fuller explanation of induced lactation should take place, which might include any or all of the other choices. (Difficulty: 2; Discipline: Psychology; Taxonomy: Goals)

7.52 **The answer is c.** This mother is showing clear, common signs of postpartum depression, and you should ensure that she is properly evaluated for depression. Many medications for depression are compatible with breastfeeding. Untreated depression can be devastating to the mother and her baby. The other suggestions are appropriate after she has been assessed and, if necessary, treated for depression. (Difficulty: 5; Discipline: Pathology; Taxonomy: Collaboration)

7.53 **The answer is c.** Babies feed for varying lengths and at varying intervals according to their hunger, emotional needs, growth and developmental stages, and other physiological factors. Placing restrictions on length or frequency, or offering substitutes disrupts the breastfeeding relationship and interferes with fulfillment of infant needs. (Difficulty: 2; Discipline: Development; Taxonomy: Goals)

7.54 **The answer is a.** The mother's milk contains rubella-specific antibodies very quickly after maternal exposure. The baby has already been exposed; therefore, continued breastfeeding helps protect the baby. Maternal rubella infection is not a contraindication for breastfeeding. (Difficulty: 3; Discipline: Pathology; Taxonomy: Plan)

7.55 **The answer is a.** Always evaluate the baby's breastfeeding technique first. This mother's baby was tongue-tied, and friction from his tongue was causing the persistent nipple wound. (Difficulty: 4; Discipline: Techniques; Taxonomy: Evaluate)

7.56 **The answer is a.** A breast abscess is usually the result of delayed or inadequate treatment for mastitis. Rarely, physical trauma may precipitate abscess formation. The baby's oral bacteria are not implicated in abscess formation in the lactating breast.

(Difficulty: 4; Discipline: Pathology; Taxonomy: Knowledge)

7.57 **The answer is b.** The crack at the base of the nipple was caused by a bacterial infection of her nipple and occurred at the same time that her baby was diagnosed with a streptococcal infection of the throat. (Difficulty: 5; Discipline: Pathology; Taxonomy: History)

7.58 **The answer is b.** This baby has oral thrush (*Candida*), which easily transfers to mother's nipples. Although a mother may have a vaginal candidal infection, it is most likely that she will have symptoms of thrush on her nipples when the baby has this fungal infection. (Difficulty: 3; Discipline: Pathology; Taxonomy: Evaluate)

7.59 **The answer is a.** Babies who sleep unattended—in a separate room, away from adult noises and activities—are at high risk of SIDS. Choice b carries no independent risk. Supine sleeping appears to be a low-risk situation related to SIDS, if the baby is in proximity to responsible adults. Sleeping next to an impaired adult puts babies at risk of smothering, not SIDS. Exclusively breastfed babies have the lowest rates of SIDS and all-cause infant mortality. (Difficulty: 4; Discipline: Psychology; Taxonomy: Goals)

7.60 **The answer is c.** If the mother's skin pigment and limited sun exposure cause a deficiency in her own vitamin D levels, then her milk will have low levels. Supplementing the mother with 2000 or more IU of vitamin D protects her own health and increases levels of D in her milk, thus protecting her and her baby. Exposing the baby and mother will help a little. The other two choices undermine the benefit of exclusive breastfeeding. (Difficulty: 5; Discipline: Pathology; Taxonomy: Plan)

7.61 **The answer is c.** Sleep training schemes create sustained, elevated cortisol levels in infants and young children. Elevated cortisol levels are known to have long-term negative consequences because babies are more sensitive to stress in the early years. Parents might or might not sleep better. Babies physiologically cannot "put themselves to sleep" in the early weeks and months. Mother's milk production hinges on frequent removal of milk including during the night; long stretches of milk stasis suppress production. (Difficulty: 5; Discipline: Development; Taxonomy: Evaluate)

CHAPTER 8

4–6 Months Questions

8.1 A mother of a 4-month-old is worried that her baby is constipated. Earlier, he stooled several times a day. Starting a few days ago, he stools 2 to 3 times in the morning only, but passes some gas during the day. What is the MOST LIKELY cause of the baby's stool pattern?

a. The mother's high-carbohydrate diet is constipating.

b. Her milk has a higher casein-whey ratio than earlier in lactation.

c. The baby absorbs over 90% of the milk components, leaving little residue to be eliminated as stool.

d. Breastfed babies of this age often pass stool less often, but the consistency remains normal.

8.2 An exclusively breastfed baby's risk of food allergies is:

a. decreased, because few food allergens pass through mother's milk.

b. decreased, because mother's milk makes passage of allergenic proteins through baby's gut less likely.

c. increased, because allergens pass readily through mother's milk.

d. increased, because mother's milk increases the permeability of the baby's gut.

8.3 The mother of a 5-month-old breastfeeding baby is MOST LIKELY to observe that the baby:

a. plays with her mother's other nipple while breastfeeding.

b. closes her eyes during breastfeeding.

c. is easily distracted while nursing.

d. does not awaken to breastfeed at night.

8.4 A mother exclusively breastfeeding her 5-month-old baby comes down with chickenpox. The BEST way she can reduce the likelihood of her child getting this disease is to:

a. wear a long-sleeved shirt to cover the lesions on her arms.

b. ask her sister to care for the baby between breastfeeds.

c. pump her milk and feed it to the baby by cup while she is sick.

d. continue breastfeeding because the baby has already been exposed.

8.5 What is the MOST LIKELY situation leading to this breast condition?

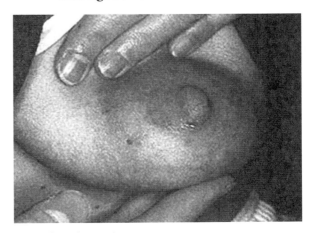

See color plate 76.

a. The child is over a year and using the mother's breast as a pacifier.

b. The mother did not wash her breasts after each nursing.

c. The child is biting during breastfeeding.

d. The child has an oral infection that was transmitted to the nipple skin.

8.6 **At what developmental age is self-feeding MOST LIKELY to begin?**

a. 3 to 4 months

b. 6 to 7 months

c. 9 to 10 months

d. 12 months and older

8.7 **The nursing baby in this picture has not yet shown any interest in eating any family foods. Your MOST APPROPRIATE response is:**

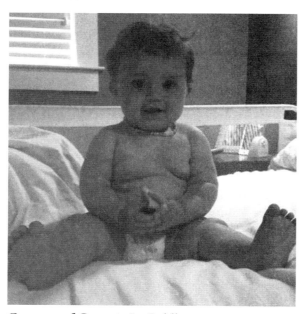

Courtesy of Cammie Jo Goldhammer.

a. He is obviously thriving. He'll soon start being interested in what your family is eating.

b. Exclusive breastfeeding for longer than 6 months is a normal and desirable behavior.

c. With your family history of allergies, it's not surprising that he's avoiding other foods.

d. Your other child is probably distracting him at mealtimes.

8.8 **A mother is planning for surgery to repair her 5-month-old child's cleft palate. What would be your FIRST suggestion to support breastfeeding?**

a. Wean your baby at least a week before the surgery.

b. Prepare to stay with your baby around the clock.

c. Practice expressing milk in case the baby cannot nurse directly.

d. Expect your baby to nurse very frequently afterward for awhile.

8.9 **This exclusively breastfed baby's mother became ill with a seasonal influenza, and her doctor suggested she stop breastfeeding. She asks you to discuss the situation with her physician. Your BEST response to the physician is:**

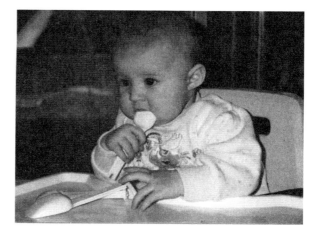

a. The baby will likely get the disease, because the virus is transmitted in breastmilk.

b. The baby is likely to get a mild case or no infection at all because of disease-specific antibodies being released into her mother's milk.

c. The mother should wean immediately to prevent the baby from becoming infected through skin-to-skin contact.

d. The medications used to treat influenza are compatible with breastfeeding.

8.10 A mother calls about her 5-month-old infant, worried that she is losing her milk because her breasts are soft and her infant no longer seems content for 2 hours after feedings. He cries frequently and puts his fists to his mouth 45 minutes after feeding. The MOST LIKELY cause for the situation she describes is:

 a. her infant is experiencing a normal growth and behavior pattern.

 b. offering bottles is interfering with breastmilk production.

 c. the development of colic in her infant.

 d. her body is adapting well to her baby's demand for milk.

8.11 A 6-month-old baby is starting to grab food off her mother's plate during meals. What would you suggest to the mother of this child?

 a. Keep your adult food out of reach because your baby will grab the wrong foods.

 b. Put some protein-rich strips of foods where she can read them easily.

 c. Start spoon-feeding her mashed vegetables and fruits.

 d. Give her a spoon or a toy to hold during your mealtimes.

8.12 Which of the following statements BEST describes the exclusively breastfed baby of this age?

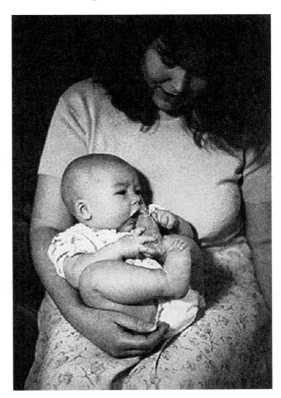

 a. Baby will need complementary (solid) food soon.

 b. Baby consumes about two-thirds of available milk over the course of a day.

 c. Baby needs vitamin D supplements.

 d. Baby is at highest risk of stunting

158 • Chapter 8: 4–6 Months Questions

8.13 This breastfed baby's mother comments that he should learn how to sleep for at least 8 straight hours at night. Your BEST response to her is:

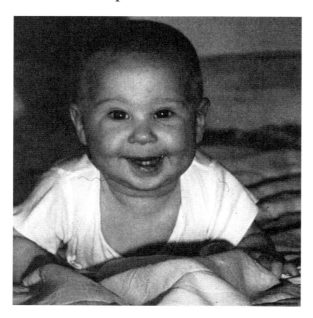

a. Most babies of this age still need to breastfeed at least once at night.
b. He is too young now, but he should be sleeping through the night soon.
c. If you don't go to him for a few nights, he will learn to sleep longer.
d. He does not need to breastfeed at night if he weighs at least 12 pounds (5.4 kg).

8.14 A mother who is becoming ill with influenza asks if she should continue breastfeeding her 5-month-old exclusively breastfed child. What is your BEST response?

a. Your milk has specific antibodies to reduce the risk that your child will get this infection.
b. Your milk is easier to digest if your baby does get sick from this infection.
c. Lactation speeds up your own production of antibodies so your illness will be less severe.
d. You will recover quicker without the additional burden of preparing artificial feeds.

8.15 This mother complains of sudden-onset sore nipples. The FIRST action you would take is to:

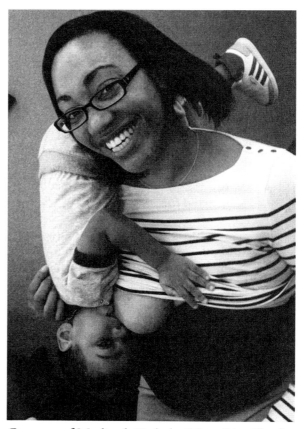

Courtesy of Mudiwah Kadeshe/Mona Lisa Hamlin.

a. ask whether her baby has teeth.
b. advise the mother to roll baby inward toward you, so her entire front side is facing yours.
c. advise the mother to pull baby's legs in closer to you.
d. ask whether she has taken an antibiotic recently.

8.16 **A 4-month-old exclusively breastfed baby feeds about 8 to 10 times per day with one or two feeds at night. His mother is concerned that she cannot make enough milk because her neighbor had to increase the amount of formula for her baby at 4 months. Your BEST response to her is:**

a. Your baby's feeding pattern indicates that he is ready for solids.

b. Your baby's milk needs are stable for at least another 2 months.

c. Your baby is clustering much of his milk intake at night, which is normal.

d. Your baby will take more milk from your breasts if he needs more.

8.17 **To relieve the condition pictured, your BEST recommendation is:**

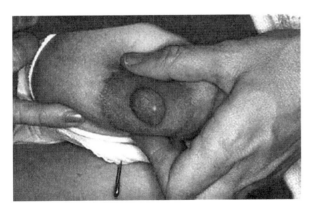

See color plate 77.

a. Hand-express for a few minutes before each feed.

b. Soak your nipples in warm water then gently massage the tip.

c. Wear breast shells between feeds.

d. Apply an antifungal preparation after each feed.

8.18 **To reduce risk of rickets in this breast-feeding child, which of the following would you recommend to the mother?**

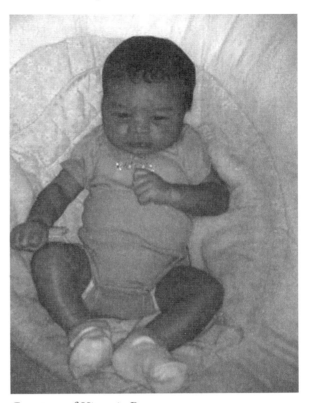

Courtesy of Kimarie Bugg.

a. Expose the child's face to sunlight for 20 minutes every day.

b. Mother should be assessed for vitamin D levels in her milk.

c. Mother should expose her face and head to sunlight for 2 hours a week.

d. Give the child a vitamin D supplement regardless of symptoms.

8.19 **This baby's mother complains that her baby keeps pulling off and looking around the room during feeds. Your BEST response to her is:**

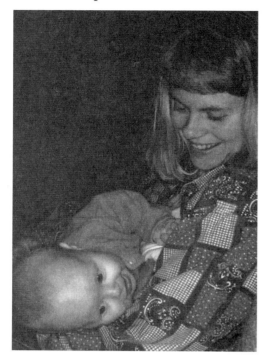

a. This is normal behavior at this age.

b. Try going to a quieter, darker place.

c. You can try feeding more family foods during the day.

d. You're creating overdependence in your baby.

8.20 **This mother's baby is teething, has recently started spending several days a week in day care, and is taking an antibiotic for strep throat. The MOST LIKELY cause of this condition is:**

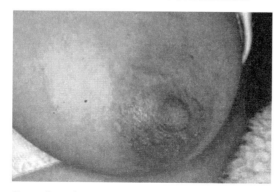

See color plate 78.

a. infection picked up from other children at the day care center.

b. allergic reaction to the medication being taken by her infant.

c. psoriasis exacerbated by the infant's saliva.

d. bacterial infection of the nipple skin.

8.21 **The child pictured has recently begun solid (complementary) foods. Which of the following foods is MOST LIKELY implicated in this condition?**

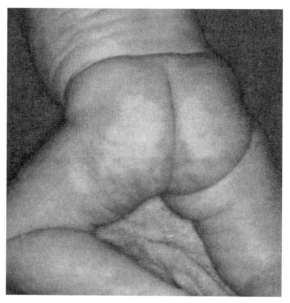

See color plate 79.

a. Carrots

b. Cantaloupe

c. Cheese

d. Chicken

8.22 **A 5-month-old breastfed baby's mother feels that she should learn how to sleep for at least 8 straight hours at night. Your BEST response to her is:**

a. She continues to need frequent contact for reassurance and comfort.

b. She is old enough to self-soothe now.

c. She has already learned how to manipulate you; you had better train her to sleep.

d. Now that she is not a newborn, you do not need to respond quickly when she cries.

8.23 This exclusively breastfed baby's physician is concerned about growth faltering based on obsolete growth standards. Which statement MOST LIKELY accurately evaluates this situation?

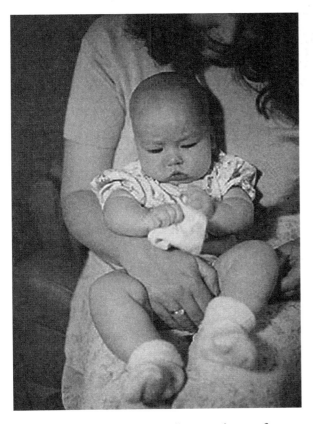

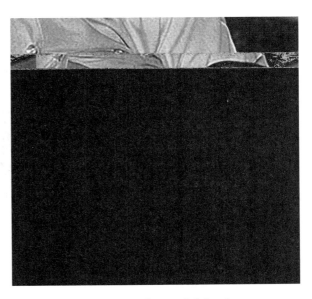

a. The mother's milk is too low in fat.
b. The baby is physiologically ready for solid foods.
c. Breastfeeding requires extra energy intake at this age.
d. Breastfed babies tend to be leaner than artificially fed babies at this age.

8.24 A relative is worried that this exclusively breastfed child is not growing appropriately. Your first action would be to recommend:

a. start giving him solid food.
b. supplement with infant formula.
c. pump your breasts after feeds to increase milk supply.
d. continue exclusive breastfeeding at least 2 more months.

8.25 You are helping a mother re-lactate after her baby became quite ill when she weaned the baby to formula at 6 months. Which of the following is the MOST LIKELY reason her baby suddenly had more illness?

a. She prepared the formula with contaminated water from her backyard well.
b. Withdrawal of the immune components in human milk left the baby with little defense against pathogens.
c. The baby was exposed to more environmental pathogens as he became more mobile.
d. The chemicals in the bottle and teat reacted with the formula to produce illness.

8.26   **A woman with a 5-month-old exclusively breastfed baby is prescribed amoxicillin for her breast infection. The MOST LIKELY possible consequence for the infant is:**

   a.   interference with bilirubin binding.

   b.   vomiting and dehydration.

   c.   none.

   d.   diarrhea or loose stools.

8.27   **A mother is exclusively breastfeeding her 5-month-old, and her menses have not yet returned. Assuming she is sexually active with a fertile male, what is her chance of conceiving another child?**

   a.   7% to 8%

   b.   5% to 6%

   c.   3% to 4%

   d.   1% to 2%

8.28   **This child's mother wonders why her child recently became ill with a respiratory illness. Your BEST response is:**

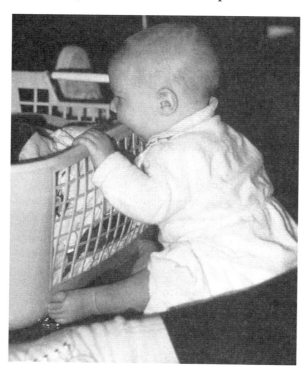

   a.   The immune factors in human milk decrease after 6 months.

   b.   As his mobility increases, he is exposed to more pathogens.

   c.   Teething lowers his resistance to infection.

   d.   Placentally acquired immunity is wearing off.

8.29   **This mother brings her baby to a well-child clinic for a routine visit and nurses in the position shown. Your FIRST response should be:**

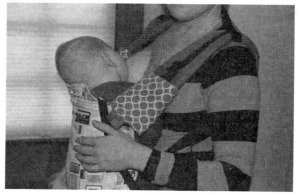

Courtesy of Ashley Franz.

   a.   How is breastfeeding going for you both?

   b.   Turn your baby's body to face your body.

   c.   Has your baby shown any interest in family foods?

   d.   What family planning method are you using or planning to use?

8.30 **This mother's baby is 4 months old. The MOST APPROPRIATE suggestion you would offer this mother is:**

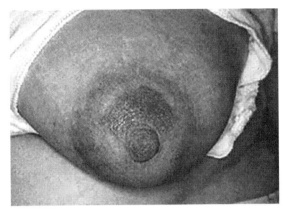

See color plate 80.

    a. Contact your doctor and the baby's doctors to rule out infections.

    b. Use an over-the-counter nipple cream 3 times a day.

    c. Keep a diary of all the foods you and your baby are eating.

    d. Start using a breast pump and feed the collected milk to the baby by another means.

8.31 **A mother complains of a sudden-onset raw sensation on this nipple. Her infant is teething, has recently started solid foods, and is taking an antibiotic for strep throat. The MOST LIKELY cause of this sensation is:**

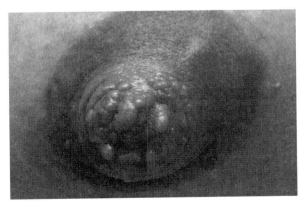

See color plate 81.

Courtesy of Carole Dobrich.

    a. an allergic reaction to a food the baby consumed.

    b. an allergic reaction to the medication being given to her infant.

    c. psoriasis that was exacerbated by the infant's saliva.

    d. a bacterial infection in the crevices of the nipple tip.

8.32 **A mother asks when she can start giving her baby bovine-based formula so she can go out to a movie. Based on your knowledge of gut closure, your BEST answer is:**

    a. After the baby is 6 months old

    b. After she breastfeeds the baby

    c. Any time, as long as a bottle is not used as the device

    d. After 1 year of age

8.33 **This baby has been spitting up after nursing a few times every day. The MOST LIKELY reason for this behavior is that the baby:**

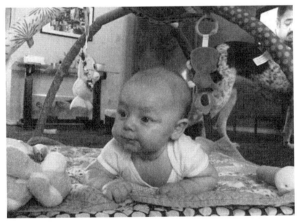

Courtesy of © Barbara Wilson-Clay.

    a. dislikes the taste of mom's milk.

    b. is feeding too frequently.

    c. has an allergy to something in mom's milk.

    d. has gastroenteritis.

8.34   The mother shown in this photograph says she sleeps with her baby like this every night and during naps as well. What is the MOST LIKELY outcome of this practice?

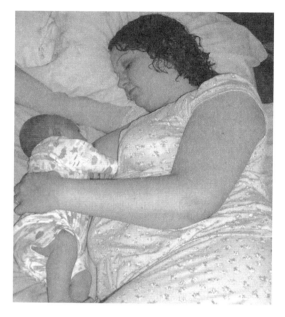

a.   Exclusive breastfeeding for at least 6 months
b.   Baby will not learn to fall asleep on her own
c.   Baby is at risk of suffocation if mother rolls forward
d.   Baby is at risk of tooth decay (dental caries)

8.35   Which statement BEST describes the reason this baby would begin reaching for table (family) food?

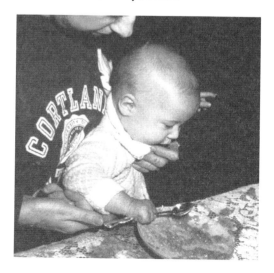

a.   The baby is developmentally ready for solid (family) food.
b.   The mother's milk supply is no longer adequate.
c.   The baby is just imitating and will not be ready for family foods for some time.
d.   The baby is jealous because everyone else is eating "real food."

8.36   Why would this baby be leaning away from his mother in the middle of a breastfeeding session?

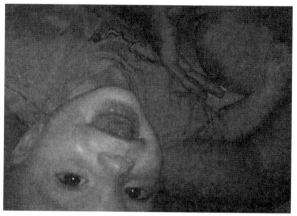

Courtesy of Erika Nehlsen.

a.   Baby is refusing because mom is forcing him to nurse.
b.   Baby is ready for solid (complementary food).
c.   Her milk is flowing too fast.
d.   This is normal behavior at this stage.

8.37   What is the MOST IMPORTANT reason that a mother with influenza should continue breastfeeding her child?

a.   Antibodies to the specific illness will appear in milk within hours.
b.   The milk is easier to digest if her baby gets sick.
c.   She will recover more quickly from the illness.
d.   It would be too tiring for her to change to artificial feeds now.

8.38 **Which of the following complementary family planning methods is MOST EFFECTIVE and compatible with breastfeeding?**
  a. Condoms
  b. Implanted progestin
  c. Combined oral contraceptives
  d. Lactational amenorrhea method (LAM)

8.39 **The condition shown in the photograph appeared when the child started taking solid foods. What would be your FIRST management strategy?**

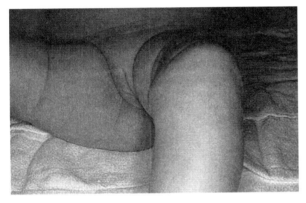

See color plate 82.

  a. Discontinue all solid food until the rash clears up.
  b. Mother should stop consuming dairy products.
  c. Take a thorough history of the mother's and baby's food intakes.
  d. Refer the dyad to a dermatologist.

8.40 **The mother of this child has been told that her baby should no longer feed at night. Your BEST response to her is:**

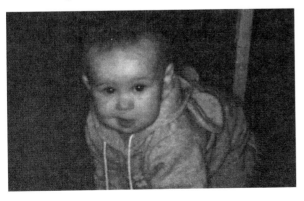

  a. It's time to begin solid foods.
  b. Try and get him to nurse more in the daytime.
  c. Use a pacifier during the night.
  d. Feeding at night is normal behavior.

8.41 **A 6-month-old baby, sitting at the family dinner table, begins reaching for food. Which statement BEST describes the reason for this behavior?**
  a. The baby is developmentally ready for solid (family) foods.
  b. The mother's milk supply is no longer adequate.
  c. The baby is imitating and will not be ready for family foods for some time.
  d. The baby is jealous because everyone else is eating "real" food.

8.42 **What is the recommended duration of exclusive breastfeeding described in the WHO / UNICEF *Global Strategy for Infant and Young Child Feeding*?**
  a. 4 months
  b. 6 months
  c. 12 months
  d. Infant self-weaning

8.43 **Giving iron-rich foods to the infant under 6 months may increase infection because:**
  a. lactoferrin is bound in solution by added foods.
  b. the foods may be contaminated with pathogens.
  c. the iron-binding function of lactoferrin is overwhelmed.
  d. iron makes the infant gut more permeable to pathogens.

8.44 **This baby's mother calls you, worried because for the past 2 days her baby has been nursing much more frequently than previously. The MOST LIKELY reason for the change in nursing pattern is:**

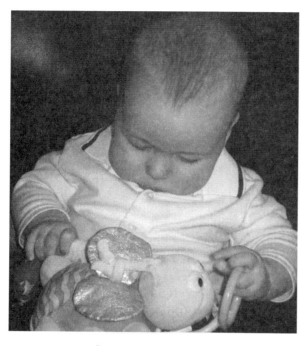

a. teething.

b. illness.

c. growth spurt.

d. need for supplemental foods.

8.45 **This child gained weight very rapidly in the first 3 months and now is lean for his length. All of his development milestones are normal. Your BEST recommendation to his mother is:**

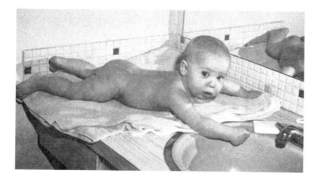

a. Continue what you are doing. His growth pattern is normal for breastfed babies.

b. Begin feeding him more solid foods to increase his weight.

c. Take away his chewing toys and pacifiers, as they are distracting him from eating.

d. Supplement with a cow's milk–based infant formula because he needs more calcium for growth.

8.46 **A mother living in a far northern latitude with limited sunlight several months a year asks about vitamin D supplements for her 5-month-old exclusively breastfed baby. Your BEST suggestion is:**

a. Mix some cod liver oil into pumped breastmilk and give it to your baby.

b. Set up several sun lamps inside your home in the darkest months.

c. Consider taking a supplement of at least 400 IU daily yourself

d. Supplement your baby with 4 oz of vitamin D–fortified formula daily.

8.47 **The mother of a 4-month-old exclusively breastfed baby wonders when her baby will sleep through the night without waking to feed. Your BEST response is:**

a. By the time he is 6 months old

b. When he has doubled his birth weight

c. When you stop nursing him as soon as he cries

d. When he is physiologically ready

8.48 **This baby breastfeeds at least 10 times a day, including 2 or 3 feeds at night. Her grandmother has advised her mother that she should be feeding her rice cereal and strained fruits. Your BEST response to her is:**

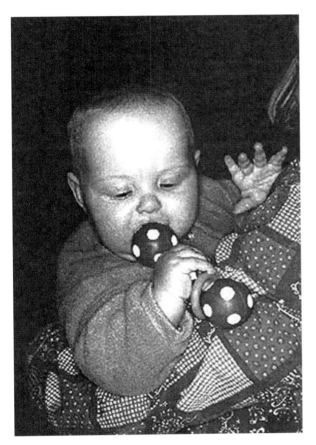

a. This pattern of breastfeeding is normal for a baby of this age.
b. If she has been nursing this frequently for several days, then you apparently cannot make enough milk for her.
c. She does not need solids, but she should be sleeping through the night.
d. If she is 4 months old, it is good to start her on supplemental foods.

8.49 **This mother tells you that her child loves the device pictured, and sleeps best this way. The MOST LIKELY reason for this is:**

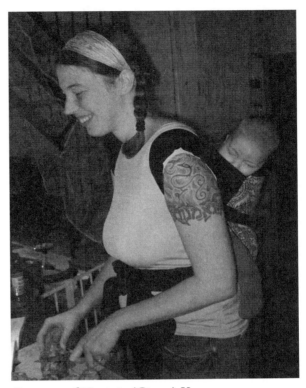

Courtesy of Virginia (Ginny) Kooyman.

a. The child has become too dependent because of prolonged breastfeeding.
b. Overuse of the baby carrier has delayed the child's ability to sleep alone.
c. The mother is using her child to meet her own needs for companionship.
d. This is normal behavior for this age child.

8.50 **What is the MOST LIKELY age of this baby?**

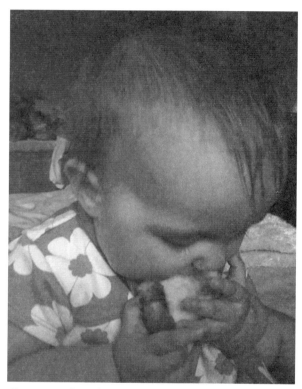

Courtesy of Cathy Norris.

    a. 4 months
    b. 6 months
    c. 8 months
    d. 10 months

8.51 **A 5-month-old exclusively breastfed baby is recovering from hernia surgery. Which is the MOST LIKELY breastfeeding pattern for this child?**
    a. The same as before the hospitalization
    b. More frequent nursing sessions to quench thirst
    c. Longer nursing sessions for the comforting of slow milk flow
    d. Less frequent sessions because milk supply has decreased

8.52 **A mother reports that her 4-month-old baby did not gain enough weight this past month. Your FIRST action should be to:**
    a. suggest she nurse her baby more frequently and weigh the baby again in a week.
    b. offer information about various galactogogues.
    c. tell her to supplement with formula until the baby's weight is appropriate for his age.
    d. take a complete history of mother's breastfeeding experience.

Answers for 4–6 Months Questions

8.1 **The answer is b.** Whey-casein ratio is high in early lactation and affects stool composition and frequency of infant elimination. The mother's short-term restricted diet has little or no bearing on milk composition or milk volume. Choices c and d are accurate but less relevant to longitudinal changes. (Difficulty: 4; Discipline: Development; Taxonomy: History)

8.2 **The answer is b.** Breastmilk optimizes the environment in the baby's gut. Allergens may be present in breastmilk and may create problems for a sensitive baby, but the risk of allergies is significantly reduced through breastfeeding. (Difficulty: 4; Discipline: Pathology; Taxonomy: Knowledge)

8.3 **The answer is c.** Distractibility is a common behavioral characteristic in the 4- to 6-month age. (Difficulty: 3; Discipline: Development; Taxonomy: Knowledge)

8.4 **The answer is d.** When a breastfeeding mother becomes ill, her body quickly begins making targeted antibodies that appear in her quickly and that protect her baby from that specific illness. None of the other suggestions are necessary. (Difficulty: 3; Discipline: Pathology; Taxonomy: Plan)

8.5 **The answer is d.** The child was diagnosed with strep throat, which caused a strep infection of the nipple and the damage shown in this picture. Ordinary breastfeeding does not cause nipple damage. Washing the breasts after every feed is impractical and unnecessary. Biting rarely causes a lesion on the areola and crack at the nipple base. (Difficulty: 4; Discipline: Pathology; Taxonomy: History)

8.6 **The answer is b.** Babies start being able to self-feed around 6 months. Offering a variety of family foods that the child can pick up and explore is appropriate. (Difficulty: 4; Discipline: Development; Taxonomy: Knowledge)

8.7 **The answer is a.** This child is clearly thriving, and his growth is not faltering. Noncoerced (baby-led) avoidance of offered family foods in the second 6 months is thought to be a possible indication of food sensitivities. (Difficulty: 4; Discipline: Development; Taxonomy: Goals)

8.8 **The answer is d.** Hospitalization is usually a traumatic experience for the child, and the emotional comfort from breastfeeding is especially important at that time. (Difficulty: 4; Discipline: Clinical Skills; Taxonomy: Goals)

8.9 **The answer is b.** The mother's body produces disease-specific antibodies that appear in milk shortly after exposure. These protect the child from the disease, either entirely or partially. There is no evidence that this viral infection is transmitted through mother's own milk, and the mother will be holding the baby skin-to-skin regardless of feeding method. The doctor did not ask you about medications, so choice d is an inappropriate response. (Difficulty: 2; Discipline: Pathology; Taxonomy: Collaboration)

8.10 **The answer is a.** Her infant is experiencing a normal growth and behavior pattern, possibly a sudden increase in appetite. Initial breast edema is resolved, and the breasts are becoming "calibrated" to produce enough milk for her baby without feeling overfull. The behavior she describes is a normal pattern for breastfed babies. (Difficulty: 4; Discipline: Development; Taxonomy: Evaluate)

8.11 **The answer is b.** Babies are developmentally ready to begin self-feeding of complementary foods around 6 months. Self-feeding allows the baby to control the type and amount of foods consumed, assuming the adult provides nutritious foods in manageable shapes. Spoon-feeding suppresses the baby's natural instincts and can result in negative attitudes toward complementary foods. Choices a and d are not appropriate or necessary. (Difficulty: 3; Discipline: Physiology; Taxonomy: Goals)

8.12 **The answer is b.** Normal 4-month-old babies take an average of two-thirds of the available milk over the course of the day. Adding complementary foods before 6 months of age is no longer recommended; neither are routine vitamin D supplements. The highest risk of stunting is between 6 and 24 months. (Difficulty: 5; Discipline: Development; Taxonomy: Knowledge)

8.13 **The answer is a.** Most babies continue waking at night for feeding throughout the first year of life and may consume up to one-third of their calories at night. (Difficulty: 4; Discipline: Psychology; Taxonomy: Goals)

8.14 **The answer is a.** The mother's milk has many disease-specific components that protect her baby from her current infection. Choice b is correct but less important. Choice c is incorrect. Choice d is correct but of minor importance. (Difficulty: 4; Discipline: Development; Taxonomy: Goals)

8.15 **The answer is b.** The most likely explanation for sudden-onset soreness is poor positioning, causing pulling or tugging on the nipple skin. The first intervention would be correcting positioning and latch. The other choices are possibilities after poor positioning has been ruled out. (Difficulty: 5; Discipline: Techniques; Taxonomy: Plan)

8.16 **The answer is d.** Babies consume about two-thirds of the available milk volume at a given feed. Milk volumes consumed are relatively stable from the first week or so until at least 6 months. The normal range varies widely. Artificially fed babies may need more milk as they get older because the nutrients are less available for growth. (Difficulty: 4; Discipline: Development; Taxonomy: Goals)

8.17 **The answer is b.** The most effective treatment for a plugged nipple pore, also known as a "bleb" or "white spot," is softening the plugged area in warm water, then massaging or expressing the duct opening. Hand-expressing before feeds is a technique for softening the entire breast; wearing shells does not treat a plugged pore, and there is no other indication of nipple thrush in this mother's situation. (Difficulty: 4; Discipline: Techniques; Taxonomy: Plan)

8.18 **The answer is b.** Maternal vitamin D levels are reflected in milk levels, so the mother should always be tested before supplementing the baby. If mother's levels are low, supplementing the mother will provide benefit to the mother and baby. Routine supplementation of all breastfed babies is not justified by the prevailing research. Supplementation should be based on history and a case-by-case basis. (Difficulty: 4; Discipline: Development; Taxonomy: Collaboration)

8.19 **The answer is a.** Distractibility is common in the 4- to 6-month period. Most babies are not yet developmentally ready for solid foods at this time. The *Global Strategy for Infant & Young Child Feeding* recommends 6 months of exclusive breastfeeding. (Difficulty: 2; Discipline: Psychology; Taxonomy: Goals)

8.20 **The answer is d.** She was diagnosed with a bacterial infection of the nipple skin, most likely streptococci transferred from the baby's mouth. The rash is exactly where the baby's mouth had come into contact with her areolar tissue. (Difficulty: 5; Discipline: Pathology; Taxonomy: History)

8.21 **The answer is c.** The cow's milk protein in cheese is the most common allergy trigger in infants. Allergy triggers are usually proteins; therefore, chicken would be the next most likely food to consider. Fruits and vegetables are unlikely to cause skin allergy signs. (Difficulty: 3; Discipline: Pathology; Taxonomy: History)

8.22 **The answer is a.** A baby's trust develops by consistently and promptly responding to her needs. Close frequent contact at night helps develop trust. Forcing a baby to "cry it out" destroys the baby's growing sense of trust. Once broken, trust is difficult to repair. Over time, her needs diminish and the baby can tolerate delays in mother's response. (Difficulty: 2; Discipline: Psychology; Taxonomy: Goals)

8.23 **The answer is d.** Pre-2000 growth curves published by the National Center for Health Statistics (NCHS) were not based on exclusively breastfed babies. The 2006 World Health Organization (WHO) Child Growth Standards clearly document that artificially fed babies are fatter (heavier) per length compared to breastfed babies in the 3- to 6-month period. The exclusively breastfed baby pictured is 4 months old and thriving. (Difficulty: 4; Discipline: Clinical Skills; Taxonomy: Collaboration)

8.24 **The answer is d.** This 4-month-old exclusively breastfed boy is completely normal and has no physiological need for solid food until about 6 months or longer. The growth standards published by the WHO in 2006 are based on normal, healthy, optimally fed breastfed children from several nations, cultures, and ethnic groups. (Difficulty: 4; Discipline: Development; Taxonomy: Goals)

8.25 **The answer is b.** Human milk contains many protective components, and the baby's immune system is still immature at 6 months. Choices a and c could have contributed to the child's illness. Chemicals in bottles and teats are being investigated for potential harmful effects. (Difficulty: 4; Discipline: Pathology; Taxonomy: Knowledge)

8.26 **The answer is d.** Even though amoxicillin is considered compatible with breastfeeding, the infant may develop diarrhea or loose stools. (Difficulty: 4; Discipline: Pharmacology; Taxonomy: Collaboration)

8.27 **The answer is d.** When baby is exclusively breastfeeding day and night without long periods away from the breast, the baby is under 6 months old, and her menses have not returned, there is only a 1% to 2% chance of pregnancy at this time. (Difficulty: 3; Discipline: Physiology; Taxonomy: Knowledge)

8.28 **The answer is b.** As this child naturally explores his environment, he is exposed to many more pathogens. Some immune components of human milk increase over time, and breastfed babies are far less likely to become ill than artificially fed children. (Difficulty: 4; Discipline: Pathology; Taxonomy: Knowledge)

8.29 **The answer is a.** Asking open-ended questions is the best way to initiate a discussion with a mother. Suggestions to correct or improve breastfeeding technique are generally not the first consideration when working with a healthy 6-month-old. Older babies can place themselves in creative postures and still breastfeed effectively. The other questions assume the normalcy of breastfeeding and provide emotional support while obtaining useful data. (Difficulty: 5; Discipline: Psychology; Taxonomy: Goals)

8.30 **The answer is a.** The rash on her breast could be a bacterial and/or yeast infection, eczema, or some other organic condition and needs evaluation by a qualified professional who can examine both the mother's breast and baby's mouth. (Difficulty: 3; Discipline: Clinical Skills; Taxonomy: Collaboration)

8.31 **The answer is d.** She was diagnosed with a bacterial infection of the nipple crevices, most likely streptococci transferred from the baby's mouth. Her nipple developed this configuration during pregnancy and posed no problem during breastfeeding. Choices a and b are possibly correct but less likely. (Difficulty: 5; Discipline: Pathology; Taxonomy: History)

8.32 **The answer is a.** Gut closure occurs around 6 months in the full-term baby. The risk of allergic sensitization from bovine protein is higher before gut closure. (Difficulty: 4; Discipline: Development; Taxonomy: Plan)

8.33 **The answer is c.** Persistent spitting up in the otherwise normal exclusively breastfed baby is most likely an allergic or hypersensitivity response to a substance in the mother's diet. Cow's milk is a highly likely cause, and cow's milk allergy may be responsible for up to 42% of gastroesophageal reflux in babies. (Difficulty: 5; Discipline: Pathology; Taxonomy: History)

8.34 **The answer is a.** Safe bedsharing, as in this photograph, has been shown to increase the likelihood of exclusive breastfeeding for the recommended first 6 months. Breastfed babies bedsharing next to a sober, nonsmoking mother on a firm flat surface are at very minuscule risk of smothering and at no greater risk of SIDS than if they were in a crib by themselves. The baby will tend to roll away onto her back when not nursing, and the nursing mother who sleeps this way is likely to get sufficient rest herself. (Difficulty: 3; Discipline: Psychology; Taxonomy: Collaboration)

8.35 **The answer is a.** Many babies show signs of developmental readiness around 6 months of age, such as reaching for family foods. Exclusive breastfeeding is recommended for about 6 months. Breastfeeding should continue with the addition of complementary foods for 2 years or longer. (Difficulty: 4; Discipline: Development; Taxonomy: Evaluate)

8.36 **The answer is d.** Distractibility is a common behavior of babies in the 4- to 6-month age. Nobody can force a baby to nurse, so choice a is incorrect. This baby could be nearly ready for complementary food, but nothing in the photograph suggests anything about other foods. Babies of this age should be able to handle mom's milk flow easily; this baby is clearly thriving. This baby is 4½ months old, and mom´s milk is leaking downward to her clothes because he needs to check what is going on around him. (Difficulty: 4; Discipline: Psychology; Taxonomy: Goals)

8.37 **The answer is a.** Targeted antibodies specific to that infection quickly appear in milk and protect the baby. Other immunofactors in milk also protect the baby. Choice b is correct as well but less important because the baby may not even get sick. (Difficulty: 4; Discipline: Pathology; Taxonomy: Knowledge)

8.38 **The answer is d.** LAM is the most compatible with breastfeeding. Condoms are also a first choice but less reliable. Progestin-only methods are second choices, and methods containing estrogen are third choices. (Difficulty: 4; Discipline: Physiology; Taxonomy: Knowledge)

8.39 **The answer is c.** Taking a thorough history of the dyad's food intake is the first step in identifying any possible allergic reactions to ingested food or allergens transferred via milk. This child's rash is an allergic reaction. (Difficulty: 4; Discipline: Pathology; Taxonomy: Document)

8.40 **The answer is d.** Feeding at night is normal and common. About two-thirds of infants 1 to 6 months old feed at night. It is always appropriate to breastfeed in response to the baby's cues 24 hours a day. (Difficulty: 3; Discipline: Development; Taxonomy: Goals)

8.41 **The answer is a.** Exclusive breastfeeding is recommended for at least 6 months. Many babies show signs of readiness at that point, such as reaching for family foods. (Difficulty: 3; Discipline: Development; Taxonomy: History)

8.42 **The answer is b.** Exclusive breastfeeding for 6 months is recommended by WHO, UNICEF, and virtually all health professional associations around the world. (Difficulty: 5; Discipline: Development; Taxonomy: Evaluate)

8.43 **The answer is c.** Lactoferrin binds iron in milk and makes it available to the infant. Adding additional sources of dietary iron overwhelms the lactoferrin, leaving the iron available to pathogenic bacteria for growth. (Difficulty: 4; Discipline: Pathology; Taxonomy: Knowledge)

8.44 **The answer is c.** This baby is 4½ months old and is most likely going through a growth spurt. He is too young to need solid foods. Teething and illness are less common reasons for a sudden change in nursing patterns. (Difficulty: 4; Discipline: Development; Taxonomy: Evaluate)

8.45 **The answer is a.** This 4-month-old boy is normal in every way. The 2006 WHO Child Growth Standards are based on healthly breastfed babies from six regions of the world. (Difficulty: 5; Discipline: Development; Taxonomy: Plan)

8.46 **The answer is c.** Supplementing the breastfeeding mother with relatively high doses of vitamin D (6400 IU or more) will raise the levels of D in her milk. Testing the child is appropriate before any direct supplements to the child are given. Local recommendations may differ; research on adequate levels of vitamin D continues to challenge our understanding of the importance of vitamin D for many health conditions. (Difficulty: 3; Discipline: Pathology; Taxonomy: Plan)

8.47 **The answer is d.** Babies have individual needs that are best met by feedings on cue, day and night, until they outgrow the need. About two-thirds of babies breastfeed at night during the first 6 months. Many babies nurse 1 to 3 times at night in the second half of the first year because the liver cannot manufacture sufficient glycogen to support the baby fasting for long periods until the latter part of the first year. (Difficulty: 3; Discipline: Psychology; Taxonomy: Goals)

8.48 **The answer is a.** This 5-month-old exclusively breastfed baby is entirely normal. The teething behavior suggests that she will soon be interested in family foods. (Difficulty: 3; Discipline: Development; Taxonomy: Goals)

8.49 **The answer is d.** This is normal behavior. Many babies and toddlers sleep better when close to their mothers or are carried on their mother's or someone else's body. (Difficulty: 2; Discipline: Psychology; Taxonomy: Evaluate)

8.50 **The answer is b.** This child is 6 months old and has been experimenting with self-feeding of cooked yams. (Difficulty: 4; Discipline: Development; Taxonomy: Evaluate)

8.51 **The answer is c.** Longer nursing sessions are most likely, although a baby who was recently hospitalized may also nurse more frequently, but not necessarily to quench thirst. It is highly unlikely that a child would want the same or less frequent breastfeeding than prior to the hospitalization. (Difficulty: 4; Discipline: Psychology; Taxonomy: Assessment)

8.52 **The answer is d.** Any suggestion may be inappropriate if you do not know the full situation. (Difficulty: 3; Discipline: Clinical Skills; Taxonomy: History)

CHAPTER 9

7–12 Months Questions

9.1 At which age is this breastfeeding behavior MOST LIKELY to occur?

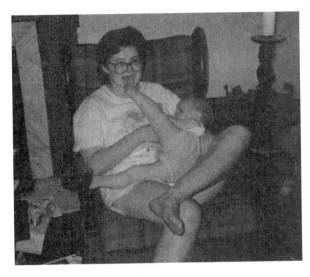

  a. 5–6 months
  b. 7–12 months
  c. 12–18 months
  d. 18–24 months

9.2 Which of the following is the MOST IMPORTANT indication of baby's readiness for solid (family or complementary) foods?

  a. Eruption of teeth
  b. Fading of tongue-extrusion reflex
  c. Baby wakes several times throughout the night
  d. Baby sits up with support

9.3 This exclusively breastfed baby suddenly begins nursing every 1–2 hours around the clock. The mother is worried that her milk supply has dried up. What is your MOST APPROPRIATE response to the mother?

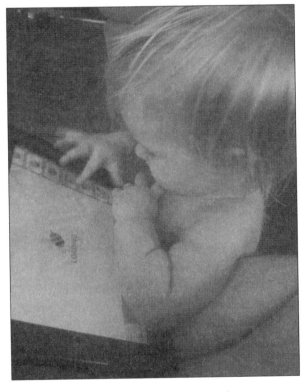

  a. Milk supply often dips at this age, so you should begin supplementing.
  b. This sounds like a typical growth spurt, which is common at this age.
  c. Babies often nurse in that pattern even when they nurse as well as your baby does.
  d. It is reassuring to see your baby gaining weight even when he seems to need to nurse that often.

9.4   At what age is a child physiologically capable of sleeping more than about 4 hours at a time?

a. 9 months
b. 6 months
c. 4 months
d. 2 months

9.5   If her mother moves the dog's water dish out of her sight, this child will probably:

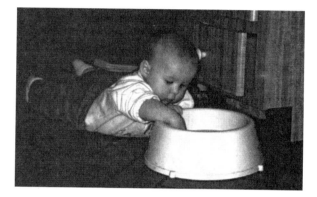

a. crawl straight to it.
b. forget it was there.
c. become confused.
d. search for it without knowing where to look.

9.6   This baby now refuses to take a bottle from her day care provider. Your BEST recommendation to her mother is that the provider should:

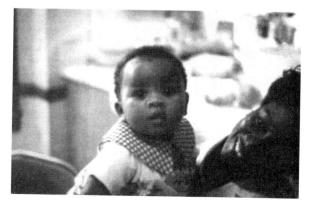

a. give milk in a cup.
b. wait until the child is really hungry.
c. try an orthodontic-shaped teat (nipple).
d. give the bottle in a dark room.

9.7   Which of the following nutrients in complementary foods is MOST NEEDED by the 6- to 12-month-old breastfed baby?

a. Carbohydrate
b. Protein
c. Fat (lipid)
d. Soluble fiber

9.8   A mother complains of sudden-onset sore nipples when her baby is 10 months old. To identify the cause, which is the MOST IMPORTANT question to ask?

a. Did you recently begin taking oral contraceptive pills?
b. Is your baby nursing more frequently than usual?
c. Have you or your baby taken an antibiotic recently?
d. Has anyone in the family been sick with an infection?

9.9   At the age shown, what is the MOST APPROPRIATE recommendation for this child's nutrition?

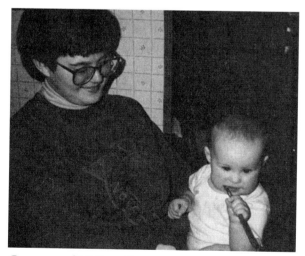

Courtesy of Melissa Courts.

a. Exclusive breastfeeding 24 hours a day
b. Breastfeeding with added carbohydrates
c. Breastfeeding with complementary family foods
d. Breastfeeding supplemented with infant formula

9.10 **In this situation, which aspect of maternal–infant bonding is MOST LIKELY to occur FIRST?**

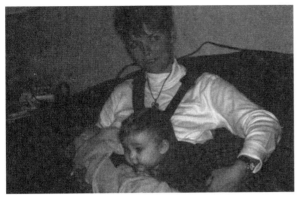

Courtesy of Erika Nehlsen.

    a. Mother bonds with the "unit"
    b. Mother bonds with the firstborn
    c. Mother bonds with the lastborn
    d. Mother has delayed bonding with all

9.11 **At the stage of breastfeeding of the older baby, which milk component is MOST LIKELY to be at a relatively low levels? (The car is stopped.)**

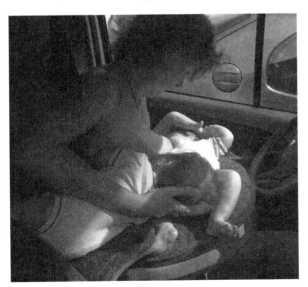

    a. Protein
    b. Lactose
    c. Zinc
    d. Lysozyme

9.12 **A breastfeeding mother is being treated for a fungal (candidal) infection on her nipples. Your BEST recommendation is:**
    a. Boil all baby's teething objects, including this toothbrush.
    b. Wash hands before and after contact with baby's mouth or diaper area.
    c. Wash bras in hot water with a small amount of bleach.
    d. Make sure your baby's mouth is being treated at the same time.

9.13 **Which is the MOST APPROPRIATE indicator that this child is ready for family (complementary) foods in addition to breastmilk?**

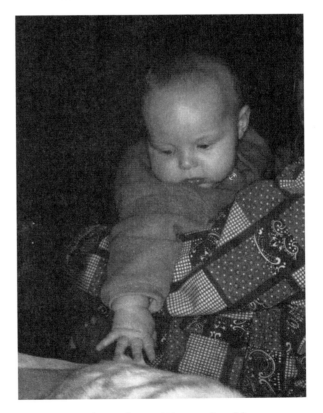

    a. She is about 6½ months old.
    b. She is reaching for table foods.
    c. The nutritional quality of mother's milk is diminishing.
    d. She enjoys the social aspects of family mealtimes.

9.14 **The condition pictured appeared suddenly several days ago, when the baby began spending several hours daily in a day care facility. The MOST LIKELY cause of the condition pictured is:**

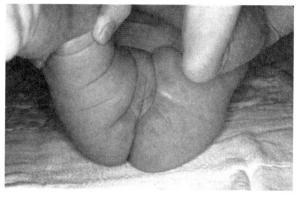

See color plate 83.

   a. The baby's mother recently began taking an antibiotic.
   b. The baby recently ingested two bottles of artificial baby milk.
   c. The baby shared teething toys with other children.
   d. The baby began using a pacifier at the day care center.

9.15 **A mother stopped breastfeeding at 6 months, but her baby could not tolerate formula and she is requesting your help with restarting to breastfeed. What is the FIRST suggestion you would make?**

   a. We can talk to your doctor about prescribing medications to resume your milk production.
   b. Start by putting your baby close to your breast, skin-to-skin, several times a day, to see how he responds.
   c. Pump with a hospital-grade breast pump with double collection kit at least 8 times a day.
   d. It is too late now—once breastfeeding is stopped, it cannot be resumed.

9.16 **Which behavior would be UNREASONABLE to expect in a child of this age?**

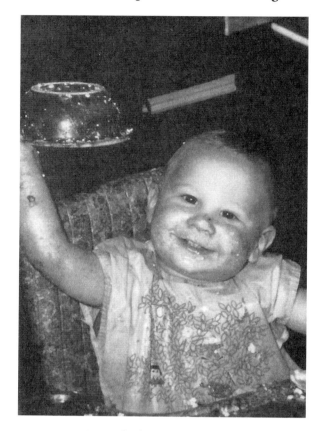

   a. Breastfeeding 8 to 12 times per 24 hours
   b. Sleeping through the night
   c. Separation anxiety
   d. Self-feeding of family foods

9.17 **Which is the MOST LIKELY risk of unplanned pregnancy for this mother?**

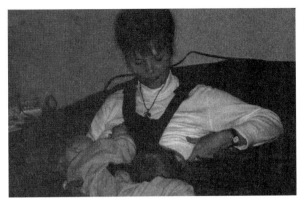

a. Low because of the estrogen-suppressing effect of nursing two children
b. High because children of this age are consuming large quantities of complementary foods
c. Not affected by her current lactation status
d. Irrelevant: there is no time for romance with two nursing babies

9.18 **Which recommendation would be the MOST APPROPRIATE for this family?**

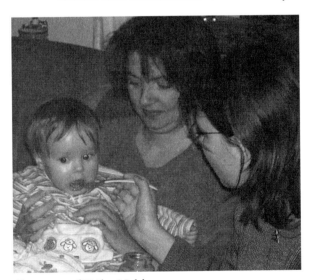

Courtesy of Erika Nehlsen.

a. Let your baby self-select some foods including strips of meat.
b. Turn the baby toward you and make eye contact during feeds.
c. Reduce the amount of mushy foods to protect his nursing skills.
d. Rice cereal would be better for him at this age.

9.19 **A mother has postponed treatment for Lyme disease for fear of the effects of long-term doxycycline on her breastfed 10-month-old baby. Your FIRST response should be:**

a. Go ahead and take the medicine. Formula would be worse than any outcome from the medication.
b. You've breastfed long enough for all the benefits to have reached your baby.
c. You sound ambivalent about these options—can we explore the risks of the disease and treatment in more detail?
d. Lyme is a terrible disease and your treatment outweighs any benefit of continuing to breastfeed your baby.

9.20 **Which immunological component of breastmilk continues to increase beyond 6 months of breastfeeding?**

a. Epidermal growth factor
b. Secretory IgA
c. Lysozyme
d. Lactoferrin

9.21 **A mother is divorcing the father of her 7-month-old breastfeeding child. The father wants her to wean immediately so the child will not miss his mother in the middle of the night. The lactation consultant (LC) has been asked by the mother to testify as an expert witness. Which is the MOST IMPORTANT aspect of the LC'S role in this situation?**

  a. Charging your usual fees for this service

  b. Preparing a written statement or deposition

  c. Giving your professional opinion about the baby's needs

  d. Encouraging the mother to comply with the father's wishes

9.22 **Which of these behaviors is this breastfeeding baby MOST LIKELY to demonstrate?**

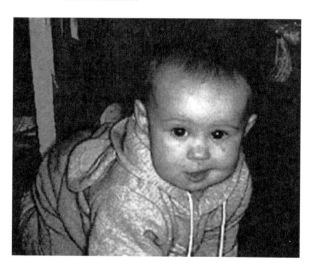

  a. Self-feed with an implement

  b. Sip liquids from an open cup that she holds

  c. Self-wean from the breast

  d. Breastfeed at least 6 times a day and night

9.23 **Which is the MOST LIKELY event to trigger a nursing strike by a 7- to 9-month-old child?**

  a. Illness in the infant

  b. Mother's reaction to baby biting during feeds

  c. Change in mother's soap, perfume, or deodorant

  d. Infant's readiness to wean

9.24 **The mother of a 9-month-old is concerned that her baby has suddenly begun waking several times at night to breastfeed. She works at a local factory 4 hours a day, leaving her child in the on-site day care center. Your FIRST response should be:**

  a. Your milk supply is faltering, so increase the amount of family foods you offer to your child.

  b. Stop into the day care center unannounced to see if any abuse is taking place.

  c. Express or pump your milk several times a day while you're at work, and feed your child that milk at night.

  d. Increased nighttime breastfeeding is common at this age. Do continue to breastfeed him on cue, and this phase will pass.

9.25 **A mother kept her 4-year-old daughter and 7-month-old baby alive by breastfeeding both children while snowbound in their car 9 days. Which component of breastmilk at this stage was HIGHER than at previous stages of lactation?**

  a. Lactoferrin

  b. Secretory IgA

  c. Bifidus factor

  d. Lysozyme

9.26 Which of the following reflexes is MOST LIKELY to have faded (integrated) in this baby?

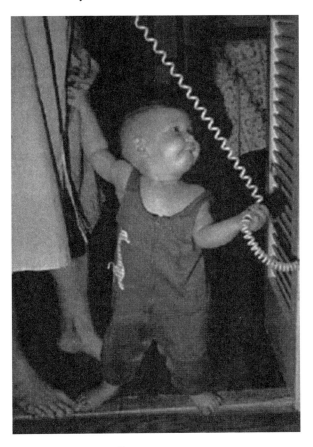

a. Gag reflex
b. Sucking reflex
c. Extrusion reflex
d. Stepping reflex

9.27 What is the MOST LIKELY nursing-related behavior pattern of a 10-month-old baby? The baby:
a. willingly goes to sleep alone in a crib.
b. prefers lumpy or mashed food from jars to common foods eaten by the family.
c. is usually negotiable about where and when to breastfeed.
d. is very social and goes quickly and readily to strangers.

9.28 This mother is getting irritated with her child's nursing habits. The child is afraid of strangers, cries when left with a caregiver, and wakes several times at night. The MOST LIKELY reason for this behavior pattern is:

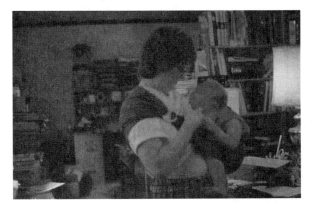

a. delayed development of autonomy caused by breastfeeding.
b. mother clinging to her child and discouraging autonomy.
c. common and normal behavior in the second 6 months of life.
d. mother's inability to set limits for the child's behavior.

9.29 **Which is the MOST COMMON feeding behavior of a baby this age?**

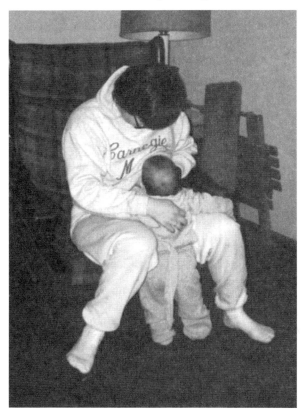

a. Can manage spoon feeding of mashed foods
b. Uses pincer grasp to pick up small pieces of food
c. Cannot hold and drink from a cup
d. Is ready to self-wean from the breast

9.30 **Which concern is the mother of this baby MOST LIKELY to share with you?**

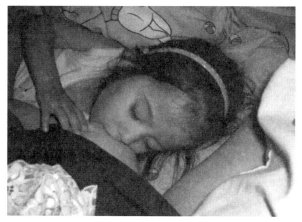

Courtesy of Sarah Hung.

a. My baby has been weaning herself—she's down to three nursings a day.
b. She just started sleeping through the night without nursing.
c. She's been so clingy lately—I can't even leave her for a moment!
d. I'm changing diapers all day—she still stools as often as she did as a newborn.

9.31 **At this stage of lactation, which of the following components of human milk is MOST INCREASED over newborn-period levels?**

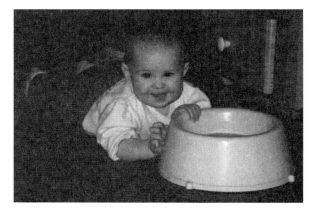

a. Lactoferrin
b. Lactose
c. Whey
d. Casein

9.32 This mother is becoming annoyed with her child's behavior during nursings, including the action shown in the photograph. Your FIRST response to her should be:

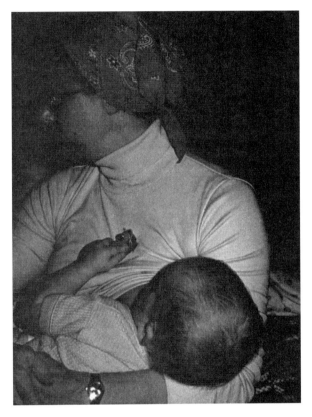

   a. Well, then it's time to think about weaning him.
   b. Many children try to nurse while they play with toys.
   c. Driving his toy truck across your chest during nursing really bothers you.
   d. Grab his hand and don't let him play with your body during feeds.

9.33 Which of the following is the MOST APPROPRIATE complementary food for a 10-month-old breastfed baby?
   a. Baked potato without salt
   b. Strips of lightly cooked pork
   c. Orange and grapefruit segments
   d. Steamed broccoli and carrots

9.34 To breastfeed successfully, it is MOST IMPORTANT for a mother of twins to:
   a. get at least 6 straight hours of sleep each night.
   b. learn to feed her babies simultaneously.
   c. use a nursing pillow.
   d. follow her babies' cues.

9.35 This baby's mother complains about clicking and smacking during breastfeeds that have continued since the baby was a newborn. She has just begun taking solid food. The FIRST action you would do is to:

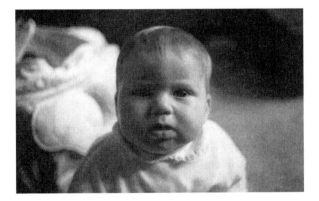

   a. check for a cleft of the soft palate.
   b. observe a full breastfeeding session.
   c. have the baby's doctor diagnose or rule out thrush infection.
   d. ask the mother to record what foods the baby has taken in the past 24 hours.

9.36 A breastfeeding mother was bitten by a tick and is being treated for Lyme disease and is worried about transmitting the disease to her baby. Which action is MOST LIKELY to protect her baby from becoming infected?
   a. Stop breastfeeding immediately.
   b. Increase family foods and decrease breastfeeding.
   c. Continue breastfeeding and take prescribed antibiotics.
   d. Continue breastfeeding and increase intake of vitamin C.

9.37 **Which is the MOST LIKELY feature of a "nursing strike"?**

a. May occur between 6 and 9 months of age

b. May coincide with infant illness

c. With patience, baby will usually return to breast

d. Baby indicating readiness to wean

9.38 **Which is the MOST LIKELY cause of sudden-onset breast pain while nursing an 8- to 10-month-old?**

a. Baby sliding down onto the nipple tip

b. Hormonally induced tenderness due to subsequent pregnancy

c. Allergic reaction to family foods that the baby is eating

d. Low milk supply due to prolonged lactation

9.39 **A 7-month-old child is beginning to turn away when her mother tries to breastfeed while eating her own dinner. Which is the MOST LIKELY explanation?**

a. The child is ready to begin self-feeding family foods.

b. Mother's milk does not provide sufficient fat and calories.

c. The child's gut has matured to handle family foods.

d. The child is bored with breastfeeding and wants to play with mother's food.

9.40 **Of the following, which is the MOST COMMON breastfeeding behavior of babies at this age?**

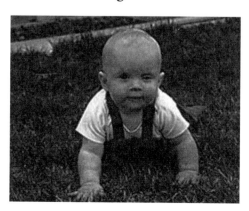

a. Mother and baby develop "code word" for nursing.

b. Baby is taking family foods well.

c. Baby has increased ability to postpone feeds.

d. Baby passes stool during most feeds.

9.41 **A child of the age shown is MOST LIKELY to be developmentally ready to:**

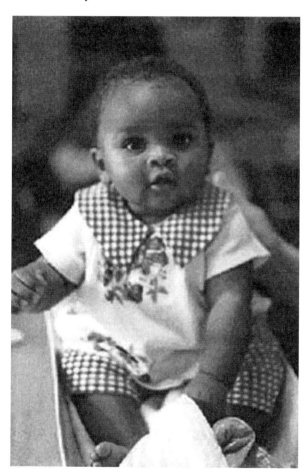

a. crawl and attempt to stand alone.

b. wean from the breast.

c. sleep through the night alone.

d. separate easily from mother.

Answers for 7–12 Months Questions

9.1 **The answer is b.** "Gymnastic" nursing, pincer grasp and self-feeding, and increased mobility are typical of the 7- to 12-month-old baby. (Difficulty: 5; Discipline: Development; Taxonomy: Knowledge)

9.2 **The answer is b.** Babies can be born with teeth but are not ready for solids. Likewise, some babies do not get their first teeth until 14 months of age, but can handle solid foods before that time. Feeding solids in the evening has not been shown to reduce nighttime feedings. Babies who can sit up alone are usually mature enough to actively participate in eating solid foods. (Difficulty: 4; Discipline: Development; Taxonomy: Assessment)

9.3 **The answer is d.** This child is about 8 months old, a time of children go through a period of "separation anxiety" and may want to breastfeed much more frequently for a while. Other babies normally and naturally nurse in that pattern. It is very unlikely that this mother's supply is reduced because the baby in the photograph is obviously thriving. (Difficulty: 4; Discipline: Psychology; Taxonomy: Goals)

9.4 **The answer is a.** The baby's liver cannot store sufficient glycogen for long sleep periods until after about 9 months. (Difficulty: 5; Discipline: Psychology; Taxonomy: Knowledge)

9.5 **The answer is a.** Object permanence emerges in the 4- to 8-month-old period. The child can remember her intention even when the object is moved out of visual range. (Difficulty: 3; Discipline: Development; Taxonomy: Assessment)

9.6 **The answer is a.** Breastfed babies are often willing to try a different feeding method when they are not ravenously hungry. (Difficulty: 3; Discipline: Techniques; Taxonomy: Plan)

9.7 **The answer is b.** Complementary feeding of the breastfed child between 6 months and 2 years should include protein-, iron-, and zinc-rich foods. Human milk is already high in carbohydrate and species-specific fats. Soluble fiber is less important than protein, iron, and zinc during this age. (Difficulty: 5; Discipline: Physiology; Taxonomy: Knowledge)

9.8 **The answer is c.** Sudden-onset sore nipples are most likely caused by yeast infection (thrush, candida) or pregnancy. Taking oral contraceptives is not likely to have caused sudden-onset sore nipples. However, if she stopped taking oral contraceptives, she could be pregnant, which could cause sudden-onset nipple pain. Choice b is an unlikely cause. (Difficulty: 5; Discipline: Clinical Skills; Taxonomy: History)

9.9 **The answer is c.** Breastfeeding with complementary family foods is recommended by UNICEF and the World Health Organization for the child in her second 6 months of life. (Difficulty: 4; Discipline: Development; Taxonomy: Knowledge)

9.10 **The answer is a.** Mothers of multiples often attach to the "unit" before the individual baby or babies. (Difficulty: 3; Discipline: Psychology; Taxonomy: History)

9.11 **The answer is c.** Zinc levels in milk decrease over time. Neither baby is likely at risk of zinc deficiency, because new lactocytes developed during her second pregnancy. Protein and lactose are stable over time. Lysozyme might even be increased at this stage. This was the middle of a traffic jam with very hot weather and a complete blocking of the limited-access highway for several hours. (Difficulty: 3; Discipline: Physiology; Taxonomy: Knowledge)

9.12 **The answer is d.** Nipple thrush is a contagious infection shared by skin surfaces. This baby's mouth should be treated simultaneously with the mother's nipples by a qualified provider. (Difficulty: 2; Discipline: Pathology; Taxonomy: Collaboration)

9.13 **The answer is b.** The child reaching for family foods is one important sign of developmental readiness. Social aspects of family mealtimes are an important developmental milestone. Age alone is not an indication of the need for complementary food. The nutritional quality of human milk does NOT diminish at 6 months. (Difficulty: 4; Discipline: Psychology; Taxonomy: Evaluate)

9.14 **The answer is b.** This is an allergic rash that began when the baby ingested cow's milk–based infant formula at day care. (Difficulty: 5; Discipline: Pathology; Taxonomy: History)

9.15 **The answer is b.** Getting the baby reinterested in the breast is the first step in resuming breastfeeding after it was stopped. If the baby will latch and attempt breastfeeding, then the other suggestions are more likely to be successful. Choice d is incorrect. (Difficulty: 4; Discipline: Techniques)

9.16 **The answer is b.** Sleeping through the night is least likely in this age child. "Gymnastic" nursing, pincer grasp and self-feeding, and separation anxiety are typical of the 7- to 12-month-old child. (Difficulty: 5; Discipline: Psychology; Taxonomy: Goals)

9.17 **The answer is a.** Nursing twins nearly always results in double the milk production over a singleton, and babies of this age frequently nurse many times day and night, thus suppressing estrogen and the return of fertility. Choices b and c are wrong. (Difficulty: 4; Discipline: Physiology; Taxonomy: Evaluate)

9.18 **The answer is a.** Babies are capable of grasping strips of foods at 9 months, which is the age of this baby. Foods high in protein, iron, and zinc are nutritionally important complementary foods, Turning the baby is appropriate, but not as important as choice a. Choices c and d are inappropriate. (Difficulty: 3; Discipline: Development; Taxonomy: Plan)

9.19 **The answer is c.** An empathetic statement is your best first response. This situation is a true dilemma because Lyme is a serious disease, and doxycycline during breastfeeding can have long-term effects on babies. A thorough exploration of risks of both the disease and its treatments in collaboration with her primary care providers is an important role of the LC. (Difficulty: 4; Discipline: Clinical Skills; Taxonomy: Goals)

9.20 **The answer is c.** Lysozyme continues to rise in the second 6 months of the baby's life. The other components decrease over time as the baby matures and can manufacture its own. (Difficulty: 5; Discipline: Development; Taxonomy: Knowledge)

9.21 **The answer is c.** The LC may be asked to serve as an expert witness in divorce and custody situations involving a breastfed baby or lactating mother. The LC should always assist the mother in maintaining an intact and appropriate breastfeeding relationship with her child. (Difficulty: 4; Discipline: Clinical Skills; Taxonomy: Collaboration)

9.22 **The answer is d.** This 9-month-old baby is likely to be nursing at least 6 and maybe many more times a day and night. She probably cannot manipulate an implement yet but may be able to sip liquids from an open cup that she holds by herself. It is unlikely that she will self-wean at this age. (Difficulty: 4; Discipline: Psychology; Taxonomy: Goals)

9.23 **The answer is b.** Nursing strikes are indications that the baby is having some difficulty with breastfeeding or the mother–baby breastfeeding relationship. Self-weaning before 12 months of age is unusual. (Difficulty: 4; Discipline: Psychology; Taxonomy: History)

9.24 **The answer is d.** Babies breastfeed at this age to reconnect with mother as much as for the milk, and giving bottles is likely to shorten the duration of breastfeeding. An empathetic response plus factual information on breastfeeding during "separation anxiety" stages is the best response. Milk supply rarely falters in the second 6 months. While abuse is a possibility, it is less likely a cause of night waking than the other responses. (Difficulty: 4; Discipline: Psychology; Taxonomy: Goals)

9.25 **The answer is d.** Lysozyme increases over the early months of lactation and is higher at 3 months than at 1 month. The other components vary less over time and are still important protective factors. (Difficulty: 5; Discipline: Development; Taxonomy: Knowledge)

9.26 **The answer is c.** The tongue extrusion reflex fades (integrates) by 6 months. The child shown is 8½ months old. Stepping at this age is not a reflex but rather a deliberate psychomotor skill. (Difficulty: 5; Discipline: Development; Taxonomy: Knowledge)

9.27 **The answer is c.** By 10 months, most breastfed toddlers are somewhat negotiable about location and timing. Their need to breastfeed is more flexible than in the first 6 months. They often breastfeed to sleep, enjoy many family foods, and may be cautious or even frightened when approached by strangers. (Difficulty: 3; Discipline: Development; Taxonomy: Plan)

9.28 **The answer is c.** These are typical and normal behaviors of breastfeeding children in the 7- to 12-month period. (Difficulty: 3; Discipline: Development; Taxonomy: Evaluate)

9.29 **The answer is b.** The 8-month-old is developmentally ready to pick up small pieces of nutritious food, chew, and swallow it regardless of whether they have teeth. Self-feeding is more appropriate than spoon feeding, and breastfeeding should continue well past 12 months. Many babies of this age can hold and drink from a small open cup. (Difficulty: 3; Discipline: Psychology; Taxonomy: Evaluate)

9.30 **The answer is c.** Separation anxiety is very common around 8 months, the age of the child pictured. (Difficulty: 3; Discipline: Psychology; Taxonomy: Goals)

9.31 **The answer is d.** Casein in milk increases in proportion to whey over time. Lactose and lactoferrin increase slightly over time. (Difficulty: 4; Discipline: Development; Taxonomy: Knowledge)

9.32 **The answer is c.** An empathetic response that clarifies the mother's feelings is the first step to establishing rapport in a counseling situation. After the mother's feelings are clearly identified, then solutions can be addressed. (Difficulty: 3; Discipline: Psychology; Taxonomy: Goals)

9.33 **The answer is b.** Nutrient-dense and iron-rich foods are the most important complementary foods for the breastfed child between 6 and 12 months. The other foods are lower in nutrient value although still important in the child's overall diet. (Difficulty: 5; Discipline: Development; Taxonomy: Knowledge)

9.34 **The answer is d.** Most mothers will produce plenty of milk for several breastfed babies, despite higher risk of early birth–related problems. (Difficulty: 3; Discipline: Development; Taxonomy: Plan)

9.35 **The answer is b.** Observing a full breastfeeding is always recommended and appropriate, especially before a more-complicated assessment is done. (Difficulty: 5; Discipline: Clinical Skills; Taxonomy: Assessment)

9.36 **The answer is c.** The many immune components in breastmilk have been shown to be protective against the spirochete that causes Lyme. Virtually all antibiotics used to treat Lyme are compatible with breastfeeding, according to several sources. (Difficulty: 3; Discipline: Pathology; Taxonomy: Collaboration)

9.37 **The answer is b.** Babies may suddenly refuse the breast if they are ill and/or breastfeeding is painful and will usually begin again when the crisis has resolved. Self-weaning is developmentally unusual and unlikely to occur before 1 year of age, at a minimum. (Difficulty: 4; Discipline: Techniques; Taxonomy: History)

9.38 **The answer is b.** Sloppy positioning, subsequent pregnancy, and allergic reactions are all possible causes of sudden breast pain at this stage, but choice b is the most likely cause. Low milk supply (choice d) is not a "given" in the second 6 months of lactation, and toddlers often wake several times at night during this age. (Difficulty: 4; Discipline: Physiology; Taxonomy: Evaluate)

9.39 **The answer is a.** Reaching for mother's food is one sign of readiness for complementary foods. Human milk contains sufficient and even increased fat and calories in the second 6 months of lactation. The other statements are true. (Difficulty: 4; Discipline: Psychology; Taxonomy: Evaluate)

9.40 **The answer is b.** This 9-month-old is eating complementary foods with his family several times a day. Some nursing dyads develop code words, and many nursing toddlers have increased flexibility in timing of feeds. Stools are usually more formed because of milk composition (higher casein-to-whey ratio) and the addition of family foods. (Difficulty: 4; Discipline: Development; Taxonomy: Goals)

9.41 **The answer is a.** The developmental milestones characteristic of the 7- to 12-month-old child include separation anxiety, sleep changes—especially increased night waking, and decreased (not increased) likelihood of self-weaning. (Difficulty: 4; Discipline: Development; Taxonomy: Assessment)

CHAPTER 10

> 12 Months Questions

10.1 A research article reports that "breast-feeding is associated with improved performance in intelligence tests 30 years later, and might have an important effect in real life by increasing educational attainment and income in adulthood." Which type of study design would give this finding the highest credibility?

a. Prospective population-based birth cohort

b. Retrospective observational analysis

c. Case-control study with a large sample size

d. Participatory action research

10.2 A breastfeeding mother resumed menstruation for the first time when her child is 16 months old. Which statement is MOST ACCURATE concerning her fertility at this time?

a. Breastfeeding at this age offers no protection against pregnancy.

b. You may experience several menstrual cycles before ovulation begins again.

c. Ovulation usually precedes the first menstrual cycle in breastfeeding women.

d. Taking a hormonal contraceptive will have no effect on lactation at this stage.

10.3 Which of the following descriptions of the protective aspects of breastfeeding is MOST ACCURATE?

a. Effective as long as baby is directly breastfeeding

b. The same whether child is directly breastfed or given breast milk in a bottle

c. Dose-related for the baby, extending well past the time of direct breastfeeding

d. Available only to the baby, not the mother

10.4 This mother is currently breastfeeding a 2-year-old. The condition pictured on her areola is MOST LIKELY:

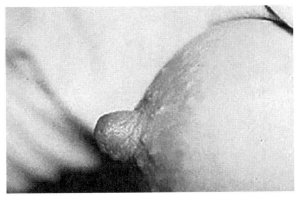

Courtesy of Greg Notestine.

a. Herpes (viral) infection.

b. Wounds from the child biting.

c. Normal Montgomery glands.

d. Urticaria (hives).

10.5 **This mother and baby are in the waiting room of a public transportation facility. What is the FIRST thing you should say to her?**

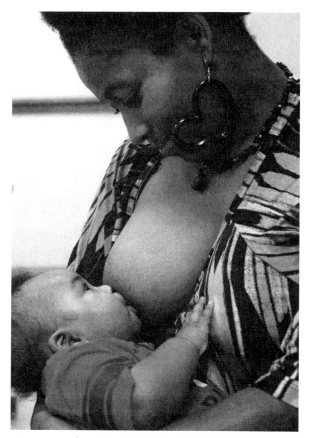

Courtesy of Kimarie Bugg.

    a. Please cover your breasts. You are making some people uncomfortable.

    b. It's mothers like you who make formula-feeding mothers feel guilty.

    c. They make covers for public breastfeeding.

    d. How wonderful to see you and your baby breastfeeding

10.6 **You are contacted by a mother who was exposed to influenza at work. Her child is 15 months old, sleeps with her, and breastfeeds several times a day and at night. Your BEST recommendation to her would be:**

    a. You should wear a face mask when breastfeeding to protect your child.

    b. Your baby has already been exposed to your illness, so keep breastfeeding so he gets some antibodies.

    c. Pump your milk while you are sick, and have someone else give it to your child by cup.

    d. Your milk can transmit the flu virus, so pump and heat-treat the milk before feeding it to your child.

10.7 **The parents of a breastfeeding 16-month-old are divorcing, and the father is arguing that breastfeeding is a control mechanism by the mother. As an expert witness for the mother, your BEST response should be:**

    a. The mother does not control the child in a breastfeeding relationship; rather, the child breastfeeds, and the mother responds.

    b. The mother could pump her milk for her child; she does not have to breast-feed directly at this age.

    c. Overnight separation from the mother at this age will not damage their breast-feeding relationship.

    d. Mothers do have strong control over the breastfeeding relationship, which can be overbearing.

10.8 **Which is the MOST COMMON experience of mothers who are breastfeeding toddler twins?**

a. Mutual enjoyment of breastfeeding

b. Sibling rivalry for the breast

c. Playfulness between children during feeds

d. Higher risk of milk stasis

10.9 **A 16-month-old breastfeeding child has severe eczema on her face. She breastfeeds several times a day and at night, and loves dairy products, which are the main part of her diet. Your FIRST suggestion should be:**

a. Cut down on her intake of dairy products to less than two servings a day.

b. Ask your pediatrician for a suitable lotion or cream for the eczema.

c. Does she rub her face on her pillow or stuffed toys?

d. Has anyone discussed the possibility of your daughter having a dairy allergy?

10.10 **The mother of a 14-month-old wants suggestions for optimizing nutrition from complementary foods. Of the following foods, which would you recommend as MOST LIKELY to fill the nutritional gap between what breastfeeding provides and the child's needs?**

a. Whole grains for their B vitamins

b. Animal products, especially red meat for iron

c. Fish or shellfish for the lipids

d. Green leafy vegetables for the fiber

10.11 **A mother is challenged to provide reasons that her 14-month-old child wants to nurse several times a day and night. The child is also eating a wide variety of family foods. The MOST LIKELY reason for the child to want to nurse into the second year or longer is:**

a. The child is seeking the immune protection found only in her mother's milk.

b. There are insufficient caloric levels in the family foods offered.

c. The child has an oral aversion to solid or lumpy foods.

d. Nursing provides emotional closeness and comfort.

10.12 **A mother asks for your help with weaning her toddler. What is your BEST suggestion for a weaning strategy?**

a. For both you and him, it is best to wean gradually.

b. Put some bitter substance on your nipples to discourage him.

c. Let's look for other ways to meet his needs for closeness.

d. Be aware that your fertility will likely return in a few weeks.

10.13 **What is the MOST IMPORTANT reason for continuing to breastfeed into the second year of life and beyond?**

a. Immune protection tailored to the child's environment

b. Nutrition and trace minerals

c. Muscular development of the jaw and mouth

d. Emotional attachment between mother and child

10.14 **Which milk component is HIGHER at 14 months postbirth than in the early weeks?**

a. Zinc

b. Lactose

c. Lysozyme

d. Alpha-lactalbumin

10.15 Which is the MOST LIKELY reason an 18-month-old child breastfeeds 4 to 8 times every day, including 1 or 2 times at night?

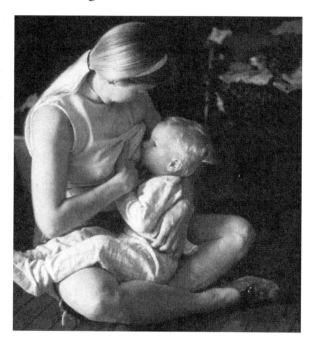

    a. Mother is pressuring the child to gratify her own desires.

    b. Child is recovering from gastroenteritis.

    c. This is normal behavior for some children.

    d. Mother is recovering from a hospital stay where the child could not visit.

10.16 A mother asks you when her baby will likely wean from breastfeeding. Your BEST response is:

    a. She should wean at 12 months to prevent dental decay.

    b. Continue to at least 24 months and as long as you and your baby desire.

    c. Your baby will begin weaning at 6 months and complete weaning by 1 year.

    d. He'll probably want to continue exclusive breastfeeding until 12 months, then begin weaning.

10.17 A mother is being pressured to wean her 16-month-old child and wants to know why continued breastfeeding is encouraged. Your FIRST response to her should be:

    a. They have a point. Breastfeeding past 12 months has little value.

    b. It's fine to continue for another few months.

    c. Would you like suggestions on discreet breastfeeding in public?

    d. Your milk continues to provide important immunity and nutrition to your child.

10.18 A mother asks about sources of vitamin D for her 16-month-old breastfeeding child. Your FIRST recommendation should be:

    a. Continue breastfeeding; you and he should get direct sunlight about 30 minutes a week.

    b. Give him two or three servings of dark-green leafy vegetables every day.

    c. An egg yolk every day will provide enough vitamin D.

    d. Start replacing breastfeeding with vitamin D–fortified cow's milk.

10.19 Which is the MOST IMPORTANT reason to continue breastfeeding for 2 or more years?

    a. Continued source of most calories in baby's diet

    b. Continued immune protection of baby

    c. Mutual pleasure in the relationship

    d. Trace nutrients

10.20 **Of the following, which is the MOST COMMON breastfeeding behavior common to a child of this age?**

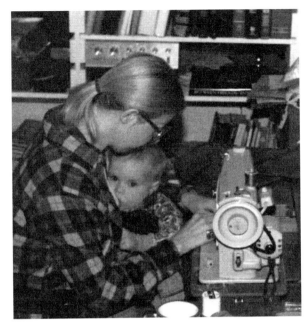

a. Playfulness at breast
b. Breastfeeding while mother is engaging in other activities
c. Persistent biting
d. Breastfeeding at night

10.21 **Which statement is MOST ACCURATE regarding breastfeeding longer than 2 years?**

a. Provides no immune protection to the child
b. Provides health benefits to mother and child
c. Prolongs the child's dependency on mother
d. Increases incidence of tooth decay

10.22 **Which immunologic component of human milk remains at high levels through this stage of breastfeeding?**

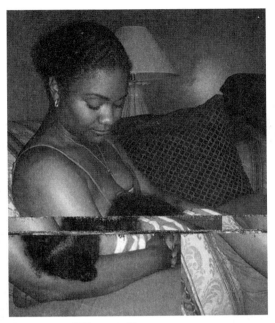

Courtesy of Kimarie Bugg.

a. Zinc
b. Leukocytes
c. Lysozyme
d. SIgA

10.23 **What is the MOST ACCURATE conclusion you could draw from the appearance of this lactating woman's breasts?**

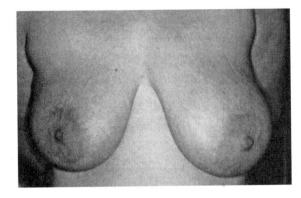

a. The smaller breast has insufficient glandular tissue.
b. The larger breast is making much more milk than the smaller breast.
c. The baby most recently nursed on the smaller breast.
d. Lactation and breastfeeding are proceeding smoothly for her and her baby.

10.24 **Which statement is MOST ACCURATE about human milk after 1 year of lactation?**

    a. Total fat is 14% lower than at 6 months of lactation.

    b. Total energy is 34% lower than at 6 months.

    c. Lactose is 8% higher in proportion to minerals.

    d. Creamatocrit (fat) levels are up to 28% higher.

10.25 **This child's mother tried unsuccessfully to breastfeed, and her child now has difficulty eating. The MOST LIKELY reason is that this child has:**

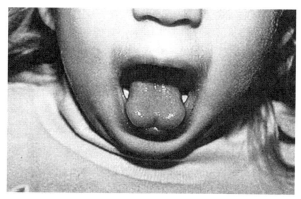

Courtesy of Greg Notestine.

    a. Ankyloglossia

    b. Macroglossia

    c. Microglossia

    d. Micrognathia

10.26 **The cause of this nursing toddler's dental condition is MOST LIKELY due to:**

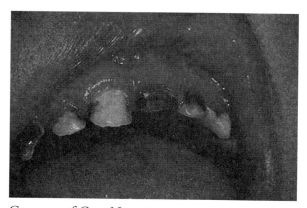

Courtesy of Greg Notestine.

    a. high intake of sweetened foods.

    b. lack of toothbrushing.

    c. congenital enamel defects.

    d. unrestricted breastfeeding at night.

10.27 **This child is nursing several times a day and often once or twice at night. Which statement BEST describes this pattern?**

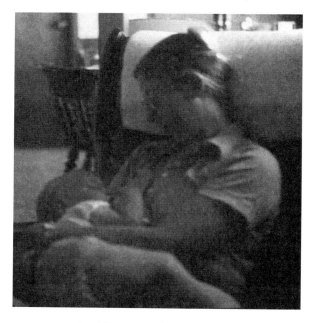

    a. highly unusual at this age.

    b. indicative of attachment disorder.

    c. normal for a child this age.

    d. likely to cause dental caries.

10.28 **At which ages/stages are babies MOST LIKELY to self-wean?**

    a. Under 12 months

    b. 12–18 months

    c. 2–2½ years

    d. 3–4 years

10.29 The nipple damage shown in this picture is MOST LIKELY due to:

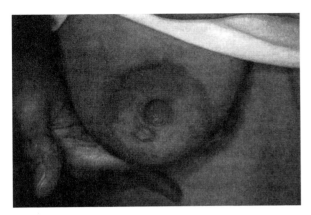

See color plate 84.

    a. poor positioning at breast.

    b. bacterial or fungal infection.

    c. tongue-tied baby.

    d. overuse of a breast pump.

10.30 This mother says she has been hand-expressing her milk as shown in the picture. Which is the MOST LIKELY result of her using the technique pictured?

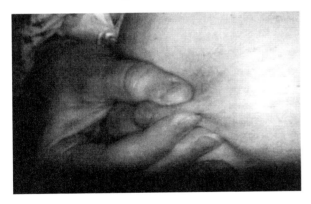

    a. Milk is easily expressed.

    b. Little or no milk flows from the nipple.

    c. The areola is bruised.

    d. The nipple and areola become more elastic.

10.31 Which of the following foods is the BEST source of calcium for a partly breastfeeding 16-month-old who cannot tolerate dairy products?

    a. Sesame seed paste

    b. Fresh oranges

    c. Spinach

    d. Oatmeal cereal

10.32 A mother is being accused of child abuse because her child is still nursing at 14 months and shares the mother's bed all night every night. What is the MOST LIKELY long-term outcome of all-night bedsharing with sustained breastfeeding?

    a. Enhanced self-esteem and confidence in the child

    b. Delayed progression to independent sleeping for the child

    c. Increased risk of maternal abuse of the child including incest

    d. Higher risk of dental caries in the child

10.33 What is the MOST IMPORTANT reason for a mother who is HIV positive to continue to breastfeed her baby past 12 months?

    a. There is a lower risk of child mortality from infectious diseases.

    b. There is stronger bonding/attachment with mother.

    c. Human milk is a reliable source of trace nutrients.

    d. There is a lower risk of diarrhea or constipation.

10.34 A mother weaned her baby at 6 months and is now trying to reestablish breastfeeding at 16 months. Which components of milk are the "last to go" during weaning and involution?

    a. Carbohydrates

    b. White cells

    c. Enzymes

    d. Immunoglobulins

10.35 **What window (age) period MOST LIKELY represents the biologic end of breastfeeding for human infants?**
   a. 9–15 months
   b. Around 18 months
   c. Around 24 months
   d. 2.5–7 years

10.36 **Which statement about complementary feeding increases nutritional risk for the child?**
   a. Feed a variety of foods including meat, poultry, fish, and eggs daily.
   b. Vegetarian diets can meet a child's nutrient needs after 12 months.
   c. Vitamin A–rich foods should be eaten daily.
   d. Whole fruits are more nutritious for children than fruit juices.

10.37 **Which of the following factors is MOST IMPORTANT for the breastfeeding child of this age?**

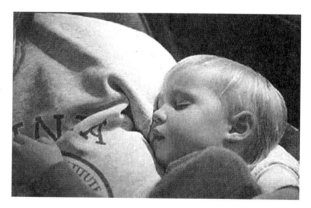

   a. Mother and child have a "code word" for breastfeeding.
   b. Child can postpone nursing for short periods.
   c. Nighttime breastfeeding increases child's risk of dental caries.
   d. Child receives substantial immune protection from breastfeeding.

10.38 **What is the MOST IMPORTANT reason that girls who consume formula by bottles are more likely to become obese later in childhood?**
   a. Bottles suppress self-regulation of feeds.
   b. Leptin levels in formula-fed children diminish rapidly.
   c. Girls consume more milk per weight than boys.
   d. Boys are unaffected by feeding methods.

10.39 **How is the nursing mother–baby relationship in the second year of breastfeeding different from any other mother–baby or parent–baby relationship?**
   a. The nursing mother's heart rate and respiratory rate continue to influence her child.
   b. A nursing toddler sleeps with her mother in a unique way, thus reducing risk for sleep-related death.
   c. Immune components in mother's own milk offer unique protection to the infant until at least age 3.
   d. Continued nursing suggests an overly dependent child or overcontrolling mother.

10.40 **The mother of a 16-month-old partly breastfed child is concerned that he started spitting up frequently and has had an itchy rash on his face ever since starting day care. His lunch meal is provided by the day care center. Which is the MOST LIKELY cause of his new spitting up and rash?**
   a. Age of the child
   b. Gastroenteritis
   c. Anxiety at being separated from his mother
   d. Allergy to a food he is eating at day care

10.41 **For an 18-month-old child, which aspect is MOST IMPORTANT to long-term well-being?**

a. Calories

b. Immunities

c. Comfort

d. Bonding

10.42 **Which of the following is the MOST COMMON breastfeeding behavior of a child at this age?**

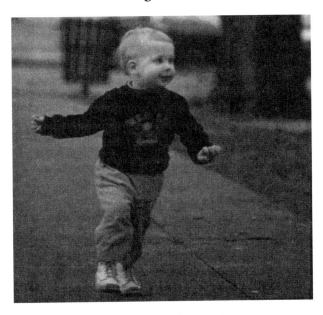

a. Biting at the end of feeds

b. Nursing strike

c. Easily distracted while nursing

d. Playfulness and vocalization during feeds

10.43 **This mother has been warned that she is spoiling her baby by using the device in the picture. What is the MOST ACCURATE statements about the relationship shown in the picture?**

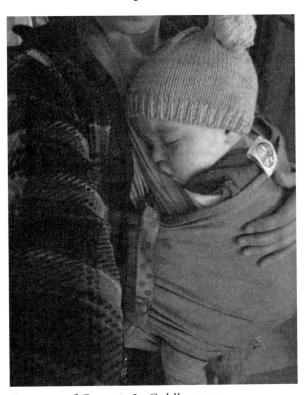

Courtesy of Cammie Jo Goldhammer.

a. Continuous body contact helps the baby maintain body temperature.

b. Carrying in a sling allows the baby easy access to breastfeeding.

c. Carrying reduces infant crying.

d. Carrying prolongs dependency of the baby on its mother.

Answers for > 12 Months Questions

10.1 **The answer is a.** Prospective population-based birth cohort studies are the highest level of evidence of the designs listed. Choices b and c are weaker evidence, and participatory action research is the least rigorous of these designs. (Difficulty: 2; Discipline: Clinical Skills; Taxonomy: Evaluate)

10.2 **The answer is b.** When a breastfeeding mother resumes menstruation after birth, even more than 12 months later, she may have several nonovulatory cycles before ovulating. The lactational amenorrhea method (LAM) is most effective when the baby is less than 6 months old. Choices a and c are incorrect. Estrogen-containing contraceptives affect lactation at all stages. (Difficulty: 2; Discipline: Physiology; Taxonomy: Knowledge)

10.3 **The answer is c.** Protection against many short- and long-term diseases is well established, even though the specific mechanisms are still poorly understood as of this writing. Understanding the public health– and population-based research is a required activity of lactation consultants (LCs). (Difficulty: 3; Discipline: Clinical Skills; Taxonomy: Evaluate)

10.4 **The answer is c.** The raised areas on her areola are normal Montgomery glands. This is a normal breast. (Difficulty: 2; Discipline: Development; Taxonomy: Assessment)

10.5 **The answer is d.** A supportive statement is the first and most appropriate statement to make to this mother. Global recommendations are to support breastfeeding to age 2 or beyond, as long as the mother and child desire. Breastfeeding in public places should be encouraged and supported. Embarrassment is a major detriment for breastfeeding mothers in many places. The other choices are inappropriate. (Difficulty: 2; Discipline: Clinical Skills; Taxonomy: Goals)

10.6 **The answer is b.** For most maternal illnesses including viruses, the child has already been exposed and mother's body is already making antibodies specific to the infectious pathogen. Choice a is rarely necessary; choice c is appropriate only if the mother is too sick to care for her child. Choice d is incorrect. (Difficulty: 4; Discipline: Pathology; Taxonomy: Plan)

10.7 **The answer is a.** When children have outgrown the need to breastfeed, they stop. Mothers cannot make their children breastfeed at any age. Pumped milk is not the same as breastfeeding, and overnight separations before the child is ready to separate can be damaging to the mother–baby relationship. Choice d is false. (Difficulty: 4; Discipline: Psychology; Taxonomy: Collaboration)

10.8 **The answer is a.** The unique closeness of nursing twins into toddlerhood is a highly motivating factor for mothers. Breastfed twins are often best friends and copy each other's breastfeeding behaviors. High milk volume may increase mother's susceptibility to milk stasis. (Difficulty: 4; Discipline: Psychology; Taxonomy: Goals)

10.9 **The answer is d.** Eczema on the face is a common symptom of food allergies, especially allergy to cow's milk protein. Cutting down on dairy will probably not help, because any amount of dairy protein may trigger a reaction. (Difficulty: 3; Discipline: Pathology; Taxonomy: History)

10.10 **The answer is b.** Complementary foods that best fill the nutritional gap between breast milk and the needs of a 12- to 24-month-old child should be nutritionally dense and high in protein, iron, and/or zinc. A variety of other foods will provide a balanced set of nutrients. B vitamins are also found in animal products. Omega-3 fats in fish are also found in human milk. Young children need less fiber than adults, although green leafy vegetables are good sources of other nutrients. (Difficulty: 5; Discipline: Development; Taxonomy: Goals)

10.11 **The answer is d.** Children who continue nursing past infancy are meeting their needs for warmth, security, emotional closeness, comfort, and more. Nursing into the second year and beyond provides some important calories to the child and important immune protection. (Difficulty: 3; Discipline: Development; Taxonomy: Collaboration)

10.12 **The answer is c.** Awareness of the mother–baby relationship is key when one party wants to end it and the other may not be ready. Application of noxious substances to the nipples to discourage breastfeeding can disrupt the trust relationship that has been carefully established via breastfeeding. (Difficulty: 4; Discipline: Psychology; Taxonomy: Goals)

10.13 **The answer is a.** The immune properties of human milk cannot be duplicated by any other source, and the protection against disease from breast milk is irreplaceable. The other choices are also important reasons to continue breastfeeding as long as the child and mother desire. (Difficulty: 5; Discipline: Psychology; Taxonomy: Knowledge)

10.14 **The answer is c.** Lysozyme increases in milk over time, providing immune protection for the breast and the nursing child. Zinc decreases over time; lactose remains stable, and proteins including alpha-lactalbumin are relatively stable over time. (Difficulty:

3; Discipline: Development; Taxonomy: History)

10.15 **The answer is c.** The breastfeeding relationship is far more than food for many nursing toddlers. Choices b and d are also common reasons for continued breastfeeding well into the second year of the child's life. Choice a is incorrect because breastfeeding cannot be forced on a child at any age. The child who does not want to breastfeed will either bite or refuse to latch on. (Difficulty: 4; Discipline: Development; Taxonomy: History)

10.16 **The answer is b.** There is no age beyond which breastfeeding is inappropriate. Complementary foods should begin some time in the second 6 months of life. (Difficulty: 4; Discipline: Psychology; Taxonomy: Knowledge)

10.17 **The answer is d.** Breastfeeding well into the second year and beyond provides important immunological components and nutrition to the child. There is no documented age beyond which breastfeeding has no value. (Difficulty: 2; Discipline: Psychology; Taxonomy: Goals)

10.18 **The answer is a.** Levels of vitamin D in mother's milk are related to the mother's own vitamin D stores. A half hour of direct sunlight ensures adequate levels of D in many locations. If direct sunlight is not available, supplements of D for the mother should be considered. Leafy vegetables for the child may help; so will egg yolk. Weaning to formula is not appropriate. (Difficulty: 3; Discipline: Pathology; Taxonomy: Plan)

10.19 **The answer is b.** Immune components and trace nutrients in milk over time are critical to the child's health and well-being. The older child is usually nursing for far more than food. Breastfeeding the older child is mutually pleasurable even when the majority of the child's calories come from other sources. (Difficulty: 4; Discipline: Development; Taxonomy: Knowledge)

10.20 **The answer is b.** Toddlers can be very creative during breastfeeding sessions. Choices a and d are also common. Persistent biting is not common in nursing toddlers. (Difficulty: 4; Discipline: Development; Taxonomy: Goals)

10.21 **The answer is b.** Breastfeeding for more than 2 years has no documented risks for mother or baby and many benefits for both. (Difficulty: 3; Discipline: Psychology; Taxonomy: Knowledge)

10.22 **The answer is c.** Lysozyme remains elevated through at least 24 months of lactation. SIgA antibodies active against *Escherichia coli* are still present into the second year as well. Leukocytes and zinc are at low levels after a few months of lactation. (Difficulty: 3; Discipline: Development; Taxonomy: Evaluate)

10.23 **The answer is d.** These lactating breasts are entirely normal. The mother's baby is 13 months old and thriving. Choice a is false. Choices b and c may be true, but cannot be determined solely from breast appearance. (Difficulty: 4; Discipline: Development; Taxonomy: Evaluate)

10.24 **The answer is d.** Fat levels, measured by creamatocrit, are up to 28% higher than levels in milk of women who lactated 2 to 6 months. Total energy contributed by fat might be significant to the infant who continues to breastfeed more than 1 year. (Difficulty: 2; Discipline: Development; Taxonomy: Knowledge)

10.25 **The answer is a.** This child is tongue-tied, often referred to as ankyloglossia. The lingual frenulum is short and/or tight, causing the heart-shaped tongue tip. Without full normal tongue mobility, breastfeeding and eating (and other activities involving movement of the tongue) are compromised. (Difficulty: 3; Discipline: Development; Taxonomy: Goals)

10.26 **The answer is a.** High intake of sweetened foods is the most common cause of dental caries in nursing children. Choices b and c are associated with caries in young children. There is no evidence that unrestricted breastfeeding at night is a cause of baby-bottle tooth decay or "nursing caries." (Difficulty: 4; Discipline: Pathology; Taxonomy: History)

10.27 **The answer is c.** This 13-month-old's nursing pattern is entirely normal. The World Health Organization recommends that breastfeeding continue for at least 2 years or longer, adding complementary food after 6 months of age. (Difficulty: 3; Discipline: Development; Taxonomy: Knowledge)

10.28 **The answer is d.** This is a period of equilibrium and many believe that babies are more likely to wean in stable ages. (Difficulty: 4; Discipline: Psychology; Taxonomy: Goals)

10.29 **The answer is b.** The damage shown is infectious in origin, not mechanical. The shape of the nipple is normal, suggesting pressure is not the cause of the damage. This mother's nursing baby is 15 months old. (Difficulty: 4; Discipline: Pathology; Taxonomy: History)

10.30 **The answer is b.** The hand is pinching the base of the nipple, cutting off milk flow. This could also bruise the areola. It is more effective to move the hand farther away from the nipple. There is no published evidence that nipple rolling will improve nipple elasticity. (Difficulty: 4; Discipline: Techniques; Taxonomy: Evaluate)

10.31 **The answer is a.** Of the foods listed, sesame seeds ground into a paste are highest in calcium. Oxalic acid in spinach binds calcium, making spinach a poor source. Oranges and oatmeal are appropriate foods for a child this age but not especially high in calcium. (Difficulty: 4; Discipline: Development; Taxonomy: Knowledge)

10.32 **The answer is a.** Children whose needs for dependency and nursing are met willingly all day and night by their mother and parents show normal, desirable outcomes in all parameters. None of the other choices are supported by research. (Difficulty: 3; Discipline: Psychology; Taxonomy: Goals)

10.33 **The answer is a.** Children of mothers who are HIV positive are at higher risk of dying from infectious diseases if they are weaned before 18 months. The other answers are all true but less important overall from a public-health perspective. (Difficulty: 5; Discipline: Clinical Skills; Taxonomy: Collaboration)

10.34 **The answer is d.** Immunoglobulins are a primary component of colostrum, the first secretion of the lactocyctes during pregnancy; the same components essentially form an "immune layer" throughout lactation. As weaning and involution progress, lactose is the first component to diminish. (Difficulty: 4; Discipline: Development; Taxonomy: Knowledge)

10.35 **The answer is d.** Anthropological evidence suggests the human infant was "designed" to breastfeed for more than 2 years. (Difficulty: 4; Discipline: Psychology; Taxonomy: History)

10.36 **The answer is b.** According to the Pan American Health Organization and World Health Organization, vegetarian diets cannot meet nutrient needs at this age unless supplements or fortified products are used. The other statements are true. (Difficulty: 3; Discipline: Development; Taxonomy: Knowledge)

10.37 **The answer is d.** The child who nurses past 12 months of age receives substantial immune protection, nutrition, and psychological benefits from breastfeeding. (Difficulty: 4; Discipline: Development; Taxonomy: Goals)

10.38 **The answer is b.** Breastfeeding mitigates the fall in leptin levels in girls. Leptin is a protein hormone that affects appetite, body weight, and metabolism. Choice a is also

true for both boys and girls. Choices c and d are false. (Difficulty: 3; Discipline: Development; Taxonomy: History)

10.39 **The answer is c.** Immune components unique to human milk protect the child until the child's immune system is fully mature at around 3 years of age. Heart and respiratory rate synchronicity occur primarily during the early days and weeks. While it is true that nursing babies and their mothers have different sleep habits than other adults, there is no evidence of elevated risk related to bedsharing after about 4 months. The last choice is false. (Difficulty: 4; Discipline: Psychology; Taxonomy: Evaluate)

10.40 **The answer is d.** Food allergy is the most likely cause of his dermatologic and gastrointestinal symptoms of allergy. The mother should investigate what foods he is being given. Gastroenteritis would not simultaneously produce a face rash. Neither his age nor any anxiety would explain both symptoms. (Difficulty: 3; Discipline: Pathology; Taxonomy: History)

10.41 **The answer is b.** The immunologic properties of human milk extend throughout the entire duration of breastfeeding. In addition, breastfeeding the child in the second year is mutually pleasurable and an important aspect of mother–baby bonding even when a portion of the child's caloric intake comes from other sources. (Difficulty: 4; Discipline: Development; Taxonomy: Knowledge)

10.42 **The answer is d.** The over-1-year-old nursing child often plays and explores mother's body during breastfeeding sessions. (Difficulty: 5; Discipline: Development; Taxonomy: Assessment)

10.43 **The answer is c.** Multiple studies have shown that carrying and holding children substantially reduces crying. Choices a and b are also true. Breastfeeding frequently on cue and continuous/frequent carrying foster all aspects of infant mental and physical development. (Difficulty: 4; Discipline: Psychology; Taxonomy: Goals)

CHAPTER 11

General Principles Questions

11.1 **According to recent studies, a woman with a history of sexual abuse**

    a. is less likely to intend to breastfeed.

    b. is more likely to initiate breastfeeding.

    c. breastfeeds at the same rate as women with no history of sexual abuse.

    d. is more likely to pump her milk and feed it by bottle.

11.2 **Which drug decreases rapidly in the breastmilk after the mother stops taking the drug?**

    a. marijuana

    b. cocaine

    c. amphetamines

    d. alcohol

11.3 **Which of the following components of human milk has the MOST IMMUNOLOGICAL IMPORTANCE?**

    a. interferon

    b. fibronectin

    c. lactoferrin

    d. secretory IgA

11.4 **Which of the following has been shown to be the MOST PREVALENT benefit to employers who adopt breastfeeding support practices?**

    a. reduced employee absenteeism

    b. increased employee productivity

    c. increased retention of employees

    d. increased employee morale

11.5 **A mother tells you that a lactation consultant (LC) in your city took a course in a manipulative therapy and used her new skills on the mother's baby, without informing the mother or the baby's primary care provider. What should you do NEXT?**

    a. Report the LC to the medical licensing board in your jurisdiction.

    b. Contact the LC and discuss what the mother reported to you.

    c. Express doubt to the mother that your colleague would ever do such a thing.

    d. Write a letter to the mother's doctor, explaining the nature of the training taken by your colleague.

11.6 **How long does it take for a baby's intestinal microflora to return to normal after being treated with an antibiotic?**

    a. Antibiotics have no effect on the infant's gut bacteria flora.

    b. One day is sufficient for the breastfed baby to recover normal flora.

    c. Seven to 10 days for the breastfed child and 2 to 3 weeks for the formula-fed child.

    d. Several weeks are necessary for the breastfed child's microflora to return to normal.

11.7 **Which of the following strategies of breastfeeding promotion has the BIGGEST EFFECT on population breastfeeding rates?**

   a. assisting in developing legislation to protect breastfeeding in public

   b. implementing the Baby Friendly Hospital Initiative (BFHI)

   c. presenting a lecture on breastfeeding to a civic organization

   d. wearing breastfeeding buttons, jewelry, or t-shirts in social situations

11.8 **Which pumping strategy is MOST LIKELY to maximize amount of milk collected?**

   a. Pump at the lowest comfortable pressure.

   b. Cycle the pump slowly at first, then faster as milk flows.

   c. Choose a flange diameter that fits the nipple snugly.

   d. Pump past two let-downs (milk ejection reflexes) or more.

11.9 **The chart presented here shows the mean axillary and skin temperatures between 15 and 90 minutes after birth in healthy, full-term babies. The closed circles are the babies cared for skin to skin with their mother. The open circles are babies who spent the time in the warming bed. Which conclusion can be drawn from this chart? At 90 minutes:**

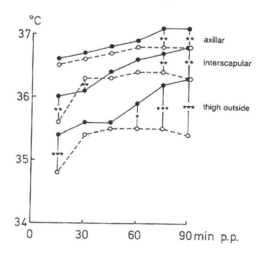

   a. there was no difference in temperature between babies cared for skin-to-skin vs. in the warming bed.

   b. all the babies were cooler as measured at all three locations—axillar, interscapular, and thigh outside.

   c. all the babies were warmer as measured at all three locations—axillar, interscapular, and thigh outside.

   d. the interscapular temperature of the skin-to-skin babies was the same as the outside thigh temperature of the warming bed babies.

11.10 **Bacterial counts 1 hour after expression are lower than immediately after collection. The MOST LIKELY explanation for this is that:**

   a. the cooler temperature in the container is unsuitable for growth of bacteria.

   b. macrophages in milk are actively phagocytic.

   c. gangliosides in milk disrupt the cell walls of bacteria.

   d. bifidus factor starves the bacteria of nutrients.

11.11 **When considering whether a breastfeeding mother should take a certain medication, which is the FIRST question to consider?**

   a. Is the drug regarded as safe in the neonatal period?

   b. How much drug would the infant receive per day via the milk?

   c. Is systemic maternal therapy needed?

   d. Is it really necessary for the mother to take this drug now?

11.12 **A client mother's nipples are healing slowly but surely. She wants to send you cellphone photographs she has taken each day, showing the progress. She will transmit them via her cellphone directly to your cellphone. The best way to protect her privacy is to:**

   a. explain that cellphone photograph transmission is not secure.

   b. delete the photograph from your phone after you look at it.

   c. refuse to accept the photographs because the mother took them, and you have no way of verifying the photograph is of her.

   d. delete them from your phone after adding the image to your password-protected secure charting system.

11.13 **Which category of drug administered to the mother is usually contraindicated during breastfeeding?**

   a. antimicrobial

   b. antihypertensive

   c. antineoplastic

   d. antidepressant

11.14 **After examining this woman's breasts, what is your FIRST suggestion?**

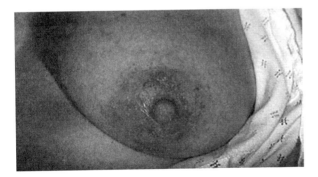

See color plate 85.

   a. Instruct her on better cleaning procedures for her breast pump.

   b. Provide her with a nipple shield to wear during feeds.

   c. Request that the primary care provider culture the baby's mouth.

   d. Recommend that she wean immediately.

11.15 **Which of the following documents applies to all health workers, including lactation professionals?**

   a. Global Strategy for Infant & Young Child Feeding

   b. IBLCE's Standards of Practice

   c. ILCA's Position Paper on Infant Feeding

   d. International Code of Marketing of Breast-milk Substitutes

11.16 **Which is the MOST IMPORTANT function of lactoferrin?**

   a. bind and deactivate pathogens

   b. nerve myelinization

   c. iron transport

   d. anti-inflammatory agent

11.17 **Why might this nonpregnant woman have trouble breastfeeding?**

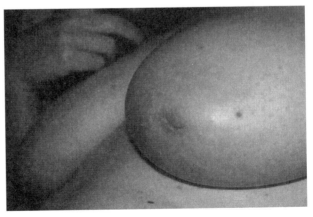

Courtesy of K. Jean Cotterman.

   a. little visible areola

   b. lack of visible blue veins

   c. large, pendulous breasts

   d. inverted/retracted nipple

11.18 **When are the fat levels in mother's milk highest?**

   a. When the milk ejection reflex is strong.

   b. During the night.

   c. After the mother eats a high-fat diet.

   d. When the breast is relatively empty.

11.19 **You have a contract to lecture and discover that the organizer of the event has created an electronic advertising flyer with a downloaded image from the Internet that links to a company that violates the International Code of Marketing of Breast-milk Substitutes. What should be your FIRST action?**

   a. Immediately cancel your contract.

   b. Insist that the organizer remove the image and issue a disclaimer immediately.

   c. Have your attorney contact the organizer regarding possible slander charges.

   d. Ignore it—most people will not click on the image anyway.

11.20 **A disgruntled family files a malpractice suit after you provided LC services to them. The FIRST thing you should do is:**

   a. call an attorney.

   b. contact your professional insurance agent.

   c. talk to the couple to find out why they are upset.

   d. speak to the couple's physician.

11.21 **Researchers have found that inguinal hernias and some other disorders of the urogenital tract are less common in breastfed babies. Which of the following components has the MOST SIGNIFICANT role in tissue maturation of the infant?**

   a. epidermal growth factor

   b. nerve growth factor

   c. secretory IgA

   d. lactoferrin

11.22 **What is the MOST LIKELY condition pictured?**

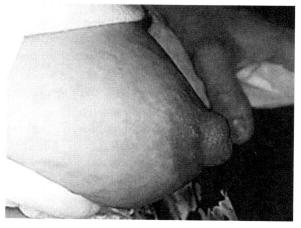

See color plate 86.

   a. candidal infection at the base of the nipple

   b. large, possibly fibrous nipple

   c. nipple edema from excessive pumping

   d. scars from breast reduction surgery

11.23 **In a lactating woman, the milk ducts act as:**

   a. secretory glands producing cleansing agents for the areola.

   b. a visual signal for the baby to latch-on.

   c. channels for the milk to flow to the nipple.

   d. milk-secreting glands.

11.24 **A mother, 4-year-old daughter, and 7-month-old baby were trapped in a snowbound car for 9 days. The mother breastfed both children after their small supply of food and liquids was exhausted. Which factor is MOST RELEVANT to milk production in this situation?**

   a. The cold temperature slowed the children's metabolism and caloric needs.

   b. Milk synthesis is mostly unrelated to maternal food or fluid intake.

   c. Water-soluble vitamins in her milk would be diminished by 9 days.

   d. The mother became malnourished and dehydrated by producing so much milk.

11.25 **Which of the following protective components of milk is destroyed by freezing?**
a. lysozyme
b. lymphocytes
c. secretory IgA
d. lactoferrin

11.26 **At what point in the suck–swallow–breathe cycle does MOST of the milk flow into the baby?**
a. when the jaw rises and collects the milk from the nipple and areola
b. as the baby draws the nipple into its mouth using negative pressure
c. as the posterior tongue and jaw drops vertically, opening the oral space
d. during the wavelike motion of the tongue stripping the milk sinuses

11.27 **What statement BEST describes the thymus gland's role in the infant's immune system?**
a. A large thymus gland may be related to increased risk of SIDS.
b. Breastfed infants have smaller thymus glands than formula-fed children.
c. The larger the thymus gland, the lower is the infant mortality rate.
d. A small thymus gland at birth is related to prematurity and prenatal nutrition.

11.28 **Which component of milk does the following: is active against inflammation, increases in milk after 6 months' lactation, destroys *Escherichia coli* and other bacteria, and is not destroyed by heat treatment?**
a. leukocytes
b. nucleotides
c. lysozyme
d. zinc

11.29 **The ease with which human milk fat is digested by the infant is BEST explained by the fact that:**
a. unsaturated fats constitute 57% of total lipids.
b. lipases are present in the milk.
c. lipids are encased in membranes (globules).
d. cholesterol is the predominant lipid in human milk.

11.30 **Which condition is MOST LIKELY to be associated with bottle-feeding?**
a. need for orthodontia
b. weak masseter muscles
c. speech and articulation disorders
d. broadly arched palate

11.31 **You are reviewing the patient handouts used in your hospital's maternity unit. Which type of handout is a violation of the International Code of Marketing of Breast-milk Substitutes?**
a. instruction sheet from a breast pump company on how to assemble, clean, and use their breast pumps
b. referenced information from a formula company on how to prepare, store, and feed their brand of formula
c. cosmetic company literature on that company's ointment marketed as a treatment for sore nipples
d. general information on breastfeeding written by a feeding-bottle company that displays the company's logo

11.32 **Pacifier (dummy, soother) use is MOST STRONGLY ASSOCIATED with:**
a. improved dental development
b. increased ear infections
c. decreased risk of SIDS
d. shorter duration of breastfeeding

11.33   **Which condition is UNRELATED to women's lactation status?**
   a. postbirth hemorrhage
   b. delayed return to prepregnancy weight
   c. menstrual irregularities and pain
   d. closely spaced pregnancies

11.34   **Which of the infant's host defense systems are MOST EFFECTIVE at birth?**
   a. ability to cough
   b. low pH of the stomach contents
   c. innate defensins in the baby's skin and vernix
   d. complement system and phagocytes

11.35   **Which statement describes the MOST RELIABLE research tool?**
   a. The tool has not broken in 5 years of continuous use.
   b. Using the tool produces the same results, even when used by different people at different times.
   c. The tool is quick to master and easy to use by multiple researchers.
   d. The tool was developed by well-known researchers at a large, prestigious university.

11.36   **You recently read a published article by an IBCLC that sounds very much like something you wrote several years ago. Comparing the two documents confirms that you were correct. What is your NEXT course of action?**
   a. The article has already been published. There is nothing further you can do.
   b. Contact the writer directly to voice your concerns.
   c. Contact the publisher of the magazine to voice your concerns and request the material be properly cited in print.
   d. Begin legal proceedings against the writer for plagiarism.

11.37   **During normal breastfeeding, where does the mother's nipple tip lie in the infant mouth?**
   a. junction of hard palate and alveolar ridge
   b. junction of hard and soft palate
   c. junction of soft palate and uvula
   d. junction of uvula and epiglottis

11.38   **If a mother says her nipples are tender and sore, which of the following is MOST LIKELY to reduce her discomfort?**
   a. wet teabags
   b. glycerin gel dressings
   c. purified lanolin
   d. expressed milk

11.39   **A mother is complaining about a red, hot, tender, wedge-shaped area on one breast. Which of the following other symptoms of this condition is she MOST LIKELY to also experience?**
   a. fatigue
   b. itching nipples
   c. stabbing pain
   d. flu-like aching

11.40 **A mother reports painful nipples and asks about this white spot that she believes is a plugged nipple pore (bleb). What is the FIRST thing you would do?**

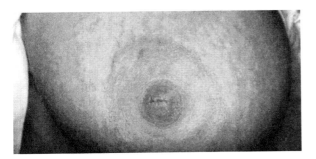

See color plate 87.

  a. Carefully observe a full breastfeed, examine her breasts, and observe the baby's mouth.

  b. Suggest she wash her nipples with warm water after every feed and massage the nipple tip.

  c. Use a sterile sharp instrument to open the plugged area of the nipple tip.

  d. Provide her with written material on plugged pores (nipple blebs) to discuss with her physician.

11.41 **Which of the following BEST describes the role of LCs in a clinical (hospital) setting?**

  a. The LC serves as a volunteer.

  b. One full-time LC position can serve about 780 hospital inpatients.

  c. The LC must work under the direct supervision of a physician

  d. LC positions must make a profit for the institution.

11.42 **This mother hopes to become pregnant soon. She has no sensation in the portion of the breast and nipple shown in the photograph. What is the major nerve supplying this part of the breast?**

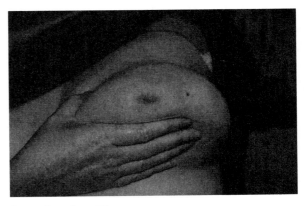

See color plate 88.

Courtesy of K. Jean Cotterman.

  a. fourth lateral intercostal

  b. brachial plexus

  c. sciatic

  d. superclavicular

11.43 **A woman had an emergency hysterectomy at 37 weeks' gestation. Which of the following statements is MOST relevant to her ability to breastfeed?**

  a. The mother may have difficulty establishing a full milk supply if she experienced excessive blood loss.

  b. The mother will be unable to produce milk if her ovaries were removed along with her uterus.

  c. The baby may nurse poorly due to the effects of the mother's anesthetics.

  d. The baby's first nursing may be delayed for several hours.

11.44 **Which component of milk VARIES MOST with maternal diet?**

  a. lactose

  b. immunoglobulins

  c. vitamins

  d. protein

11.45 **Which aspect of lipid composition VARIES MOST in human milk?**

   a. ratio of unsaturated to saturated fats

   b. profile of fatty acids (chain length)

   c. percentage of fat in a given feed

   d. ratio of triglycerides to cholesterol

11.46 **Which body system is MOST AFFECTED by breastfeeding?**

   a. orofacial musculature

   b. gastrointestinal functioning

   c. urogenital system

   d. speech and language

11.47 **What is the MOST LIKELY reason this device is being used?**

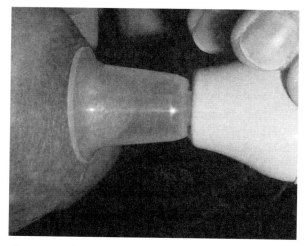

Courtesy of K. Jean Cotterman.

   a. pumping colostrum

   b. drawing out inverted nipple

   c. pressing back into the areola to reduce edema

   d. applying antiseptic liquid to nipple skin

11.48 **This child's imitative behavior suggests which of the following?**

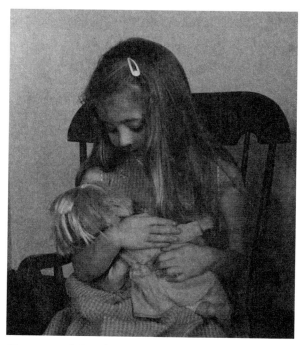

Courtesy of Carol Narigon/Sophie Holquist.

   a. latent homosexuality

   b. normal behavior modeling

   c. deviant behavior

   d. precocious sexuality

11.49 **This woman is planning to become pregnant. She is concerned about her nipple size and worried that her baby will have difficulty breastfeeding. Your BEST response to her is:**

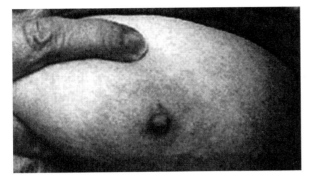

See color plate 89.

   a. Yes, your small nipple may be a problem.

   b. Normal nipples vary in size, and your nipple appears normal.

   c. Be sure to pull and roll your nipples daily throughout pregnancy.

   d. Wear breast shells during your pregnancy to increase eversion.

11.50 **A breastfeeding infant has been diagnosed with oral thrush. What is your FIRST recommendation?**

   a. Begin simultaneous treatment of the baby and mother's breasts.

   b. Unless the mother has signs of infection, treat only the baby's mouth with an antifungal medication.

   c. Check mother's nipples for signs or symptoms of infection.

   d. Assume that mother's nipples, all infant sucking objects, and possibly other infant areas are infected until proved otherwise.

11.51 **A mother is planning to return to full-time employment after her baby is born. Which suggestion for feeding her baby BEST supports breastfeeding?**

   a. Practice using a bottle before going back to work.

   b. Safely bedshare and breastfeed all night long.

   c. Have the caregiver feed your baby with slow-flow nipples.

   d. Prepare storage containers with 6 oz of milk for the caregiver.

11.52 **A researcher plans to study the effect of giving breastfeeding mothers an herbal preparation to increase milk supply. The mothers are all from the same community, and their babies are in the same age range. Which of the following is the DEPENDENT variable in this study?**

   a. use of the herbal preparation

   b. milk volume intake of the babies

   c. amount of milk pumped

   d. use of a placebo preparation

11.53 **How would you document the visual appearance of this lactating mother's nipple?**

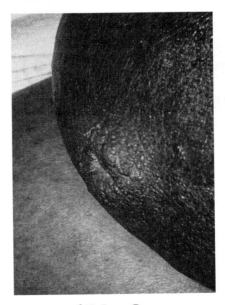

Courtesy of K. Jean Cotterman.

   a. inverted

   b. flat

   c. folded

   d. everted

11.54 **Why is it vital for the baby to breastfeed immediately postbirth, before any other substance is ingested?**
a. The gut is relatively high in pH.
b. The newborn gut is sterile and permeable.
c. To neutralize any residual amniotic fluid remaining.
d. The baby needs caloric support as soon as the cord is cut.

11.55 **Which hormone in the milk is MOST RESPONSIBLE for anti-inflammation activity?**
a. prolactin
b. prostaglandins
c. oxytocin
d. relaxin

11.56 **This mother's condition has persisted for 2 weeks despite correcting the baby's positioning and latch. What is the MOST LIKELY strategy to resolve this condition?**

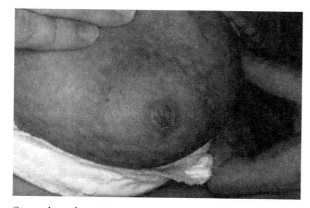

See color plate 90.
Courtesy of Catherine Watson Genna.

a. Apply a nipple shield during feeds to protect the area.
b. Massage some expressed milk into the area to speed healing.
c. Coat the area with a thick ointment to prevent scab formation.
d. Rinse the area with clean water, then apply an antifungal ointment

11.57 **The standard temperature and time for Holder pasteurization used in donor human milk banks is:**
a. 87°C for 10 minutes
b. 70°C for 25 minutes
c. 62.5°C for 30 minutes
d. 60°C for 60 minutes

11.58 **The FIRST thing that the LC should do for this mother's nipple condition is:**

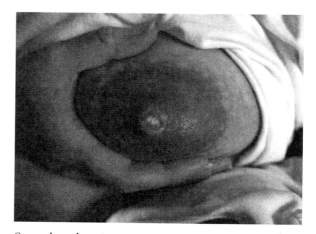

See color plate 91.
Courtesy of Catherine Watson Genna.

a. Request that the primary provider culture the skin for infection.
b. Wash off the white substance to examine the underlying skin.
c. Position the baby deeper onto the breast to prevent friction on the nipple tip.
d. Instruct the mother to massage expressed milk into the nipple tip.

11.59 **Which statement about the effect of human milk on the child's immune system would be MOST IMPORTANT to medical students?**
  a. Human milk stimulates baby to begin making his own SIgA and other antibodies.
  b. Exclusively breastfed babies have poorer response to immunizations.
  c. Mother's own milk provides passive immunity between placentally acquired immunity and autonomous immune protection.
  d. The breastfed baby is at higher risk of infection because he relies on mother's immune protection during breastfeeding

11.60 **Which of the following components found in breastmilk may be particularly important as an energy source for the rapidly developing brain of the infant?**
  a. lactose
  b. taurine
  c. choline
  d. iron

11.61 **When revising or creating policies relating to breastfeeding, which of the following provides the STRONGEST evidence for the policy?**
  a. meta-analyses
  b. randomized controlled trials
  c. case-control studies
  d. case reports

11.62 **Which of the following situations DO NOT REQUIRE written documentation?**
  a. phone calls from clients
  b. bedside contacts with mothers in a hospital
  c. clinic or office visits when the primary care provider also sees the client
  d. telephone inquiries about business hours or prices

11.63 **This mother complains of increasingly sore nipples and this rapidly growing condition on her nipple. What would be your BEST course of action?**

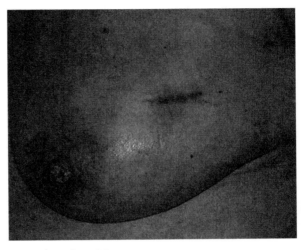

See color plate 92.
Courtesy of Catherine Watson Genna.

  a. Give the mother information on candidal infections of the nipple.
  b. Refer her to a qualified medical care provider immediately.
  c. Suggest she wash her nipples with water after each feed.
  d. Inquire about the red line on the lateral side of the breast.

11.64 **To minimize your legal risk when practicing as an LC, it is MOST IMPORTANT for you to:**
  a. keep accurate financial records.
  b. obtain detailed information from the primary care provider(s).
  c. establish a respectful rapport with open communication.
  d. accept the client's health insurance payment plan.

11.65 **Which statement regarding depression in breastfeeding mothers is MOST ACCURATE?**
a. Mothers must avoid treatment with antidepressants during breastfeeding.
b. Depression is higher in breastfeeding mothers than in formula-feeding mothers.
c. Breastfeeding mothers have suppressed cellular immunity when exposed to stress.
d. Breastfeeding protects maternal health by downregulating the stress response.

11.66 **The condition pictured outside the nipple and areola on this woman is very sensitive about once a month. She has two similar areas on her torso. What is this condition MOST LIKELY to be?**

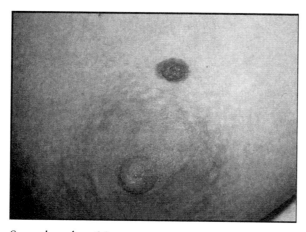

See color plate 93.
Courtesy of Carole Dobrich.

a. warts
b. hyperpigmented moles
c. skin cancer
d. accessory nipples

11.67 **Which aspect of maternal–infant bonding with mothers of multiple infants is most likely to occur FIRST?**
a. Mother bonds with the unit.
b. Mother bonds with the firstborn.
c. Mother bonds with the lastborn.
d. Mother has delayed bonding with all babies.

11.68 **Which breast structure contains muscle fibers?**
a. lactiferous sinuses
b. nipple–areola complex
c. Montgomery tubercles
d. lactocytes

11.69 **A research article reports that giving a baby one bottle of formula daily between the 2nd and 6th weeks postbirth had no effect on breastfeeding outcomes at 6 weeks. Which aspect of the study would MOST CAUSE you to question its conclusions?**
a. The planned-bottle group gave an average of five to nine bottles per week.
b. From 45% to 70% of the total breast-feeding group gave up to two bottles per week.
c. No in-person, skilled follow-up care was provided to either group of mothers and babies.
d. The content of the bottles used (whether formula or mother's own milk) was not consistently documented.

11.70 **Of the following, which is the MOST SIGNIFICANT risk when a breastfeeding mother who smokes tobacco sleeps next to her baby?**
a. Nicotine inhibits her let-down response.
b. Secondhand smoke triggers respiratory illness.
c. Exhaled carbon monoxide reduces oxygen to the baby.
d. Particles of tobacco residue on her clothing are irritants.

11.71 **What is thought to be the PRIMARY function of the Montgomery glands?**
a. pigmented marker for visual targeting
b. to lubricate the skin of the areola
c. to secrete antibiotic substances
d. change elasticity of areolar skin

11.72 **Which cranial nerve is responsible for the gag response and, if triggered, may inhibit the infant's deep latch at breast?**
a. hypoglossal (C XII)
b. vagus (C X)
c. trigeminal (C V)
d. glossopharyngeal (C IX)

11.73 **Which of the following respiratory conditions is MOST serious condition related to infant feeding?**
a. otitis media (ear infections)
b. bronchitis and bronchiolitis
c. asthma
d. wheezing/reactive airway disease

11.74 **The MOST IMPORTANT determinant of drug penetration into milk is the mother's:**
a. plasma level
b. body weight
c. blood type
d. milk storage capacity

11.75 **Which maternal medication is MOST LIKELY to require temporary discarding of the mother's milk?**
a. tetracycline
b. iodine-131
c. diazepam
d. prednisone

11.76 **Which statement is MOST ACCURATE about the variation in composition of human milk?**

a. Fat levels vary within a feed.
b. Zinc levels increase over time.
c. Lactose levels are related to time of day.
d. Vitamin K is lowest in colostrum and then increases.

11.77 **Which of the following statements regarding the relationship between breastfeeding and postpartum depression is the MOST ACCURATE?**
a. Breastfeeding mothers do not get postpartum depression.
b. Breastfeeding increases the risk of postpartum depression
c. Breastfeeding problems increase the risk for postpartum depression
d. Breastfeeding has no relationship to mother's mental health.

11.78 **Which would be the MOST HELPFUL activity for celebrating World Breastfeeding Week?**
a. Setting up a display showing environmental hazards associated with formula manufacturing.
b. Instituting a hospital policy that all mothers must breastfeed their babies at least once before the hospital staff will assist them with formula feeding.
c. Compiling a printed and online directory of local lactation support services in the community.
d. Printing "Breastfeeding Welcome Here" stickers/signs for local businesses and employers.

11.79 **Which practice is MOST LIKELY to suggest that a health care provider is unsupportive of breastfeeding?**
a. breastfeeding texts on office shelves
b. providing formula samples or coupons
c. LC on staff
d. list of mother support groups provided to all clients

11.80 **What is the LC's MOST IMPORTANT role in helping this mother and baby?**

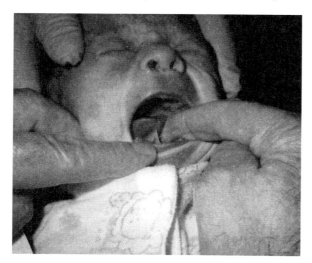

Courtesy of K. Jean Cotterman.

a. Learn to perform the procedure that will increase mobility of the tongue.

b. Hold the baby steady while the clinician performs a frenotomy.

c. Teach the mother to hand-express her milk while the baby's suck improves.

d. Help the mother position the baby with deep latch immediately after frenotomy.

11.81 **Which contraceptive method is MOST LIKELY to inhibit breastfeeding?**

a. barrier methods

b. progestin methods

c. intrauterine devices

d. estrogen patches

11.82 **Which is the primary or main immuno-globulin found in human milk?**

a. IgA

b. IgE

c. IgG

d. IgM

11.83 **A baby begins sucking on his fists about 45 minutes after the last feed ended. His mother should:**

a. give the baby a pacifier.

b. nurse the baby again.

c. change the baby's diaper.

d. wait until he cries, then feed him.

11.84 **Some women who have experienced childhood sexual abuse (CSA) by family members do choose to breastfeed their babies. Research shows that, compared with breastfeeding mothers who have not experienced such abuse, which of the following are CSA survivors LESS LIKELY to experience?**

a. lack of pleasure and sexual response while breastfeeding

b. heightened concern about controlling where breastfeeding occurs and being able to cover up

c. difficulty establishing an emotional bond with her baby

d. belief that her breasts cannot be trusted to make nutritious breastmilk in adequate amounts

11.85 **Which organization fostered and financially supported the development of the LC profession?**

a. International Lactation Consultant Association

b. La Leche League International

c. American Academy of Pediatrics

d. International Board of Lactation Consultant Examiners

11.86 **Tail of Spence is mammary glandular tissue that:**

a. is present only with supernumerary nipples.

b. does not produce milk.

c. extends into the axilla.

d. is not connected to the breast's duct system.

11.87 **A mother asks how to maximize the amount of milk connected with an automatic-cycling electric breast pump. Your BEST suggestion is to:**

a. pump for 10 minutes on the first breast, then 10 to 15 minutes on the other breast.

b. use the maximum tolerable vacuum pressure.

c. set the speed to cycle as fast as possible.

d. use a narrow-diameter flange for maximum nipple stimulation.

11.88 **What is the function of the infant's epiglottis during swallowing?**

a. prevents milk from entering the trachea

b. prevents air from entering the esophagus

c. propels the bolus of milk to the back of the mouth

d. traps the bolus of milk, triggering a swallow

11.89 **A research study found that when a baby has been given a pacifier for every sleep but does not get one on a particular night, the baby may be more likely to die from Sudden Infant Death Syndrome (SIDS). Which conclusion can accurately be made from that report?**

a. All babies should get pacifiers for every sleep to prevent SIDS.

b. Pacifiers do not interfere with breastfeeding.

c. If a mother begins giving a pacifier, she may need to continue doing so.

d. Breastfed babies are protected from SIDS if they breastfeed all night long.

11.90 **Which statement is TRUE about experimental research designs?**

a. Controls receive the intervention; subjects do not.

b. The independent variable is manipulated to see what happens to the subjects.

c. The dependent variable is manipulated to test the hypothesis.

d. Confounding variables do not affect the results of the experiment.

11.91 **A speaker's lecture title is very similar to a lecture you have prepared and presented at a large conference recently. You have not given anyone else permission to use your particular lecture material. What is the FIRST action you should take?**

a. Report the speaker to the Ethics Committee of IBLCE.

b. Contact the speaker and find out if proper attribution is being made in the presentation.

c. Contact your attorney to investigate whether the speaker violated copyright laws.

d. Ignore the situation under the assumption that LCs may independently create similar material.

11.92 **A mother requests your help with her faltering milk supply. After ruling out breastfeeding management, which of the following would be MOST APPROPRIATE?**

a. Loan her a book about herbal preparations.

b. Tell her to buy domperidone from an online pharmacy.

c. Recommend that her physician conduct metabolic and endocrine tests.

d. Suggest she discuss alternative therapies with her primary care provider.

11.93 **Which of the following actions by a health care worker is a violation of the International Code of Marketing of Breast-milk Substitutes?**

a. Accepting a carton of a new specialized formula for research at the institutional level.

b. Distributing generic volu-feed bottles to parents whose babies are in the neonatal intensive care unit.

c. Teaching formula-feeding parents how to safely prepare formula on a one-to-one basis.

d. Giving samples of two competing brands of formula to non-breastfeeding mothers so they can test them.

11.94 **You work in a clinic with an LC who advises mothers to "toughen up" their nipples by rubbing them with a rough washcloth during pregnancy. The FIRST action you should take is to:**

a. immediately lodge a complaint with the IBLCE Discipline Committee.

b. bring in research evidence of the harmful nature of this practice, and discuss it with the LC.

c. form a committee to develop written protocols on all aspects of lactation practice for your clinic.

d. try to intercept all of the clients seen by this LC and correct the misinformation.

11.95 **Which of the following is considered "fair use" of published written material according to International Copyright Law?**

a. downloading or photocopying one copy of a published research article for your personal use

b. making copies of a research article for all participants in your for-profit breastfeeding course

c. using pictures downloaded from the Internet in your presentations or lectures

d. making lecture handouts that include reproductions of copyrighted images that you purchased

11.96 **Which type of bacteria are MOST DANGEROUS for the newborn?**

a. anaerobic bacteria in the gut

b. enterococcal bacteria in the feces

c. *Staphylococcus epidermis* on the skin

d. aerobic bacteria on the mucous membranes

11.97 **Which component of human milk is MOST IMPORTANT in preventing neonatal septicemia?**

a. lysozyme in colostrum

b. SIgA antibodies

c. oligosaccharide receptor analogues

d. lactoferrin protein

11.98 **What effect does at least 7 months of breastfeeding have on urinary tract infections?**

a. higher risk of infections unless water is given, because less urine is produced by the breastfed child

b. lower risk of infection for up to 2 years because of SIgA antibodies and lactoferrin in milk

c. no difference in the risk of infection after supplements and family foods are started

d. no difference in boys, but breastfed girls have increased risk after 6 months of breastfeeding

11.99 **Banking of donated human milk has been practiced since the early 1900s. Which factor is MOST IMPORTANT in dispensing banked donor milk?**

a. being financially able to afford its purchase

b. acquiring a prescription from the physician

c. being under the age of 3

d. Socio-economic status of the family

11.100 **Which of the following situations is a VIOLATION of the ethical principle of role fidelity?**

a. An IBCLC in private practice tells her clients to take fenugreek to increase milk supply.

b. A physician/IBCLC prescribes metoclopramide for low milk supply.

c. An IBCLC instructs a mother on methods to increase a low milk supply and helps her to rent an electric breast pump.

d. A nurse/IBCLC assists the mother of a premie to increase her milk supply by increasing frequency of pumping and refers her to a physician for a prescription.

11.101 The UNICEF/WHO Ten Steps to Successful Breastfeeding (Baby-Friendly Hospital Initiative) includes which one of the following steps?

a. Train all maternity staff with 3 hours of breastfeeding education.

b. Give only breastmilk to premature infants under 37 weeks' gestation.

c. Use at-breast supplementers for supplementing breastfed infants.

d. Encourage feeding on cue for all parents regardless of feeding method.

11.102 Which maternal prenatal factor is MOST LIKELY to compromise lactation?

a. three previous closely spaced pregnancies

b. maternal underweight

c. maternal obesity

d. mother older than 35 years

11.103 A pregnant woman taking phenobarbital for several years asks about the safety of this medication when breastfeeding. Where would you find the BEST source of information on drug compatibility with breastfeeding?

a. a neighborhood pharmacist

b. the drug package insert

c. her obstetrician or midwife

d. published current breastfeeding text

11.104 Your hospital is working toward Baby-Friendly designation but is currently giving out discharge bags donated by a formula company. Why does this violate the International Code of Marketing of Breast-milk Substitutes?

a. Mothers are more likely to start early formula use if they get a free sample.

b. Brand-name formula is more expensive than generic (store) brand products.

c. The International Code prohibits distributing free samples to new mothers.

d. The samples contain powdered formula, which is never sterile and possibly contaminated.

11.105 Which one of the following is a core component of the Lactational Amenorrhea Method (LAM) of contraception?

a. Baby must be less than 12 months old.

b. There should be no more than 2 hours between feedings during the day.

c. All sucking is at the breast; no pacifiers or bottles are used.

d. Mother has no vaginal bleeding after the 36th day postpartum.

11.106 Which description of oral function of the baby during breastfeeding is the MOST IMPORTANT?

a. sense of taste and smell of milk

b. pressure of the breast against the oral tissues

c. tactile sensation of breast filling the infant's mouth

d. ability of infant to control shape of breast

11.107 When a breastfeeding baby has this condition, the FIRST thing you would do is:

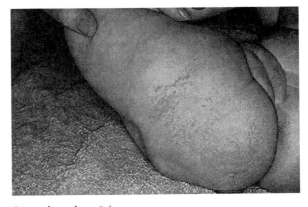

See color plate 94.

a. Treat the baby and mother's breast for a fungal infection

b. Check the child for other manifestations of allergic responses

c. Advise the mother to change the baby's diaper more frequently

d. Have the mother apply a cortisone ointment on the rash

11.108 **What is the MOST IMPORTANT function of lactose in human milk?**

a. supplies of 40% of infant's energy needs

b. aids absorption of phosphorus and manganese

c. protects the gastrointestinal tract from pathogens

d. supports the central nervous system (CNS) and cognitive development

11.109 **A mother is adamant about not wanting to breastfeed or provide her pumped milk or to obtain donor human milk. She asks which manufactured formula would be next safest for her baby. Your BEST suggestion is:**

a. soy-based liquid

b. goat's milk

c. cow's-milk–based powdered

d. cow's milk–based liquid

11.110 **A mother expressing milk for premature twins notices that her milk is slightly green colored on the second day post-birth. What should she do with the milk?**

a. Ask the laboratory to run bacteriological tests.

b. Examine her diet for the presence of foods high in chlorophyll.

c. Discard the milk until the greenish color is no longer present.

d. Feed it to her baby as usual.

11.111 **Which of the following components of human milk protects the baby by binding nutrients needed by pathogens in the baby's gut?**

a. lactoferrin

b. lysozyme

c. mucins

d. oligosaccharides

11.112 **The FIRST thing you would suggest to the mother whose nipple looks like this is:**

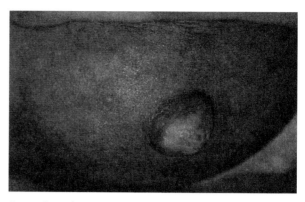

See color plate 95.

Courtesy of Catherine Watson Genna.

a. Have your doctor culture the nipple skin for thrush.

b. Wash your nipple with plain cool water after feeding.

c. Use a nipple shield for the next day or two.

d. Keep the nipple warm, especially after feeds.

11.113 **Which of these sets of symptoms is MOST LIKELY to culture positive for mammary candidiasis?**

a. deep aching pain

b. itching on the areola

c. achy breast pain

d. shiny nipple skin

11.114 **A research study is designed to determine whether breastfeeding decreases the incidence of asthma in 5-year-olds. Pregnant women are asked whether they plan to breastfeed. Five years later, the children are examined for signs and symptoms of asthma. This type of research design is called**

a. intent to treat.

b. double blind.

c. crossover.

d. meta-analysis.

11.115 **Which maternal factor is MOST RESPONSIBLE for the amount of milk consumed by a baby at a feed?**
   a. size of the breast
   b. number of milk ejections
   c. number of milk ducts
   d. amount of fat in the breast

11.116 **In a Baby-Friendly Hospital, which of the following is a standard care practice?**
   a. All mothers and babies room-in 24 hours per day.
   b. Infant formula is never administered to breastfed babies.
   c. All physicians and staff are competent in teaching hand expression of breastmilk.
   d. Mothers need to bring their own formula.

11.117 **A research study examined the effectiveness of supplemental feeding away from the breast compared with supplemental feeding at the breast. Women were randomly selected to participate ($N = 258$). Feeding-tube devices were used to supplement at the breast, and cup feeders were used to supplement away from the breast. The results demonstrated that supplementing at the breast was more effective than supplementing away from the breast ($p < 0.02$). What is the MOST SIGNIFICANT flaw in this study?**
   a. The participants were not selected with breastfeeding experience as a criterion.
   b. The independent variables were inconsistent.
   c. The probability was not significant.
   d. There are no significant flaws in this study.

11.118 **You are planning to stock several kinds of breastfeeding equipment in your private practice. Which item MOST INCREASES your liability?**
   a. cloth baby slings made by a commercial manufacturer
   b. 30-mL syringes that have been altered for use as nipple-pulling devices
   c. manual breast pumps distributed by a formula company
   d. small plastic cups made for storing food

11.119 **Which component of human milk is active against at least 40 tumors?**
   a. alpha-lactalbumin
   b. beta-lactoglobulin
   c. lactoferrin
   d. gangliocides

11.120 **A breastfeeding mother with type 1 (insulin-dependent) diabetes melliltus (IDDM) is at increased risk for which of the following conditions?**
   a. insufficient milk supply
   b. mastitis
   c. oversupply
   d. plugged milk ducts

11.121 **You are helping a woman who has a documented allergy to dairy products (cow's milk). Which of the following foods would provide many of the nutrients contained in dairy products?**
   a. rice and potatoes
   b. almonds and cashews
   c. spinach and onions
   d. corn tortillas soaked in lime

11.122 **Which statement MOST ACCURATELY documents this mother's breast and nipple?**

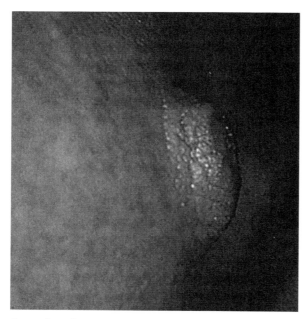

See color plate 96.

Courtesy of Greg Notestine.

  a. The nipple is short and somewhat flat.
  b. The nipple–areolar complex has poor elasticity.
  c. The nipple tip is very soft and pliable.
  d. The nipple inverts between feeds.

11.123 **At what point during gestation does the mammary ridge form?**
  a. 4–5 weeks
  b. 14–15 weeks
  c. 24–25 weeks
  d. 34–25 weeks

11.124 **A mother was given 40 mg of a drug with a half-life of 4 hours. How much of the drug is left in her system after 4 half-lives have elapsed?**
  a. 20 mg
  b. 10 mg
  c. 5 mg
  d. 2.5 mg

11.125 **Cholecystokinin, which is released by sucking, has which of the following effects?**
  a. arousal
  b. satiety
  c. agitation
  d. depression

11.126 **Which term refers to the middle score in a range of scores?**
  a. mean
  b. median
  c. mode
  d. meridian

11.127 **You think you are seeing a certain phenomenon in your clients. In order to study this more thoroughly, the FIRST kind of research study you might design or undertake would be**
  a. observational study.
  b. qualitative survey.
  c. case reports.
  d. clinical trial.

11.128 **Which statement describes a false-negative (Type II) error in a breast-feeding research study?**
  a. deciding there is a difference between groups when there is no real difference
  b. deciding there is no difference between groups when there is a real difference
  c. failure to include a control group
  d. using too small a sample size to detect differences between groups

11.129 **What's the MOST IMPORTANT difference between pasteurized donor milk and mother's own milk?**
  a. species specificity
  b. allergy prevention
  c. bioavailability
  d. potential HIV exposure

11.130 **Which relationship between postpartum depression and breastfeeding is MOST COMMON?**

a. Depression precedes breastfeeding cessation.

b. Breastfeeding cessation can lead to depression.

c. Depression is not related to breastfeeding.

d. Depressed mothers should not breastfeed.

11.131 **Which breast structure contains the cells that secrete milk?**

a. lactiferous ducts

b. lobules

c. alveoli

d. nipple

11.132 **Which of the following is an example of a QUALITATIVE research design?**

a. What are mothers' experiences of breastfeeding after cesarean birth?

b. How many mothers in Norway gave birth by cesarean section in 2003?

c. Is there a relationship between cesarean birth and infant suck dysfunction?

d. What percentage of babies are helped by LC contact 3 days after a cesarean birth?

11.133 **When selecting a device to assist breastfeeding, which is the MOST IMPORTANT principle to consider?**

a. Use a device authorized by your employer.

b. Select the least expensive device.

c. Use the least intervention for the shortest time.

d. Obtain informed consent from both parents.

11.134 **What is a clinically appropriate use of a nipple shield?**

a. feels like the breast in the baby's mouth

b. therapeutic changes in baby's oral-motor response

c. enhances milk transfer in some babies with weak suck

d. extends duration of breastfeeding

11.135 **You work in a public health department that is developing a vitamin D policy for pregnant women, breastfeeding mothers, and infants. Your BEST recommendation based on global research is to:**

a. screen all mothers and babies, and supplement those who are at risk or have low levels.

b. supplement all pregnant women, breast-feeding mothers, and breastfed babies.

c. warn all mothers to avoid using sun-screen on babies under 6 months old.

d. provide vitamin D supplements to dark-skinned mothers and babies.

11.136 **Which of the following is an example of mutual interdependency during breastfeeding?**

a. Baby's gut closure occurs around the time he is ready for solid foods.

b. Mother's milk contains environmental chemicals, triggering baby's immune system.

c. Skin contact during breastfeeding helps regulate baby's temperature.

d. Sucking at breast triggers release of gut hormones in mother and baby.

11.137 **A lactating mother noticed two raised bumps on her areola that drip milk when her baby is nursing on the other breast. These bumps are MOST LIKELY:**

a. Montgomery glands.

b. milk duct pores.

c. warts.

d. insect bites.

11.138 **You are working with a mother who complains of sore nipples. When you observe her breasts, you see the condition pictured. What should be your NEXT action?**

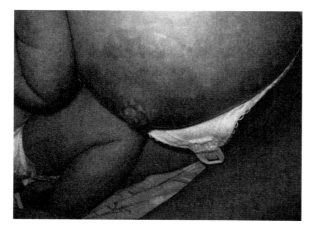

See color plate 97.
Courtesy of Catherine Watson Genna.

   a. Tell her to stop breastfeeding on that breast immediately.
   b. Give her a tube of antibacterial ointment.
   c. Wash your hands, put on sterile gloves, and wipe off the nipple with gauze.
   d. Contact her primary care provider and request diagnosis and treatment of the condition.

11.139 **During breastfeeding, how long does the nipple extend beyond its resting length?**

   a. one-quarter resting length (25%)
   b. half again (50%)
   c. twice its length (100%)
   d. it does not extend at all (0%)

11.140 **Which muscle is responsible for closing the lips around the nipple or other object?**

   a. masseter
   b. temporal
   c. orbicularis oris
   d. internal pterygoid

11.141 **Which property of maternal medications INCREASES the amount of the drug that gets to the breastfeeding baby via breastmilk?**

   a. short half-life
   b. no active metabolites
   c. high oral absorption
   d. high gut destruction

11.142 **A mother calls you, frustrated because her 3-week-old baby's preference for nursing at the right breast is so strong that she is unable to get him to nurse on her left side. What is the MOST LIKELY explanation for this baby's nursing behavior?**

   a. There is a subtle positioning difference in the mother's hold on her left side.
   b. The mother is making much more milk in the right breast.
   c. The mother has an undetected breast cancer in her left breast.
   d. The baby has a birth injury affecting his neck and shoulders.

11.143 **A mother has been having migraine headaches and asks about various remedies and their effect on her nursing 3-week-old. The remedy MOST LIKELY to affect her baby is:**

   a. acetaminophen
   b. an herbal preparation
   c. a homeopathic remedy
   d. a caffeinated beverage

11.144 **A breastfeeding mother must receive a radioactive isotope for diagnostic testing. How long should she wait before breastfeeding her baby again?**

   a. 5 days
   b. 48 hours
   c. 5 half-lives
   d. she must completely wean

11.145 **Which conclusion can be drawn from Chart 1?**

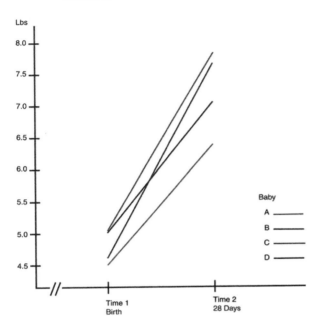

a. Baby A will always be smaller than baby D.

b. Baby B gained weight faster than the others.

c. Baby C is failing to thrive.

d. Baby D gained the most weight in 1 month.

11.146 **Which nutritional recommendation is MOST RELEVANT to a breastfeeding mother?**

a. Drink a large glass of water whenever she breastfeeds.

b. Avoid spicy or gas-producing foods.

c. Increase her caloric intake to make enough milk.

d. Follow her usual dietary practices.

11.147 **You are helping a mother 3 days after a surgical procedure to drain a breast abscess. Her breast is firm, and milk is leaking from the incision, which is on the lateral side of the breast near her chest wall. What is the FIRST action she should take?**

a. Put the baby to breast on the affected side to relieve milk stasis.

b. Express or pump milk from the affected breast and discard the milk.

c. Massage the affected breast to push milk out of the incision and out of the nipple.

d. Apply cold packs to the affected side and continue to feed on the other breast.

11.148 **Why is human milk often a bluish-white color?**

a. The whey:casein ratio of human milk is 80:20.

b. The whey:casein ratio of human milk is 20:80.

c. Secretory IgA is a blue color.

d. Human casein does not bind calcium.

11.149 **Where is MOST of the glandular tissue of the breast located?**

a. deep in the breast, close to the chest wall

b. clustered on the distal ends of the milk ducts

c. interspersed throughout the breast fairly evenly

d. within a 30-mm radius of the nipple base

11.150 **Mother support groups are MOST EFFECTIVE for which of the following reasons?**

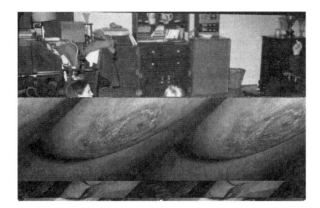

a. Groups meet in members' homes.
b. The group leader is highly trained.
c. Cost for support groups is usually low.
d. Mothers hear other mothers' ideas.

11.151 **The risk of which of the following maternal reproductive cancers is MOST INCREASED in women who do not breastfeed after pregnancy?**

a. cervical cancer
b. premenopausal breast cancer
c. ovarian cancer
d. endometrial cancer

11.152 **A research article claims that bottle-feeding results in the need for fewer orthodontic corrections than breastfeeding. The sample size was 438 children, the standard deviation was 0.7, and breastfeeding was defined as feeding at the breast at least once a day. What is the MOST SERIOUS flaw in this study?**

a. the sample size
b. the standard deviation
c. the definition of breastfeeding
d. there are no obvious flaws in this study

11.153 **How long does it take the infant gut to recover its normal flora after ONE bottle of artificial baby milk?**

a. two feedings
b. 2 days
c. 2 weeks
d. 2 months

11.154 **A research study was conducted in which cholesterol levels were examined in breastfeeding women and women who were not breastfeeding. An analysis of the statistics from the study resulted in a standard deviation of 0.6 for the breastfeeding cohort and 1.2 for the non-breastfeeding cohort. What can we learn from this distribution of data?**

a. The breastfeeding mothers had more similar cholesterol levels.
b. The non-breastfeeding mothers had more similar cholesterol levels.
c. The breastfeeding mothers had better cholesterol levels than the non-breastfeeding mothers.
d. The non-breastfeeding mothers had better cholesterol levels than the breastfeeding mothers.

11.155 **You are writing a pamphlet on breastfeeding for new mothers. The BEST advice on whether to use one or both breasts is:**

a. Use only one breast per feed.
b. Be sure to use both breasts per feed.
c. Let the baby finish one breast before switching to the second breast.
d. Switch breasts several times per feed.

11.156 **A research report indicates that a sample of breastfed infants had no differences in illness rates from a comparable sample of artificially fed infants. While reading this report, the MOST IMPORTANT point to look for is:**

a. the type of study used.
b. operational definitions.
c. the sample used.
d. the review of the literature.

11.157 **Where is the BEST placement for the examiner's fingers when testing a nipple-areola complex for inversion?**

a. at the base of the nipple

b. at the edge of the areola

c. 3 inches back from the nipple tip

d. on the nipple itself, touching the nipple base

11.158 **What is the MOST LIKELY number of milk ducts terminating on the nipple?**

a. fewer than 6

b. 9 or 10

c. 15 to 20

d. more than 20

11.159 **You are visiting this mother in her home and observe this situation on her breast. What is the FIRST thing you should do?**

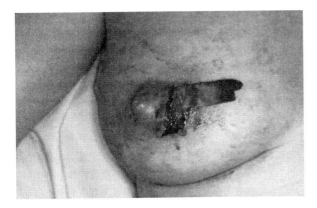

a. Document her history leading up to this situation.

b. Wearing gloves, assess the degree of milk stasis in the breast tissue.

c. Clean the incision and surrounding skin with an antiseptic solution.

d. Gently teach or assist in expressing milk from the injured breast.

11.160 **What is the MOST LIKELY outcome when a breastfeeding mother becomes ill?**

a. her milk supply often decreases.

b. she can transmit many diseases to her baby via her milk.

c. she can usually continue breastfeeding.

d. she is likely to be more sick than if she were not breastfeeding.

11.161 **Which of the following designations is considered legally valid in the United States?**

a. certified lactation educator

b. certified lactation nurse

c. breastfeeding peer counselor

d. International Board Vertified Lactation Consultant

11.162 **This condition has not improved with the application of antifungal ointment, antibacterial ointment, and several non-medicated nipple creams. What is your NEXT course of action?**

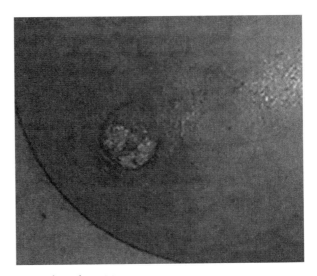

See color plate 98.

Courtesy of Catherine Watson Genna.

a. Suggest the mother wear a silicone nipple shield during feeds.

b. Examine the baby's mouth for signs of infection.

c. Recommend breast shells between feeds to keep the sore area from crusting over.

d. Refer the mother for a medical evaluation of the white areas on her nipple.

11.163 **You agreed to give a lecture presentation on breastfeeding to health care professionals. When you arrive for the event, you discover that the program is funded by a company that violates the International Code of Marketing of Breast-milk Substitutes in advertising their products. What is your MOST ETHICAL course of action?**

   a. Present the lecture without mentioning the Code or the funding from the company for the event.

   b. Give the lecture but donate your honorarium to a suitable charity that is not related to infant feeding or care.

   c. During your presentation, disclose to the participants that you were unaware of the funding and have refused the honorarium.

   d. Refuse to give your presentation, and walk out without explaining your reason for leaving to the event organizers.

11.164 **What is the MOST LIKELY reason this device is being used?**

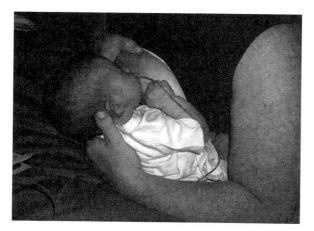

Courtesy of Catherine Watson Genna.

   a. Baby has a weak suck and cannot stay latched at breast.

   b. Mother adopted this baby 3 weeks ago and is building up her supply.

   c. Baby has a cardiac defect and tires easily when breastfeeding.

   d. Mother is giving a prescribed medication during each feed.

11.165 **An adopting mother is exploring maternal factors that may influence her ability to induce lactation. Which of the following factors or conditions is MOST LIKELY to reduce her chances of inducing lactation?**

   a. clinical depression

   b. mild anemia

   c. polycystic ovary syndrome

   d. hypertension

11.166 **A 16-month-old partly breastfed child has been diagnosed with food allergies. Which of the following is the MOST LIKELY allergy trigger?**

   a. rice

   b. cow's milk

   c. soy

   d. cabbage

11.167 **What is the MAIN function of the lymphatic system in the lactating breast?**

   a. drains extracellular fluid from breast tissue

   b. filters bacteria that have entered ducts

   c. provides local responses to infection

   d. supplies lymphocytes present in milk

11.168 **A research study claims no difference in prevalence of asthma between breastfed and formula-fed infants. Which aspect of the study would MOST CALL the findings into question?**

   a. All subjects were living in poverty conditions.

   b. All subjects were born by cesarean section.

   c. All subjects were given a latex pacifier for more than 1 hour per day.

   d. All subjects were given a bottle of formula in the first 48 hours.

11.169 **Why is the appearance of this breast MOST LIKELY to be caused by a condition in the infant's mouth?**

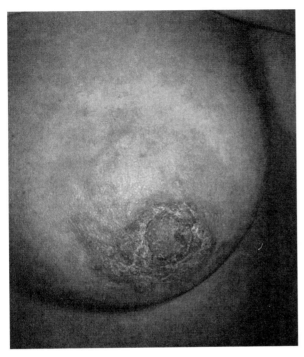

See color plate 99.

Courtesy of Catherine Watson Genna.

 a. The yellow areas around the nipple are probably infant saliva.

 b. The reddened area is asymmetric and mostly below the nipple.

 c. The baby recently had an oral candidal infection.

 d. There is no visible darkened areola.

11.170 **When is the equipment shown in this picture MOST APPROPRIATE?**

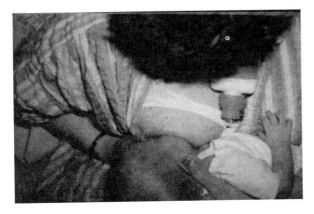

 a. inducing lactation when the baby is adopted

 b. supplementing an impaired baby at breast

 c. correcting a baby's dysfunctional sucking pattern

 d. aiding the mother to reestablish breast-feeding after an interruption

11.171 **Which of the following designations is the globally recognized credential for LCs?**

 a. IBCLC

 b. CLC

 c. CLE

 d. BFC

11.172 **A breastfeeding mother calls to report waking up with a high fever, chills, and flu-like aches. Her left breast is red and painful. Which is the MOST LIKELY condition causing these symptoms?**

 a. blocked milk duct

 b. inflammatory mastitis

 c. infectious mastitis

 d. breast abscess

11.173 **A woman who took phenobarbital (carbamazepine) during pregnancy to control seizures wants to exclusively breastfeed. Which of the following infant signs is MOST LIKELY to be related to this drug transferring to her milk and should be reported to the primary care provider(s)?**

 a. facial rash

 b. sedation or drowsiness

 c. vomiting or spitting up

 d. fussiness, excessive crying

11.174 **A 22-year-old woman has had bilateral breast reduction surgery. After the surgery, her surgeon reported that he believes he had been very successful in not severing many, if any, lactiferous ducts. The surgical technique performed was the "Round Block" pedicle procedure, wherein the only incision is around the perimeter of the areola with the areola and nipple still attached to a pedicle of tissue that is moved into a higher position. What effect on her future milk production can she expect?**

    a. It is impossible to estimate what her milk supply will be.

    b. It is unlikely that there will be a diminished milk supply.

    c. It is likely there will be diminished milk supply.

    d. Other factors have a greater bearing on her milk supply.

11.175 **Which of these research designs has the HIGHEST internal validity?**

    a. quasi-experimental group studies

    b. case-control studies

    c. cross-sectional surveys

    d. pre-test followed by post-test

11.176 **Training expenses for Step 2 are sometimes a barrier for some facilities working toward Baby-Friendly designation. Which of these sources of funding is unethical?**

    a. hospital or private charitable foundations with humanitarian missions

    b. government-funded grants, stipends, or budget-line allocations

    c. formula company–sponsored training courses

    d. religious institutions affiliated with the hospital

11.177 **Which product does NOT fall within the scope of the International Code of Marketing of Breast-milk Substitutes and subsequent World Health Assembly resolutions?**

    a. breast pumps

    b. infant formula

    c. feeding bottles and teats

    d. weaning foods

11.178 **Fresh human milk can be instilled in the eye to treat infections. Which component of milk is MOST LIKELY to be therapeutic?**

    a. casein

    b. fatty acids

    c. lysozyme

    d. mucins

11.179 **The MOST IMPORTANT deficit of all artificial feeding products is:**

    a. calcium.

    b. lactose.

    c. protein.

    d. leukocytes.

11.180 **A breastfeeding mother is prescribed fluconazole to treat a vaginal infection. She asks the LC whether it is safe to take this drug while breastfeeding. Which is your BEST response?**

    a. Yes, it's safe to take fluconazole while breastfeeding.

    b. What has the baby's pediatrician said?

    c. I would be glad to look it up in reference books.

    d. What is your baby's age and health status?

11.181 **A mother is concerned about an "odd smell" in a container of milk that she pumped 2 days ago and that has been stored in her refrigerator in a closed container. The milk smelled normal when she collected it. The MOST LIKELY cause of this odd smell is that:**

    a. the protein has been changed by amylase.

    b. the minerals have been changed by bile salt–stimulated lipase.

    c. the fats have been changed by lipase.

    d. the lactose has been changed by lysozyme.

11.182 **You want to document how a mother's nipples are healing under your care plan by taking a photograph at today's appointment. What permission is required?**

    a. The mother's verbal consent, during the consult, is sufficient.

    b. No permission is required; photographs allow you to chart clinical progress.

    c. Written permission from the mother, prior to your taking the photograph.

    d. Written permission from the mother, at the conclusion of the consult.

11.183 **Which of the following is a description, not a marketing statement, and thus meets the criteria of the International Code of Marketing of Breast-milk Substitutes and subsequent World Health Assembly resolutions?**

    a. Brand AA's Stage One foods for babies 4 months and older gently introduce single-ingredient pureed fruits and vegetables.

    b. Breast milk is the first choice for your infant's growth and development. But if you choose formula, Brand BB provides organic infant formulas that contain all the nutrients your baby needs.

    c. Brand CC bottle is the perfect product for babies of all ages, and this makes it easy for them to learn how to drink.

    d. Brand DD milk storage containers are compatible with most breast pumps, dishwasher-safe, leak-proof, and made of food-grade polypropylene.

11.184 **Which action is prohibited by the International Code of Marketing of Breast-milk Substitutes?**

    a. factual descriptions of a product that falls within the scope of the International Code

    b. company logo on instructions for using that company's breastmilk substitute

    c. a health care worker at a large institution accepting supplies for research and evaluation within their institution from a company does not meet their obligations under the Code

    d. no use of space, equipment, or education materials sponsored or produced by companies when teaching mothers about infant feeding

11.185 **Which product falls within the scope of the International Code of Marketing of Breast-milk Substitutes?**

    a. swaddling blankets

    b. breast pumps

    c. feeding bottles

    d. diapers

11.186 **Which of these statements BEST describes the mucosal defense system?**

a. A microbe is taken up by the mother's B cells and passed to M cells.

b. Helper T cells break down the pathogens.

c. The mother's secretory immune system provides targeted protection.

d. The infant's mucosal membranes provide passive immunity.

11.187 **A 27-year-old woman had breast augmentation surgery when she was 18. A 37-year-old woman had similar surgery when she was 33. The same surgeon performed both surgeries, using the same saline implant with a periareolar incision. What is the likely outcome for each woman's milk production?**

a. They are likely to have similar milk production, given that all other factors are similar.

b. The 37-year-old woman is likely to have greater milk production because she is older and has had more years of breast development.

c. The 27-year-old woman is more likely to have greater milk production because the longer interval of time has permitted more extensive recanalization and reinnervation.

d. It is impossible to estimate the milk supplies of these two women based on the facts presented.

11.188 **Sexual assault has a pervasive, negative effect on women's health and well-being. It can also influence her experience as a new mother. In a 2013 article in *Breast-feeding Medicine*, Kendall-Tackett et al. found that breastfeeding had which of the following impact on the effects of sexual assault?**

a. no effect on women's experiences

b. increased their risk of postpartum depression

c. breastfeeding lessened their risk of sleep problems

d. reduced their overall sleep quality

11.189 **To help this mother sustain exclusive breastfeeding for 6 months and continue breastfeeding for 2 years or more, which of the following would be the MOST IMPORTANT action that you could take?**

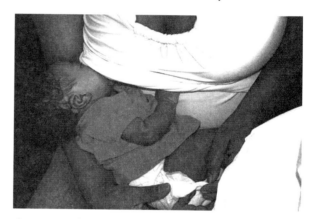

Courtesy of Kimarie Bugg.

a. Teach her to hand-express her milk so her family can help with the baby.

b. Refer her to a local mother-support or peer-support group.

c. Schedule monthly follow-up appointments in a lactation clinic.

d. Advise her to avoid pacifiers, bottles, and teats for the first 2 months.

11.190 This woman says the condition pictured on her inner thigh becomes tender about once a month. It is MOST LIKELY a (an):

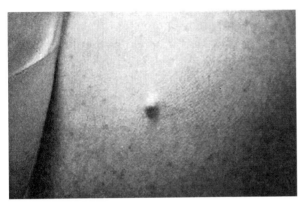

See color plate 100.

    a. skin tag responding to varying estrogen levels.

    b. wart that is sensitive to her clothing.

    c. mole that should be examined by a dermatologist.

    d. accessory nipple with sensitivity paralleling menstrual cycles.

11.191 Banked donor human milk has been used clinically to treat many diseases and conditions. Which of the following is the MOST COMMON and TRADITIONAL use of banked donor milk?

    a. treatment of adult gastrointestinal problems such as ulcers or colitis

    b. treatment for infantile botulism

    c. nutrition and immunological therapy for premature infants

    d. therapy for inborn errors of metabolism

11.192 A mother had surgery to drain a breast abscess. What is the MOST IMPORTANT contributing factor for breast abscess?

    a. partial formula-feeding

    b. mother had influenza

    c. sore nipples

    d. prolonged milk stasis

11.193 When selecting a drug to be given to a breastfeeding woman, which of the following drug properties is MOST IMPORTANT to consider?

    a. absorption from the gastrointestinal (GI) tract

    b. protein binding

    c. milk:plasma ratio

    d. pediatric half-life

11.194 Which statement BEST describes the role of the father of a exclusively breast-fed baby?

    a. Breastfeeding increases the father's jealousy of the mother–baby relationship.

    b. Fathers of breastfed babies miss out on the opportunity to bond during feeding.

    c. Breastfeeding is not a barrier to father–child bonding.

    d. The baby may attempt to feed from the father's breasts.

11.195 A research study concludes that an event happened purely by chance. Which probability value is MOST LIKELY to show an effect by chance?

    a. $p < 1.0$

    b. $p < .10$

    c. $p < .01$

    d. $p < .001$

11.196 Which of the following actions by LCs is unethical and PROHIBITED under the International Code of Marketing of Breast-milk Substitutes?

    a. Selling infant formula to mothers in your practice who are unable to produce enough milk

    b. Discussing preparation, storage, and safe bottle-feeding with individual mothers who need that information

    c. Purchasing several brands of formula, bottles, and teats for your clinical practice

    d. Distributing free samples of a new bottle that is marketed for breastmilk feeding to all prenatal clients

11.197 **Which statement about breastfeeding related to multiple sclerosis (MS) is MOST ACCURATE?**

a. Use extra household help whenever you can.

b. Many medications used for MS are compatible with breastfeeding.

c. Breastfeeding lowers the risk that her baby will develop (MS).

d. Breastfeeding decreases the likelihood of acute episodes of MS during the early postbirth period.

11.198 **On day 5 postbirth, a mother who has had breast reduction surgery notices that she has hard lumps in her breast that do not soften when the breast is drained. She is not currently experiencing fever or flu-like symptoms. What is your explanation and recommendation?**

a. Those are glands connected to ducts that have been severed. Because the milk has nowhere to go, the glands will quickly atrophy and the milk will be reabsorbed. .

b. Those are glands connected to ducts that have been severed. Because the milk has nowhere to go, the milk will stagnate and may become infected.

c. It is possible that the ducts connected to those glands may still be intact.

d. All nursing mothers normally have hard lumps in their breasts. The baby cannot drain all glands at each feeding.

11.199 **Which nodes collect MOST of the lymph drainage from the lactating breast?**

a. axillary nodes

b. intermammary nodes

c. subclavicular nodes

d. mesenteric nodes

11.200 **Which is the MOST IMPORTANT factor in how breastfeeding protects the infant against allergy?**

a. preventing the baby from exposure to nonhuman proteins

b. slowing or preventing the absorption of allergens through the baby's gut

c. protecting the baby's gut from inflammation, which weakens the mucosal barrier

d. providing white cells in milk, which attack the allergens directly

11.201 **You are aware of research that reports that chronic wounds can heal with topical use of manuka honey, which is (U.S.) FDA approved for its inherent antibacterial properties. To avoid ethical concerns about discussion of the product as part of a mother's care plan for her cracked nipples, you should:**

a. carry the product with you, to show how it is properly applied. Leave the sample with your client.

b. tell the mother about how the product works, and ask her to discuss with her primary healthcare provider whether it is appropriate for her use given her medical history.

c. discuss a variety of topical products that the mother might use to speed nipple healing, and ask her to consult with her primary health care provider first about which one to use.

d. ask the mother if she has any allergy to honey first.

11.202 **Which factor is MOST IMPORTANT in regulating the short-term rate of milk production?**

a. mother's intake of fluids

b. degree of breast fullness

c. maternal serum prolactin level

d. age of baby

11.203 **Breastfeeding care in a modern industri- alized health care system is IMPEDED MOST by its:**

   a. heightened emphasis on the baby at the expense of the mother.

   b. heightened emphasis on the mother at the expense of the baby.

   c. failure to consider the breastfeeding dyad as a unique biological unit.

   d. failure to consider the role of the father in solving breastfeeding problems.

11.204 **What is the MOST ACCURATE visual documentation of this woman's breasts?**

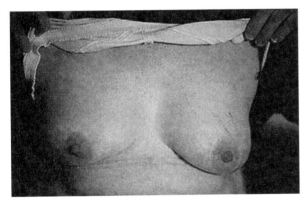

See color plate 101.

   a. Breasts are asymmetric with a pinkish nipple–areola complex.

   b. Right beast is very small; left breast is moderate size and pendulous.

   c. Both breasts have scant palpable glandular tissue.

   d. Right breast has insufficient glandular tissue for lactation.

11.205 **Which of the following has the STRONGEST evidence as an outcome of Implementation of the Baby-Friendly Hospital Initiative (BFHI)?**

   a. decreased rates of infant abandonment during the hospital stay

   b. decreased risk of upper respiratory tract infection in the first year of life

   c. increased rates of breastfeeding initia- tion, duration, and exclusivity

   d. decreased risk of gastrointestinal infec- tion in the first year of life

11.206 **Which component is found in the fatty (lipid) component of milk?**

   a. SIgA

   b. lactoferrin

   c. docosahexaenoic acid

   d. bifidus factor

11.207 **Which component of human milk is destroyed by freezing?**

   a. lactoferrin

   b. macrophages

   c. lysozyme

   d. SIgA

11.208 **A mother is coping with persistently sub- optimum milk production, despite nurs- ing her baby frequently with supplemental pumping. She asks about beverages, foods, or herbs to increase milk production. Of the following, which might have a positive effect on her milk production?**

   a. electrolyte-replacing fluids

   b. beer

   c. fenugreek tea

   d. sage infusion

11.209 **According to the Global Strategy for Infant and Young Child Feeding, what is the safest technique or device for feeding a baby who cannot feed directly at breast?**

   a. wide-base teat (nipple)

   b. slow-flow teat (nipple)

   c. tube-feeding device

   d. open cup or spoon

11.210 **Which policy document was adopted on August 1, 1990, in Florence, Italy, and contains specific national action steps to promote, protect, and support breastfeeding?**

    a. Innocenti Declaration

    b. International Code of Marketing of Breast-milk Substitutes

    c. Convention on the Rights of the Child

    d. Baby-Friendly Hospital Initiative

11.211 **A mother contacts you for help weaning her baby because she's going back to work and has no place to express and store her milk. Your FIRST response should be:**

    a. discussion of milk expression techniques and/or equipment.

    b. information on storing milk at room temperature.

    c. encouragement to wean completely.

    d. how to negotiate with her employer for reasonable accommodation.

11.212 **A mother, 4-year-old daughter, and 7-month-old baby were trapped in a snowbound car for 9 days. The mother breastfed both children after the small supply of food and liquids was exhausted. Which lactation-related hormone helped reduce stress in this mother?**

    a. estrogen

    b. progesterone

    c. prolactin

    d. placental lactogen

11.213 **What is the approximate risk reduction for leukemia conferred by breastfeeding?**

    a. 10% to 15%

    b. 20% to 30%

    c. 40% to 55%

    d. greater than 60%

11.214 **Which breast surgery technique is MOST LIKELY to preserve lactation function?**

    a. inferior pedicle reduction mammoplasty

    b. superior pedicle reduction mammoplasty

    c. periareolar incision

    d. lumpectomy

11.215 **Which falls outside the IBCLC scope of practice?**

    a. providing newsletters from the local mother-support group to mothers in your practice

    b. working closely with a dietitian in the case of a baby diagnosed with phenylketonuria (PKU)

    c. obtaining a referral from a surgeon before providing breastfeeding help to the mother of a newborn with an unrepaired cleft palate

    d. discussing a feverish mother's inflamed breast with her physician to develop an appropriate care plan that preserves breastfeeding

11.216 **"Exclusive breastfeeding" means that the baby:**

    a. breastfeeds directly and without restriction day and night.

    b. receives expressed or pumped breast-milk plus supplemental vitamins.

    c. receives less than 2 oz (60 mL) of other fluids per day.

    d. receives no formula or solid foods but is given a pacifier daily.

11.217 Your client's baby is having problems breastfeeding and appears to have oral thrush. She requests that you NOT report your findings to the baby's primary care provider. Your BEST response is to:

a. inform her that LCs are required to communicate relevant information to the primary health care provider(s).

b. agree to keep this information confidential.

c. provide information on over-the-counter treatments for oral thrush.

d. immediately discontinue providing breastfeeding care to this mother.

11.218 Which of the following components of mother's milk VARIES the MOST with the infant's feeding pattern?

a. proteins

b. minerals

c. fat-soluble vitamins

d. lactose

11.219 What is the MOST LIKELY reason this device is being used?

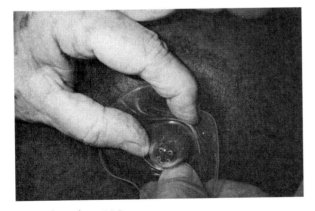

See color plate 102.

a. The mother's baby is premature and has a weak suck.

b. The mother is experiencing very painful nipples.

c. To help evert a flat or inverted nipple.

d. The baby is transitioning from bottle to breast.

11.220 Which of the following drug properties results in MORE transfer into milk?

a. low pH

b. highly protein bound

c. high milk:plasma ratio

d. low lipid solubility

11.221 The mother of a healthy 10-month-old must take tetracycline for 2 weeks and asks about possible effects on her baby. Your FIRST response should be:

a. Tetracycline is considered compatible with breastfeeding by the American Academy of Pediatrics.

b. Your baby will likely have diarrhea for the duration of your treatment.

c. Ask your doctor for an antifungal for your nipples to prevent thrush.

d. Offer more family foods to your baby while you are taking this medicine.

11.222 A mother saw a television advertisement for infant formula with added long-chain fatty acids, claiming the product would "result in early mental development scores." Why is this ad a violation of the International Code of Marketing of Breast-milk Substitutes?

a. No manufactured product made from animal milk can replicate human milk.

b. Long-chain fatty acids are not associated with early mental development.

c. The International Code forbids advertising of products covered by the Code to the general public.

d. The International Code requires television stations to give equal air time to breastfeeding promotion.

11.223 You are about to assess a breastfeeding mother–baby dyad. What should you do FIRST?

a. Obtain written consent from the mother.

b. Weigh the baby on a sensitive scale.

c. Examine the mother's breasts.

d. Wash your hands for 2 minutes.

11.224 **Which of the following educational opportunities violates the International Code of Marketing of Breast-milk Substitutes?**

   a. conferences sponsored by breastfeeding mother-support organizations or LC professional associations

   b. college courses in lactation management

   c. short courses and distance-learning programs run by lactation education organizations

   d. in-service programs presented by scientists employed by formula or feeding-bottle manufacturers

11.225 **A cultural attitude that emphasizes the sexual nature of breasts is MOST LIKELY associated with:**

   a. harassment for breastfeeding in public.

   b. increased breast augmentation surgery.

   c. mothers enjoying the attention created by larger breasts during lactation.

   d. conflicts in custody disputes involving breastfeeding babies.

11.226 **Breastfeeding rates are MOST AFFECTED by which health policies?**

   a. food security

   b. environmental protection

   c. reduction in family violence

   d. maternity protection

11.227 **Some brands of artificial baby milk produced in the 1980s lacked one essential mineral, causing brain damage and learning disabilities in the children who received this product exclusively. Absence of which of the minerals listed would have that effect?**

   a. sodium

   b. chloride

   c. potassium

   d. calcium

11.228 **Why would a professional organization issue a position paper on a topic?**

   a. directive that members of the association are required to follow

   b. has no influence on practices of members of the association

   c. represents the official position of the association to the public and its members

   d. marketing/publicity piece to increase prestige of the association

11.229 **A LC can BEST empower a mother by:**

   a. helping the mother meet her own breastfeeding goals.

   b. strengthen the mother's relationship with her partner.

   c. helping the mother meet her family's expectations.

   d. informing her that she is meeting public health recommendations.

11.230 **Your client is a 19-year-old mother with her first baby, new to the community, and away from all family support. Which strategy would be MOST SUPPORTIVE of her breastfeeding goals?**

   a. Schedule professional visits monthly.

   b. Connect her with a mother-to-mother support group.

   c. Tell her about classes available in the community.

   d. Help her find appropriate social media sites.

11.231 **What is the MOST LIKELY consequence of this hospital's Baby-Friendly policies?**

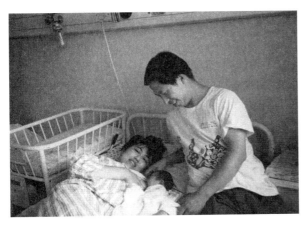

Courtesy of Mary Kroeger.

    a. The father can start bonding with his newborn daughter.

    b. The father can bottle-feed his daughter with infant formula if mother is too tired.

    c. The mother gets more rest because her baby is rooming-in with her around the clock.

    d. The hospital can employ fewer staff members because fathers provide much of the care.

11.232 **An exclusively breastfed baby needs surgery that must be performed under anesthesia. How long must breastfeeding be withheld before administration of anesthesia?**

    a. 30 minutes

    b. 2 hours

    c. 4 hours

    d. 6 hours

11.233 **What is the MOST IMPORTANT function of viral fragments that appear in human milk?**

    a. often cause infant illness

    b. act as a "vaccination" against disease

    c. digested by the infant as food

    d. can be killed by heat treatments

11.234 **Which operational target is included in the Innocenti Declaration of 1990?**

    a. developing a national infant and young child feeding policy

    b. adoption of the WHO Growth Standards in all health care settings

    c. implementation of the International Code of Marketing of Breast-milk Substitutes

    d. passage of legislation protecting a mother's right to breastfeed in public

11.235 **As part of BFHI training for maternity staff, what is the MOST IMPORTANT reason that the person on the left (in the white shirt) would be doing this to the person on the right?**

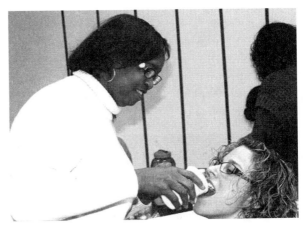

Courtesy of Kimarie Bugg.

    a. The person on the right is thirsty.

    b. Cup-feeding is an essential skill for maternity staff.

    c. In emergency situations, cups are safer than bottles.

    d. The training is being conducted in a low-resource setting.

11.236 **Which of the following features is MOST IMPORTANT in a pamphlet promoting breastfeeding?**

    a. listing advantages of breastfeeding

    b. comparison of breastfeeding with artificial feeding

    c. information about making enough milk

    d. local sources of breastfeeding help

11.237 The existing policy on the maternity unit at your hospital is to supplement all breastfeeding babies with 1 oz (30 mL) glucose water by bottle after every breastfeed. Which strategy is MOST LIKELY to be effective in changing this policy?

a. Include pediatricians, nursing staff, and neonatologists on the policy planning committee.

b. Distribute copies of research articles from peer-reviewed journals on the subject.

c. Plan a series of in-services for all affected staff to carefully educate them on the risks and benefits of supplementing breastfeeding babies.

d. Develop the new policy with a small core group, then tell the staff that they must follow the new policy.

11.238 This mother is concerned about the condition on her breast, which suddenly appeared when her baby was 4 months old. Which is the FIRST action you should take?

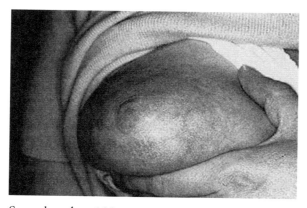

See color plate 103.

a. Visually examine the baby's mouth and throat.

b. Take a thorough history of the mother and baby.

c. Give her a topical steroid cream to reduce inflammation.

d. Recommend that she get a medical evaluation.

11.239 Which of the following activities is permissible under the terms of the World Health Organization's International Code of Marketing of Breast-milk Substitutes?

a. Discharge bags containing samples and coupons for formula are given to new mothers at hospital discharge.

b. Detailed information on product composition is provided to health workers.

c. Advertisements for toddler formula appear on local television stations.

d. A picture of a happy baby appears on the label of infant formula containers.

11.240 An article published in a women's magazine says that women who breastfeed feel better bonded to their infants compared with women who do not breastfeed. The article concludes that breastfeeding is desirable because of the effect of breastfeeding on the mother's attitude. Because women choose whether to breastfeed, the conclusion may be considered flawed because of:

a. sociocultural influences

b. confounding variables

c. lack of a placebo group

d. sample size

11.241 What is the FIRST step in developing and implementing evidence-based policies in your institution?

a. Gather research evidence for future use in policy development.

b. Convince the top administration to issue orders of the new policies.

c. Prohibit formula representatives from visiting the maternity floors.

d. Form a team of 5 to 12 representatives from all affected departments.

11.242 **Why might this mother use this technique?**

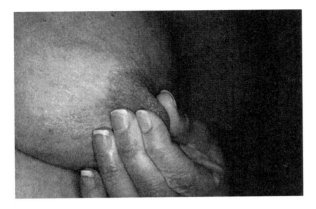

a. to massage a plugged nipple pore
b. to firm the nipple tip before feeding
c. to express milk
d. to increase tissue elasticity

11.243 **After appropriate treatment of infectious mastitis, a mother reports that a well-defined area of her breast remains red, hard, and tender. What should be your NEXT action?**

a. Encourage her to nurse her baby or hand-express frequently.
b. Teach her breast massage in the area of the lump.
c. Refer her to her primary care provider to rule out or confirm an abscess.
d. Suggest that she gradually reduce nursing to prepare to wean her child.

11.244 **Which is the MOST PREVALENT antibody on mucosal membranes and in human milk?**

a. IgA
b. IgE
c. IgG
d. IgM

11.245 **What is the MOST APPROPRIATE documentation of the appearance of this woman's breast?**

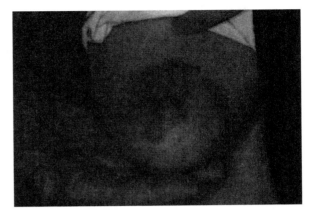

a. red circular area on the areola near the nipple margin
b. red lesion 0.5-in. (1-cm) diameter on the areola at the 7:00 position
c. bacterial infection on the areolar skin in the lower, outer quadrant
d. painful nipples with reddened area below the nipple base

11.246 **You have been collaborating with a physician regarding a breastfeeding mother who experienced a psychotic episode. The question is whether she should continue to breastfeed during drug treatment. The drug prescribed is considered compatible with breastfeeding. Your BEST response is:**

a. Breastfeeding may be healing for her under carefully controlled conditions.
b. Breastfeeding is contraindicated for mothers with mental illnesses.
c. Her baby is in great danger and should be kept away from her at all costs.
d. The hormones of breastfeeding will exacerbate her illness.

11.247 **Guidelines from the U.S. Centers for Disease Control and Prevention state that health care workers should wear gloves when assisting breastfeeding mothers in which of the following situations?**

a. touching a mother's breast

b. positioning a baby at breast

c. helping a mother pump her milk

d. processing donor human milk

11.248 **You are employed by a community rescue squad and are establishing a large shelter for victims of a devastating hurricane. To BEST prepare for a sudden influx of young families, your MOST IMPORTANT action should be to:**

a. use bottled water for preparing donations of powdered formula.

b. create private areas for pregnant and breastfeeding mothers.

c. stock plenty of ready-to-feed formula.

d. purchase hand-operated breast pumps to help re-lactation efforts

11.249 **Which drug taken by a breastfeeding mother is MOST LIKELY to have an effect on her baby?**

a. insulin

b. digoxin

c. caffeine

d. warfarin

11.250 **A primapara mother has had bilateral breast reduction surgery, with the inferior pedicle technique and 800 mL of breast tissue removed. On day 7, her baby is gaining well (30 g per day). What recommendation to the mother is MOST APPROPRIATE?**

a. No recommendation is necessary, as the mother has a full milk supply.

b. The mother should be encouraged to continue to track stool output for the next month and have the baby weighed regularly.

c. The mother should be advised to pump after every feeding to ensure that her milk supply remains as high as possible.

d. Information about herbal supplements should be given, as galactagogues are appropriate in order to maximize her milk supply

11.251 **Which type of cell in human milk gives rise to antibodies targeted against specific microbes?**

a. neutrophils

b. B-lymphocytes

c. macrophages

d. granulocytes

11.252 **Which of the following citations is a PRIMARY reference or source?**

a. DeCoopman, JM. Pacifier Use in Breastfed Infants: Review and Recommendations. (Masters' Thesis). Ann Arbor: University of Michigan, 1996.

b. Als H, Lester BM, Tronick E, and Brazelton TB. Manual for the assessment of preterm infants' behavior (AFPB). In Fitzgerald JE, Lester BM, Jogman MW, eds. Theory and Research in Behavioral Pediatrics, Vol. 1, New York: Plenum, 1982, 64–133.

c. Fildes V. Breasts, Bottles and Babies: A History of Infant Feeding. Edinburgh: Edinburgh University Press, 1986.

d. Aarts C, Hornell A, Kylberg E, et al. Breastfeeding patterns in relation to thumb sucking and pacifier use. Pediatrics 1999;104(4).

11.253 You are working to implement the Baby-Friendly Hospital Initiative (BFHI) in your facility. Scheduled feeds are often recommended for outdated and incorrect reasons. Your FIRST strategy should be to :

a. design charting forms with at least 8 to 12 spaces to record number of feeds per day.

b. during Step 2 training, explore and correct all the reasons that are given for scheduling feeds.

c. develop disciplinary measures for staff who continue to advise scheduled feeds.

d. meet with the prenatal class teachers and provide accurate patient handouts.

11.254 What is the MOST IMPORTANT feature when selecting a device like the one pictured?

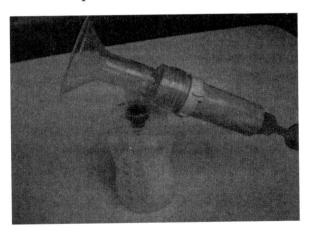

a. can cycle 40 to 60 times per minute

b. creates vacuum pressure in the range of 100 to 300 mm Hg

c. flange diameter easily accommodates the mother's nipple

d. requires sterilization after every use

11.255 What is the average percentage of a drug administered to a lactating woman that actually reaches the breastfeeding baby?

a. 0.01%

b. 0.1%

c. 1.0%

d. 10%

11.256 Which aspect of breast anatomy has been studied because of its role in breast cancer?

a. nervous system

b. lymph system

c. blood vessels

d. connective tissues

11.257 The mother of this baby is having difficulty latching on. How would you document what you see in this photograph?

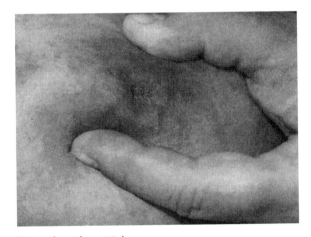

See color plate 104.

Courtesy of K. Jean Cotterman.

a. flat nipple with infection in the center

b. nipple appears inverted with crater in the middle

c. normal nipple pigment with pale areola

d. nipple is so inverted baby will never latch

11.258 **Which description BEST describes the configuration of milk ducts in the lactating breast?**

a. deep in the breast, like the core of an apple

b. branching begins posterior to the areolar margin

c. bulbous pea-shaped swellings near the areolar margin

d. superficial and easy to compress

11.259 **International Board Certified LCs are expected to recertify under the following circumstances:**

a. every 3 years

b. every 5 years

c. every 10 years

d. recertification is not required

11.260 **Manufacturers of artificial feeding products have attempted to increase the protective properties in their products by adding which of the following non-protein nitrogen compounds found in human milk?**

a. polyamines

b. nucleic acids

c. nucleotides

d. creatinine

11.261 **A breastfeeding mother should ensure that her diet includes:**

a. additional B vitamins.

b. plenty of liquids to ensure sufficient milk volume.

c. an extra 1000 calories per day.

d. her normal intake of food and drink.

11.262 **A 4-month-old exclusively breastfed baby requires surgery under general anesthesia. Which statement is MOST ACCURATE about fasting related to medical procedures?**

a. Withhold breastfeeding for 4 hours before the procedure.

b. Continue clear fluids up to 1 hour before the procedure.

c. Wait to begin breastfeeding until 2 hours after the procedure.

d. Give formula up to 2 hours before the procedure.

11.263 **Which drug property results in MORE transfer of the drug into mother's milk?**

a. Milk:plasma ratio <1.0

b. molecular weight >300

c. high protein binding

d. lipid solubility

11.264 **What is the MOST IMPORTANT function of SIgA in mother's milk?**

a. protects mucosal membranes

b. actively destroys bacteria

c. enhances inflammation

d. suppresses infant's immune system

11.265 **Which of the following ALWAYS occurs in the processing of banked donor human milk WORLDWIDE?**

a. pasteurization of milk prior to dispensing

b. bacteriological screening of milk

c. screening milk for environmental contaminants

d. serum screening of all donors

11.266 **Which study design presents the STRONGEST evidence for Kangaroo Mother Care?**

    a. Influence of feeding patterns and other factors on early somatic growth of healthy, preterm infants in home-based kangaroo mother care: A cohort study. J Pediatr Gastroenterol Nutr. 2005 Oct;41(4):430–437.

    b. Implementation of kangaroo mother care: A randomized trial of two outreach strategies. Acta Paediatr. 2005 Jul;94(7):924–7.

    c. Getting to know you: Mothers' experiences of kangaroo care. MCN Am J Matern Child Nurs. 2005 Sep–Oct;30(5):338.

    d. Early skin-to-skin contact for mothers and their healthy newborn infants. Cochrane Database Syst Rev. 2003;(2): CD003519.

11.267 **A breastfeeding mother sustained a broken pelvis in an accident. Which of the following actions is MOST SUPPORTIVE of breastfeeding after acute care is finished?**

    a. Provide her with a hospital-grade electric breast pump.

    b. Encourage family to bring her baby to her for feeding.

    c. Collaborate in selecting pain-relief medications compatible with breastfeeding.

    d. Help the family select an infant formula to use during her hospitalization.

11.268 **A research study of questionnaires given to 1000 women when their babies were 8 months old found that an increase in the breastfeeding rate at 6 months was correlated with the use of breast pumps. What conclusions can be drawn from this study?**

    a. Mothers breastfeed longer when they use breast pumps.

    b. Breast pumps facilitate breastfeeding.

    c. The sample size is insufficient to prove the relationship of breast pump use to breastfeeding duration.

    d. This study does not demonstrate that breast pump use fosters breastfeeding.

11.269 **A breastfeeding mother who follows a strict vegetarian diet (no animal protein whatsoever) should take a supplement containing which of the following vitamins?**

    a. vitamin A

    b. vitamin B_{12}

    c. vitamin C

    d. vitamin K

11.270 **Which is the MOST PREVALENT medical use for donor human milk?**

    a. postsurgical nutrition

    b. cancer treatment

    c. solid organ transplants

    d. allergies and feeding intolerance

11.271 **Which is the MOST IMPORTANT feature of an effective breast pump?**

    a. transfers milk effectively

    b. painless for mother

    c. from 20 to 40 cycles per minute

    d. from −100 to 250 mm Hg pressure

11.272 **The MOST EFFECTIVE educational strategy for prenatal teaching is:**

    a. including grandparents with new parents.

    b. teaching fathers (male partners) separately.

    c. using videos and DVDs in group settings.

    d. having nursing mothers talk about their experiences.

11.273 **Which of the following statements is an example of idealizing artificial feeding?**
   a. "Our teat has a flow rate similar to the breast."
   b. "Container is made of food-grade polypropylene."
   c. "Clear sides with quantity marking."
   d. "Cycles at 40 to 60 times per minute."

11.274 **Which trace element found in human milk substantially reduces the term newborn's risk of anemia for at least 6 months?**
   a. manganese
   b. fluoride
   c. iodine
   d. iron

11.275 **Lack of sensation in the nipple and areola is MOST LIKELY caused by damage to the**
   a. fourth intercostal nerve.
   b. supraclavicular nerve.
   c. thoracic intercostal nerve.
   d. spinal accessory nerve.

11.276 **Which of the following diseases is MOST LIKELY to be related to artificial feeding?**
   a. childhood obesity
   b. sudden infant death syndrome (SIDS)
   c. eczema (atopic dermatitis)
   d. gastrointestinal infections

11.277 **A mother asks why she can express an ounce of milk even after her baby finishes feeding. The MOST LIKELY explanation for this is that:**
   a. the baby is not feeding effectively.
   b. babies normally do not take all of the milk available at a given feeding.
   c. she has an oversupply of milk.
   d. her baby does not like the taste of her milk.

11.278 **Which of the following provisions IS part of the International Labor Organization (ILO)'s Maternity Protection Convention of 2000?**
   a. 4 weeks' maternity leave
   b. three or more nursing breaks per day
   c. on-site (workplace) child care
   d. job protection after maternity leave

11.279 **Which family planning (contraceptive) method is MOST COMPATIBLE with breastfeeding?**
   a. progestin-only oral contraceptives
   b. "combined" hormonal contraceptives
   c. barrier methods
   d. emergency contraceptives

11.280 **After giving your first lecture at a professional conference, you learn that the luncheon will be provided by an infant formula company. Your BEST response is to:**
   a. eat the lunch quietly with other participants, because raising the issue would embarrass the conference sponsor.
   b. refuse to eat the luncheon, and find another source for your food for that meal.
   c. announce from the speaker's stand that you are offended and refuse to give the rest of your lectures.
   d. thank the formula company publicly from the podium for their support of the conference.

11.281 **You suspect the mother and baby's breast-feeding situation will rapidly improve if the baby has the lingual frenulum revised or surgically released. To best meet your ethical obligations, you should:**

a. inform the mother of your diagnosis of ankyloglossia.

b. provide several options of health care providers who can examine for and diagnose ankyloglossia

c. explain how the baby's tongue is used during normal feeding and the impact of any anatomic restrictions

d. discuss use of breast compression during feeds to maximize flow and intake.

11.282 **Which of the following actions by an IBCLC is OUTSIDE the LC scope of practice?**

a. examining a breastfeeding mother's breast

b. developing supplementing policies for the NICU

c. dispensing and instructing on the use of breast pumps

d. advising a mother that prescribed medication is safe to use during breastfeeding

11.283 **A mother tells you, "Breastfeeding has been so wonderful! Now I want to talk to every pregnant woman and tell her to breast-feed!" This statement is an example of**

a. overenthusiasm

b. empowerment

c. delusion of grandeur

d. self-actualization

11.284 **When doing a review of the literature for a research study, which sources are MOST IMPORTANT to include?**

a. review articles that analyze several studies

b. textbooks that explain basic concepts

c. peer-reviewed journal report of research, written by the researcher

d. lectures given at large conferences by well-known speakers

11.285 **When are the levels of SIgA highest in human milk?**

a. in the second year of lactation

b. when the mother's own SIgA is highest

c. during the first 24 hours after birth

d. levels of SIgA are stable throughout lactation

11.286 **Which of the following actions is a violation of the International Code of Marketing of Breast-milk Substitutes?**

a. providing free samples of formula to all mothers who visit your clinic

b. teaching formula-feeding individually to mothers who have made the decision to not breastfeed

c. including bottles with the breast pump kits you sell to mothers who are returning to work

d. recommending a teat-style feeding device for a baby with a sucking disorder

11.287 **Which components of human milk are MOST STABLE to pasteurization and freezing?**

a. proteins

b. lipids

c. cellular components

d. minerals

11.288 **Which research study design is considered to be the MOST RIGOROUS?**

a. case-control

b. randomized controlled trial

c. quasi-experimental

d. observational

11.289 **Which situation is MOST LIKELY to cause the condition shown?**

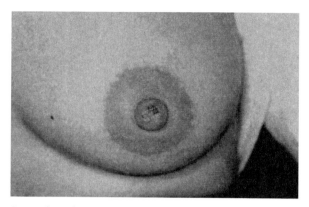

See color plate 105.

   a. baby has a short, tight frenulum
   b. shallow latch
   c. flat, inelastic nipple tissue
   d. biting during nursing

11.290 **Which component of human milk is MOST VARIABLE?**

   a. proteins
   b. lipids
   c. carbohydrates
   d. minerals

11.291 **When would this mother's baby receive milk with the highest fat content?**

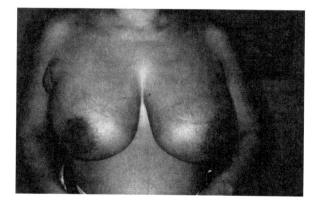

   a. the last 5 minutes of each feed on either breast
   b. after nursing several times on one breast
   c. in the middle of the night
   d. when mother is eating a high-fat diet

11.292 **A mother is concerned that her baby has suddenly lost interest in breastfeeding. Your BEST response is:**

   a. Do nothing. Breastfeeding mothers are usually overprotective.
   b. Reassure her that baby's appetite may change abruptly.
   c. Carefully investigate the situation.
   d. Instruct her how to give her milk in a bottle.

11.293 **A breastfeeding mother asks about taking an herbal remedy for migraine headaches. Your BEST response is:**

   a. Herbs do not pass into milk, so whatever you take should be safe.
   b. Comfrey is a good choice.
   c. Please discuss this with your physician and a qualified herbalist.
   d. Migraines are best treated with prescription drugs.

11.294 **About an hour after collection, bacterial counts in freshly expressed human milk are lower than immediately after collection. The MOST LIKELY explanation for this is that:**

   a. the cooler temperature in the container is unsuitable for growth of bacteria.
   b. macrophages in milk are actively phagocytic.
   c. gangliosides in milk disrupt the cell walls of bacteria.
   d. bifidus factor starves the bacteria of nutrients.

11.295 **When are the growth factors MOST CONCENTRATED in human milk?**

   a. 38 weeks' gestation
   b. 2 days postbirth
   c. 2 months postbirth
   d. 7 months postbirth

11.296 **A mother in Western industrialized cultures is MOST LIKELY to continue breastfeeding past 1 year if she has the support of:**

   a. her male partner.

   b. her father.

   c. her doctor.

   d. her sister.

11.297 **Which of the following components of bovine milk is MOST LIKELY to cause an allergic reaction in babies?**

   a. lactose

   b. beta-lactoglobulin

   c. alpha-lactalbumin

   d. lactoferrin

11.298 **Which drug property results in MORE transfer of the drug into mother's milk?**

   a. milk:plasma ratio <1.0

   b. molecular weight >500

   c. high protein binding

   d. lipid solubility

11.299 **Which product falls within the scope of the International Code of Marketing of Breast-milk Substitutes?**

   a. breast pumps

   b. milk storage bags

   c. pacifiers/dummies

   d. feeding bottles

11.300 **Which component of human milk affects stool composition and frequency in the baby?**

   a. whey:casein ratio

   b. soluble proteins

   c. lactose

   d. lipids

11.301 **You're assisting in an emergency shelter after a hurricane. What should you do with unsolicited donations of powdered infant formula?**

   a. Lock them up until legitimate need is determined.

   b. Prepare only with boiled water.

   c. Feed the donated products to adults.

   d. Rejoice at the generosity of the donor.

11.302 **Which carbohydrate is absent in human milk?**

   a. lactose

   b. oligosaccharides

   c. sucrose

   d. gluconjugates

11.303 **You are asked to help develop treatment policies that support breastfeeding for maternal infectious diseases in a family/general medical practice office. Which statement is MOST ACCURATE concerning risk to the breastfed baby of maternal infectious diseases?**

   a. Most maternal infections are passed to the baby through her milk, therefore immediate weaning is advised.

   b. Antibiotics for maternal infections are likely to cause severe problems in the breastfed baby.

   c. Babies can continue to breastfeed during maternal bacterial infections, but not viral infections.

   d. Mother's immune system makes specific antibodies to infections acquired during breastfeeding, so breastfeeding should continue.

11.304 **What is the name of the string-like structure under this baby's tongue?**

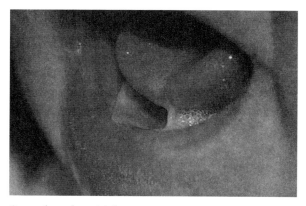

See color plate 106.

Courtesy of Greg Notestine.

    a. labial frenulum
    b. incisive papilla
    c. lingual frenulum
    d. mucous membrane

11.305 **Of the following options for mothers returning to work, which is the MOST PROTECTIVE of the breastfeeding relationship?**

    a. on-site child care
    b. paid maternity leave
    c. flexible working hours
    d. facilities for collecting and storing milk

11.306 **This mother is concerned about the condition shown in this picture. Which of the following is the MOST APPROPRIATE response?**

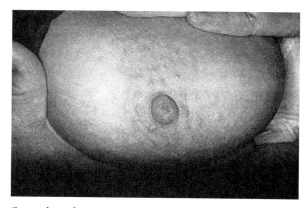

See color plate 107.

    a. You may have Reynaud syndrome. Keep the room warm when you breastfeed.
    b. The lumps are Montgomery glands, which help lubricate the skin. They're normal.
    c. This appears to be an allergic reaction. Did you recently start wearing a new bra?
    d. May I check your baby's mouth to see if he has a thrush infection?

11.307 **Which of the following substances accumulates in breastmilk if taken by the mother?**

    a. nicotine
    b. alcohol
    c. methadone
    d. *Cannabis* (tetrahydrocannabinol [THC])

11.308 **A baby's tongue is pressing a mother's nipple against the baby's hard palate. Which cranial nerve is MOST RESPONSIBLE for this tongue movement?**

    a. spinal accessory (C XI)
    b. vagus (C X)
    c. hypoglossal (C XII)
    d. trigeminal (C V)

11.309 **This mother wants to know if her breasts and nipples are normal. Which of the following is the MOST APPROPRIATE response?**

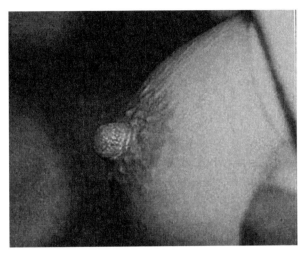

Courtesy of Greg Notestine.

    a. Your breasts are entirely normal.

    b. Your nipple is slightly retracted.

    c. Your areola is slightly narrow in diameter.

    d. Your large nipple will likely be a problem for your baby.

11.310 **What is the MOST LIKELY reason you would recommend this technique?**

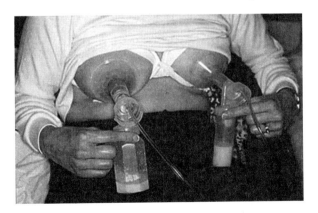

    a. premature baby

    b. separation of mother and baby for any reason

    c. mother taking a contraindicated medication

    d. mother has a history of sexual abuse

11.311 **What is the MOST ACCURATE description of this nipple shape?**

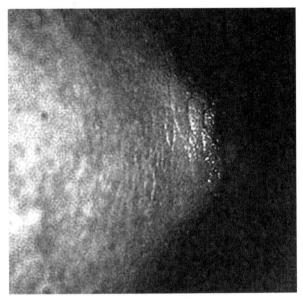

Courtesy of Greg Notestine.

    a. normal

    b. flat

    c. conical

    d. inverted

11.312 **This breastfeeding mother says that this condition appeared when her baby was about 4 months old. Which is the MOST LIKELY cause of the condition shown?**

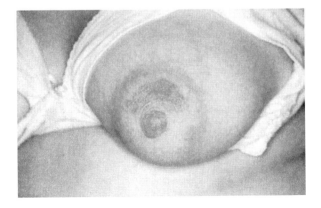

    a. atopic dermatitis

    b. fungal infection

    c. eczema

    d. psoriasis

11.313 **Which of the following is a result of pasteurizing donor human milk?**

a. concentration of lipids

b. reduction in lactose

c. inactivates viruses and eliminates bacteria

d. diminishes lactoferrin

11.314 **If a mother cannot provide her milk to her baby, the World Health Organization (WHO) recommends that the NEXT BEST food for her baby is:**

a. soy-based formula

b. cow's-milk–based formula

c. banked donor human milk

d. milk of another woman

11.315 **Additional body contact, as when the mother uses a soft tie-on type carrier, is MOST LIKELY to have which of the following effects?**

a. decreased total crying

b. increased dependency

c. delayed walking

d. more night waking

11.316 **What is the primary reason that the Baby Friendly Hospital Initiative Step 8 requires avoiding teats and pacifiers?**

a. Artificial teats have chemicals that can be toxic.

b. The liquid can flow too rapidly.

c. Artificial teats are hard to clean.

d. Teats can change oromotor patterning.

11.317 **In disasters and emergencies, what is the MOST IMPORTANT reason that a small open cup or spoon should be used to feed non-breastfed babies?**

a. inexpensive; readily available

b. deprives baby of comfort from sucking

c. avoids bottle/teat use

d. easy to clean

11.318 **Which of the following conditions is MORE common in children who were never breastfed?**

a. obesity

b. lower respiratory tract diseases requiring hospitalization

c. diarrhea and vomiting

d. asthma

11.319 **The pale-colored lumps on this mother's breast are MOST LIKELY:**

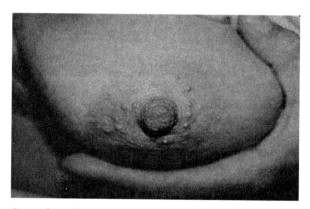

See color plate 108.

Courtesy of Greg Notestine.

a. lipomas.

b. plugged pores.

c. Montgomery's tubercles.

d. warts.

11.320 **If an LC sees this condition in a breast-feeding mother, which is the MOST IMPORTANT course of action to take?**

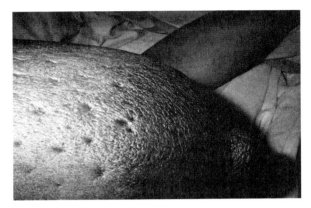

See color plate 109.

Courtesy of K. Jean Cotterman.

    a. Instruct the mother to use a lotion or oil to lubricate her skin.

    b. Apply cold green cabbage leaves.

    c. Contact her primary care provider to rule out cancer.

    d. Ask about any history of polycystic ovary syndrome (PCOS).

11.321 **Which is the MOST EFFECTIVE technique for hand expression of milk?**

    a. Compress the breast behind the areola, then slide the fingers toward the nipple.

    b. Pinch the base of the nipple.

    c. Press deeply at the nipple–areolar juncture.

    d. Position fingers at the edge of the areola, press inward, and roll toward the nipple.

11.322 **What is the reason that professions develop theoretical frameworks?**

    a. to keep graduate students busy

    b. to establish a systematic point of view

    c. to systematize their policies

    d. to establish standards of practice

11.323 **Which of the following psychosocial effects are breastfeeding mothers MOST LIKELY to experience?**

    a. depressing effect of lactation hormones

    b. enhanced fulfillment of their maternal role

    c. more work time lost because of babies' needs

    d. lower stress hormones

11.324 **The management of mother–baby couples addressed in the WHO/ UNICEF Baby Friendly Hospital Initiative (Ten Steps to Successful Breastfeeding) applies to:**

    a. all babies, no matter how fed

    b. all artificially fed babies

    c. only breastfed babies

    d. breastfed babies who room-in

11.325 **Which attribute of immunofactors in human milk is MOST ACCURATE?**

    a. decrease over the duration of lactation

    b. remain stable over the duration of lactation

    c. are all stable to heating or freezing

    d. are all acquired prenatally

11.326 **Which of the following is the MOST IMPORTANT impact of this practice on the infant's physiology?**

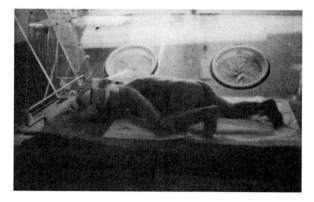

a. higher risk of infant suffocation
b. reduces infant pain
c. stabilizes infant temperature
d. increases infant oxygen saturation

11.327 **Which preparation would be MOST LIKELY to increase milk production?**

a. metronidazole
b. beer
c. domperidone
d. theophylline

11.328 **Which maternal disorder can negatively affect breastfeeding?**

a. Crohn's disease
b. polycystic ovary syndrome (PCOS)
c. dwarfism
d. epilepsy

11.329 **Which drug property is MOST LIKELY to permit high passage into milk?**

a. high lipid solubility
b. high pH
c. large molecular weight
d. high protein binding

11.330 **An LC working on a postpartum unit notices that a physician routinely prescribes medroxyprogesterone acetate (Depo-Provera) for all of "his" patients to prevent pregnancy before the 6-week postpartum return visit. The IBCLC knows that this drug may inhibit establishment of adequate and abundant milk supply. Ethically, the LC should:**

a. Follow the doctor's orders and assume he has told each patient about the potential hazards of the medication.
b. Discuss potential side effects on the milk supply with each mother prior to her receiving the injection.
c. Ask breastfeeding mothers if they know the potential problems with milk supply that may be related to this medication.
d. Report the physician to the ethics committee of the hospital for not using a medication according to the package insert.

11.331 **Which drug would MOST LIKELY inhibit lactation?**

a. bromocriptine
b. metoclopramide
c. domperidone
d. cimetidine

11.332 **During breastfeeding, where is the infant's tongue USUALLY placed?**

a. resting behind the alveolar ridge
b. covering the alveolar ridge
c. spread flat across the floor of the mouth
d. extended past the lower lip

11.333 **Research has shown that babies who received human milk have higher scores in cognitive development and vision. Which of the following milk components is MOST LIKELY to explain this difference?**

a. long-chain fatty acids
b. short-chain fatty acids
c. phospholipids
d. sterols

11.334 **Which infant reflex, if lacking, is an indicator that the child may have feeding problems?**
   a. rooting
   b. startle (Moro)
   c. Babinski
   d. tonic neck

11.335 **Of the following conditions, which is MOST LIKELY to result in this pattern of growth?**

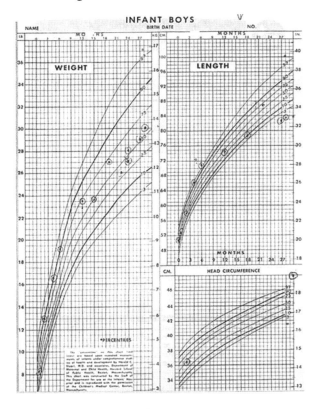

   a. Down syndrome
   b. exclusive breastfeeding
   c. premature baby
   d. exclusive formula feeding

11.336 **The mother in this picture says nursing her younger baby has been surprisingly uncomfortable right from the start. Her older child nurses briefly a few times day and night. Which factor is the MOST LIKELY reason for her discomfort?**

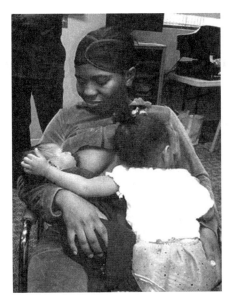

   a. Ambivalent feelings about nursing two siblings who are not twins.
   b. Oral structural anomaly in the younger child.
   c. Older child distracts the younger baby during nursing sessions.
   d. Low milk supply due to the demands of two nursing babies of different ages.

11.337 **A cohort of 300 pregnant women were asked the following question: "In light of the fact that breastfeeding increases children's intelligence, do you plan to breastfeed or bottle-feed?" The results reported that breastfeeding rates rose 48% since a similar survey was conducted 10 years earlier. Why would you question the reported result of this study?**
   a. The survey question began with a leading question.
   b. That amount of increase in rates is unlikely.
   c. The methods are not the same in the two studies.
   d. Pregnant women often change their minds after giving birth.

Answers for General Principles Questions

11.1 **The answer is c.** Although some assume that women with a history of sexual abuse or assault would want to avoid breastfeeding, research studies have found the opposite to be the case. Women with a history of abuse/assault breastfeed at the same rates as women without a history of assault. Those women are also more likely to intend to breastfeed and initiate breastfeeding. There is currently no research on why some women elect to pump their milk and feed it in a bottle. (Difficulty: 5; Discipline: Psychology; Taxonomy: Evaluate)

11.2 **The answer is d.** Alcohol in milk is directly related to levels in maternal serum and does not accumulate in milk. (Difficulty: 4; Discipline: Pharmacology; Taxonomy: Knowledge)

11.3 **The answer is d.** Secretory IgA is the predominant antibody in human colostrum and milk. The other components also have immunologic importance. SIgA is especially important to the infant in the first few days and weeks after birth. (Difficulty: 5; Discipline: Development; Taxonomy: Evaluate)

11.4 **The answer is c.** Employee retention has been shown to be the most prevalent benefit seen by employers who adopt breastfeeding support practices. The others are also true. Employee productivity is actually increased when mothers are enabled to continue breastfeeding their babies. (Difficulty: 5; Discipline: Psychology; Taxonomy: Collaboration)

11.5 **The answer is b.** First, discuss the mother's accusations with the LC in question. If the mother's report is accurate, the LC is violating the International Board Certified LC (IBCLC) Code of Professional Conduct and Standards of Practice and a complaint should be lodged with IBLCE. (Difficulty: 3; Discipline: Clinical Skills; Taxonomy: Plan)

11.6 **The answer is d.** Antibiotic treatments severely reduce the number of anaerobic bacteria, allowing the growth of pathogenic aerobic strains including *Klebsiella* and *Enterobacter*. It takes several weeks for the breastfed child's gut to recover, and much longer for the child who is deprived of human milk. (Difficulty: 4; Discipline: Pathology; Taxonomy: Knowledge)

11.7 **The answer is b.** Strong evidence supports evidence-based maternity care practices (BFHI) as having strong positive influence on breastfeeding rates. The others are positive but with weaker evidence. (Difficulty: 5; Discipline: Clinical Skills; Taxonomy: Collaboration)

11.8 **The answer is d.** Pumping through two let-downs often collects about 76% of available milk. The first let-down collects about 45% of available milk. More milk flows with higher pump pressure; a faster pattern at first followed by a slower pattern during let-down collects more milk; and tight flanges restrict duct expansion and therefore restrict milk release. (Difficulty: 2; Discipline: Techniques; Taxonomy: Evaluate)

11.9 **The answer is c.** Comparing the lines with the closed circles with the lines with the open circles, the closed-circle lines (representing skin-to-skin babies) represent higher temperature at all three places where the temperature was measured. (Difficulty: 3; Discipline: Clinical Skills; Taxonomy: Evaluate)

11.10 **The answer is b.** Macrophages and possibly neutrophils and T-lymphocytes actively kill microbes by phagocytosis. (Difficulty: 5; Discipline: Development; Taxonomy: History)

11.11 **The answer is d.** The first question should be, "Is it really necessary to take this drug at all, or at this time?" If the answer is clearly yes, then the other questions are appropriate in selecting a compatible medication for the mother's condition. (Difficulty: 5; Discipline: Pharmacology; Taxonomy: Collaboration)

11.12 **The answer is d.** See 3.1 of IBLCE's Code of Professional Conduct regarding preserving confidentiality. The duty of obtaining prior written permission for photographs is when the LC takes the picture, not the mother. But the LC has an overall duty of care to preserve confidentiality if the mother decides to take and send a photograph. (Difficulty: 4; Discipline: Clinical Skills; Taxonomy: History)

11.13 **The answer is c.** Antineoplastics, often called chemotherapy agents, are used in treating malignant tumors. Breastfeeding is usually contraindicated because of the potential risk to the infant. (Difficulty: 4; Discipline: Pharmacology; Taxonomy: Knowledge)

11.14 **The answer is c.** This was diagnosed by a physician as a bacterial infection of the nipple skin. Immediate weaning is not appropriate, because the baby has already been exposed and may even have caused the infection. A nipple shield may provide some comfort, providing it is thoroughly cleaned between uses. (Difficulty: 4; Discipline: Clinical Skills; Taxonomy: Collaboration)

11.15 **The answer is d.** The International Code applies to all health workers, including lactation professionals. (Difficulty: 4; Discipline: Clinical Skills; Taxonomy: Collaboration)

11.16 **The answer is a.** Pathogen finding is the most important function of lactoferrin. It is also an iron transport agent and reduces/prevents inflammation. Lactoferrin has no known function relative to nerve myelinization or growth. (Difficulty: 4; Discipline: Development; Taxonomy: Knowledge)

11.17 **The answer is d.** Her inverted or retracted nipple may be difficult for the baby to find and latch onto. Since she is not yet pregnant, the color of her areola, vein development, and breast size are not relevant to her potential ability to breastfeed. (Difficulty: 5; Discipline: Development; Taxonomy: Plan)

11.18 **The answer is d.** Research in Australia has found that the relative fullness of the breast accounts for about 70% of the fat variation in milk. (Difficulty: 4; Discipline: Development; Taxonomy: Evaluate)

11.19 **The answer is b.** IBCLCs are governed by the Code of Professional Conduct (CPC). Cooperating in an event where intellectual property laws regarding images on the Internet were probably violated and permitting a fraudulent link to a code-violating company could put the IBCLC in violation of the CPC. (Difficulty: 3; Discipline: Clinical Skills; Taxonomy: Document)

11.20 **The answer is b.** Professional malpractice insurance companies have access to qualified attorneys for their clients in ethical and legal matters. (Difficulty: 3; Discipline: Clinical Skills; Taxonomy: Collaboration)

11.21 **The answer is a.** Epidermal growth factor plays a major role in gut maturation. Lactoferrin also promotes tissue maturation. (Difficulty: 5; Discipline: Development; Taxonomy: Evaluate)

11.22 **The answer is b.** This is a large nipple with no abnormal conditions. A fibrous texture became apparent when the mother's breast was physically examined. (Difficulty: 4; Discipline: Development; Taxonomy: Assessment)

11.23 **The answer is c.** The milk ducts are channels that collect milk and direct it to the nipple. The ducts dilate during the milk-ejection reflex. Milk-secreting cells are in the alveoli; the areola is possibly a landmark for the baby, and the Montgomery glands (tubercles) secrete a substance that cleanses the areola. (Difficulty: 3; Discipline: Development; Taxonomy: Evaluate)

11.24 **The answer is b.** Maternal hydration and nutritional status are relevant to lactation capacity only if the mother is nearly in starvation herself. A well-nourished mother can produce large volumes of milk at little metabolic cost to herself, as in this true situation. (Difficulty: 3; Discipline: Development; Taxonomy: Knowledge)

11.25 **The answer is b.** Freezing destroys living white cells such as T- and B-lymphocytes. The other components are not significantly affected by freezing. (Difficulty: 5; Discipline: Development; Taxonomy: Evaluate)

11.26 **The answer is dc.** Ultrasound studies confirm that the tongue's wavelike peristaltic motion strips and gathers the milk and propels it to the posterior oropharynx. The droppping of the jaw and posterior tongue assist this process. (Difficulty: 5; Discipline: Development; Taxonomy: Knowledge)

11.27 **The answer is c.** A fully breastfed baby's thymus gland is twice the size of a formula-fed baby's. A small thymus at birth is related to low birth weight, malnutrition, and higher infant mortality. An old and false myth alleged that SIDS was due to a large thymus. Prenatal infections are a common cause of fetal death and are associated with smaller thymus glands. (Difficulty: 4; Discipline: Development; Taxonomy: Knowledge)

11.28 **The answer is c.** Lysozyme is the only of these components that meets all of these criteria. The others are vital anti-infective components. (Difficulty: 2; Discipline: Development; Taxonomy: Knowledge)

11.29 **The answer is b.** Lipase is secreted at the same time as lipids. Triglycerides are the predominant lipids in human milk. Human milk fat is far more easily digested, especially by premature babies, than any other source of lipids. (Difficulty: 4; Discipline: Development; Taxonomy: Knowledge)

11.30 **The answer is a.** Bottle fed children are more likely to need orthodontia and have weakened masseter muscles, more speech disorders, and a narrower palate. Bottle-feeding is not associated with normal broad palate configurations. (Difficulty: 4; Discipline: Pathology; Taxonomy: Knowledge)

11.31 **The answer is d.** Any marketing literature about products covered by the International Code must be scientifically accurate and factual and be limited to information on the use, composition, and other facts regarding that specific product. Information on general breastfeeding issues produced by companies manufacturing products covered by the InternationalCode are prohibited from being distributed in hospitals designated as Baby-Friendly Hospitals. Nipple treatment products are not covered by the code. (Difficulty: 3; Discipline: Clinical Skills; Taxonomy: Document)

11.32 **The answer is d.** Numerous studies report that pacifier use decreases breastfeeding. Children who use pacifiers have higher rates of ear infections than do those who do not use pacifiers. The evidence that pacifier use decreases risk of SIDS is weak. Some allege that "orthodontic shape" pacifiers improve dentition, but research reveals more orthodontic problems in children who use pacifiers. (Difficulty: 4; Discipline: Clinical Skills; Taxonomy: Evaluate)

11.33 **The answer is c.** Menstrual irregularities and pain are not known to be related to whether the woman breastfed her children. (Difficulty: 2; Discipline: Physiology; Taxonomy: Assessment)

11.34 **The answer is c.** Innate defensins on the baby's skin and in the vernix provide a measure of protection to the newborn. The other systems are not fully mature at birth. Breastmilk compensates for and enhances the development of other host defense systems. (Difficulty: 5; Discipline: Development; Taxonomy: Knowledge)

11.35 **The answer is b.** Reliability of a test instrument means that the instrument produces consistent results regardless of user, time of use, use over a duration of time, and when applied to different subjects. (Difficulty: 2; Discipline: Clinical Skills; Taxonomy: Knowledge)

11.36 **The answer is c.** Contacting the publisher is the next appropriate step to take. If the publisher does not respond, further legal action may be an option. Meanwhile, you may elect to lodge a formal complaint with IBLCE for violation of intellectual property laws. (Difficulty: 5; Discipline: Clinical Skills; Taxonomy: Document)

11.37 **The answer is b.** At rest, the nipple tip is slightly anterior to the juncture of the hard and soft palates. (Difficulty: 5; Discipline: Development; Taxonomy: Knowledge)

11.38 **The answer is b.** Conclusive evidence on remedies for nipple pain is lacking, although a review of clinical trials reported some pain relief from glycerin gel pads. Anything applied to the skin of the nipple will get into the baby's mouth. Rubbing anything into the nipple should be attempted only with freshly washed hands to prevent massaging any pathogens into the skin. Other causes of nipple pain should be explored and ruled out before considering any topical treatment. (Difficulty: 5; Discipline: Pathology; Taxonomy: Goals)

11.39 **The answer is d.** Infectious mastitis often presents with flu-like aching, fever and/or chills, and a red, tender area on one breast. Redness, pain, and heat may be present with noninfectious or infectious mastitis. If there is aching or fever and/or chills, she is more likely experiencing infectious mastitis and should be referred to a physician. Fatigue may be a contributing factor. Stabbing pain or itching nipples are not common during mastitis. (Difficulty: 3; Discipline: Pathology; Taxonomy: History)

11.40 **The answer is d.** Providing printed information on pathological conditions is always appropriate. It is not within the scope of practice of LCs to perform procedures, diagnose illnesses, or prescribe medications, even over-the-counter preparations. (Difficulty: 4; Discipline: Clinical Skills; Taxonomy: Plan)

11.41 **The answer is b.** It is estimated that one full-time equivalent LC position is needed for every 780 live births for postbirth inpatient care. Mannel and Mannel calculated full-time equivalent requirements for a large maternity hospital in the United States. (Difficulty: 5; Discipline: Clinical Skills; Taxonomy: Collaboration)

11.42 **The answer is a.** The fourth lateral intercostal nerve supplies the nipple and areola and is central to breastfeeding. The brachial plexus and the superclavicular nerve do not supply the breast. The sciatic nerve is in the hip and leg. (Difficulty: 2; Discipline: Development; Taxonomy: History)

11.43 **The answer is a.** Excessive blood loss may trigger pituitary shock and Sheehan syndrome, which suppresses prolactin response to sucking. Ovarian function postbirth is not related to lactation. (Difficulty: 4; Discipline: Physiology; Taxonomy: History)

11.44 **The answer is c.** Water-soluble vitamins vary with maternal intake. Fat-soluble vitamins vary slightly with maternal intake and exposure to sunlight. Deficiencies are rare except for vitamin B_{12} in mothers who consume no animal products, and vitamin D in women who lack sunlight exposure. Supplementing the mother in both cases increases these components in her milk. (Difficulty: 3; Discipline: Development; Taxonomy: Knowledge)

11.45 **The answer is c.** The major variation in fat content is related to the relative emptiness of the breast. The proportion of fat increases as the breast drains. Ratios of unsaturated to saturated fats and triglycerides to cholesterol are relatively stable. Fatty-acid profiles change slightly with changes in maternal diet. (Difficulty: 4; Discipline: Development; Taxonomy: Knowledge)

11.46 **The answer is b.** Breastfeeding profoundly affects gastrointestinal functioning and facial development, speech, and language. It is least related to urogenital development. (Difficulty: 4; Discipline: Physiology; Taxonomy: Knowledge)

11.47 **The answer is b.** This kind of device could be used to draw out an inverted nipple or press into the areola to reduce edema, or possibly to collect colostrum. This nipple puller is not being used and should not be used to squirt antiseptic liquid onto the nipple skin. (Difficulty: 4; Discipline: Clinical Skills; Taxonomy: Plan)

11.48 **The answer is b.** Young children imitating breastfeeding with a doll is a common and normal occurrence in most cultures worldwide. (Difficulty: 2; Discipline: Psychology; Taxonomy: Assessment)

11.49 **The answer is b.** Small nipples work just fine for breastfeeding. This woman's breast is entirely normal. (Difficulty: 5; Discipline: Development; Taxonomy: Goals)

11.50 **The answer is d.** Assume that the mother's nipples are also infected with the same organism, as well as other infant body parts and any/all sucking objects. Mother–baby cross-infection is likely when the baby has an oral infection. (Difficulty: 4; Discipline: Pathology; Taxonomy: Evaluate)

11.51 **The answer is b.** The most successful strategy of those listed is to breastfeed intensively when she is with the baby. Mothers should only breastfeed; other caregivers can give open cups or bottles with teats. Storage containers should have 2 to 3 oz per container: 6 oz is too much because babies typically take 2 to 3 oz per feed, and a larger amount would encourage waste. (Difficulty: 4; Discipline: Psychology; Taxonomy: Goals)

11.52 **The answer is c.** Amount of milk pumped is the dependent variable. Use of the herb or a placebo is the independent variable. Weight gain of the babies is a confounding variable, since milk volume intake by the baby may not reflect actual milk volume produced. (Difficulty: 3; Discipline: Clinical Skills; Taxonomy: Evaluate)

11.53 **The answer is b.** This nipple appears flat at rest. Visual appearance alone is an important part of a thorough evaluation, along with physical examination. (Difficulty: 4; Discipline: Pathology; Taxonomy: Document)

11.54 **The answer is b.** The newborn gut is sterile and should be protected by colostrum before anything other is ingested or inhaled. Colostrum paints the gut, sealing it from potential pathogens. (Difficulty: 4; Discipline: Pathology; Taxonomy: Knowledge)

11.55 **The answer is b.** Prostaglandins in the milk have anti-inflammatory properties which protect all tissues, especially the infant gut. (Difficulty: 4; Discipline: Development; Taxonomy: Evaluate)

11.56 **The answer is d.** Cracks at the base of the nipple plus shiny, reddened skin are most likely due to yeast (*Candida*) infection. Rinsing with clean water then applying an antifungal ointment with clean hands is most likely to resolve the infection. Choices a, b, and c are ineffective in the presence of a yeast infection. (Difficulty: 5; Discipline: Pathology; Taxonomy: Plan)

11.57 **The answer is c.** Holder pasteurization used by donor human milk banks raises the temperature of milk to 62.5°C for 30 minutes. (Difficulty: 5; Discipline: Clinical Skills; Taxonomy: Collaboration)

11.58 **The answer is a.** This is a bacterial infection of the nipple; therefore, the LC should arrange for a medical provider to properly diagnose the infection. Washing with water and positioning the baby more deeply onto the breast are reasonable actions after medical diagnosis is in progress. Massaging expressed milk into the nipple is inappropriate because there is no benefit, and it could exacerbate the infection. (Difficulty: 4; Discipline: Clinical Skills; Taxonomy: Plan)

11.59 **The answer is c.** Mother's own milk is an important passive immune system for the infant which dynamically changes as the dyad is exposed to pathogens. Human milk also stimulates and supports active immune system development in the infant (choice a). Choices b and d are false—breastfed babies have stronger positive responses to immunizations and lower risks of infections. (Difficulty: 3; Discipline: Development; Taxonomy: Collaboration)

11.60 **The answer is a.** Lactose is an especially important carbohydrate needed for brain development and is found in abundance in human milk. The other components are also found in milk and have importance to the infant. (Difficulty: 5; Discipline: Development; Taxonomy: Knowledge)

11.61 **The answer is a.** Systematic reviews and meta-analyses are the strongest forms of evidence for a policy or practice. Case reports are the weakest form of evidence. (Difficulty: 4; Discipline: Clinical Skills; Taxonomy: Evaluate)

11.62 **The answer is d.** Inquiries about price, hours, or other business transactions do not require written documentation. All clinical contacts, including by phone, should be documented. (Difficulty: 2; Discipline: Clinical Skills; Taxonomy: Collaboration)

11.63 **The answer is b.** This mother has Paget disease, a form of nipple cancer. She had "sore" nipples for several months and then noticed this lesion, which continued growing rapidly until a breast surgeon performed a mastectomy. The scar on her breast is from a tumor that was removed, probably the original site of the cancer. (Difficulty: 5; Discipline: Pathology; Taxonomy: Collaboration)

11.64 **The answer is c.** The most effective protection against legal actions is establishing a mutually respectful relationship and rapport. (Difficulty: 4; Discipline: Clinical Skills; Taxonomy: Collaboration)

11.65 **The answer is d.** Breastfeeding protects maternal mental health in multiple ways, including downregulating the stress response. The other choices are false. Most drugs for depression are compatible with breastfeeding; formula-feeding mothers have higher rates of depression, and cellular immunity is enhanced during breastfeeding. (Difficulty: 2; Discipline: Pathology; Taxonomy: Knowledge)

11.66 **The answer is d.** Accessory or supernumerary nipples and/or mammary tissue may be found along the "milk lines," which run from the upper inner arm to the inguinal region. Accessory mammary tissue develops during fetal development. The red area outside the nipple and areola is an accessory nipple with small areola. (Difficulty: 3; Discipline: Development; Taxonomy: Assessment)

11.67 **The answer is a.** Mothers of multiples are more likely to attach to the unit before the individual children. (Difficulty: 4; Discipline: Psychology; Taxonomy: Assessment)

11.68 **The answer is b.** Smooth muscle fibers are found in the nipple–areola complex. (Difficulty: 3; Discipline: Development; Taxonomy: Knowledge)

11.69 **The answer is b.** Both groups gave bottles. The majority of subjects (the total breast-feeding group) and controls (the planned-bottle group) gave bottles every week; therefore, the variable of bottle use cannot be compared accurately. (Difficulty: 4; Discipline: Clinical Skills; Taxonomy: Assessment)

11.70 **The answer is c.** Exhaled carbon monoxide is the most significant risk of anyone smoking near the baby, especially all-night bedsharing, and may be a factor in higher rates of SIDS among parents who smoke. The other choices are significant risks as well. Nevertheless, the baby of a mother who smokes is better off being breastfed than being artificially fed. Efforts to help the mother stop smoking are appropriate. (Difficulty: 5; Discipline: Pharmacology; Taxonomy: Collaboration)

11.71 **The answer is b.** The Montgomery glands are sebaceous glands that produce oil to lubricate the nipple and areolar skin, and they may have other functions. (Difficulty: 4; Discipline: Development; Taxonomy: History)

11.72 **The answer is d.** The glossopharyngeal nerve (cranial nerve IX) controls the gag response in the soft palate and posterior tongue. (Difficulty: 5; Discipline: Development; Taxonomy: Knowledge)

11.73 **The answer is c.** Asthma in babies who are not breastfed is the most serious of the conditions listed and most prevalent. The other diseases are strongly associated with artificial (formula) feeding. (Difficulty: 5; Discipline: Pathology; Taxonomy: History)

11.74 **The answer is a.** The concentration of drug in the milk is nearly always proportional to the level in maternal plasma (blood). (Difficulty: 2; Discipline: Pharmacology; Taxonomy: Knowledge)

11.75 **The answer is b.** Iodine-131 is a radioactive isotope requiring temporary cessation of breastfeeding. Mother should express her milk to maintain supply until the isotope is out of her system. (Difficulty: 5; Discipline: Pharmacology; Taxonomy: Knowledge)

11.76 **The answer is a.** Fat levels vary within a feed, between feeds, and in proportion to the relative fullness or emptiness of the breast. The other statements are false. Zinc levels decrease over time; lactose levels are unrelated to the time of day, and vitamin K is highest in colostrum. (Difficulty: 3; Discipline: Development; Taxonomy: Evaluate)

11.77 **The answer is c.** Breastfeeding difficulties, particularly pain, increase mothers' risk for depression. If breastfeeding is going well, mothers have lower risk of depression. (Difficulty: 2; Discipline: Psychology; Taxonomy: History)

11.78 **The answer is c.** World Breastfeeding Week themes focus on benefits of breastfeeding and positive changes to facilitate breastfeeding. Forcing mothers to breastfeed is inappropriate. World Breastfeeding Week celebrates the signing of the Innocenti Declaration on the Protection, Promotion and Support of Breastfeeding on August 1, 1990. (Difficulty: 4; Discipline: Clinical Skills; Taxonomy: Collaboration)

11.79 **The answer is b.** Giving formula samples sends the message that the mother will need formula, thereby undermining breastfeeding. (Difficulty: 2; Discipline: Clinical Skills; Taxonomy: Collaboration)

11.80 **The answer is d.** Helping the mother with positioning and latch is always appropriate. The baby is being evaluated for tongue-tie and readied for a frenotomy procedure performed by a credentialed professional. Choice a is inappropriate and beyond the scope of practice of an IBCLC. Choice b is not specified in the scope of practice. Teaching hand expression is always appropriate but may not be necessary in this situation. (Difficulty: 3; Discipline: Clinical Skills; Taxonomy: Plan)

11.81 **The answer is d.** Estrogen-containing options are more likely to inhibit lactation and entail other risks to the mother. Progestin-containing products may inhibit lactation in some women if prescribed too early in the postbirth period. Intrauterine devices without hormones have no known impact on lactation. Barrier methods have no impact on lactation. (Difficulty: 4; Discipline: Pharmacology; Taxonomy: Collaboration)

11.82 **The answer is a.** Secretory IgA is found in large quantities in human milk, protecting the entire gastrointestinal tract. The other immunoglobulins are also present in human milk, in lower proportions. (Difficulty: 5; Discipline: Development; Taxonomy: Knowledge)

11.83 **The answer is b.** Sucking on fists is a feeding cue, which should be responded to by offering the breast. (Difficulty: 2; Discipline: Development; Taxonomy: Plan)

11.84 **The answer is c.** Surviving sexual abuse can cause a woman to feel her body is dirty (need to keep covered) or inadequate (fear of inadequate or nonnutritious milk). She needs to separate anything sexual from the task of breastfeeding, viewing breastfeeding more like a chore. But it does not seem to affect her ability to bond with her baby. (Difficulty: 4; Discipline: Psychology; Taxonomy: Plan)

11.85 **The answer is b.** La Leche League created the LC Department to develop the idea and loaned IBLCE money to develop the first examination. JoAnne Scott was the department director, and Linda Smith was the assistant director. (Difficulty: 4; Discipline: Clinical Skills; Taxonomy: Knowledge)

11.86 **The answer is c.** The tail of Spence is normal mammary glandular tissue extending into the axilla. (Difficulty: 3; Discipline: Development; Taxonomy: History)

11.87 **The answer is b.** The higher the vacuum pressure, the more milk collected during the let-down (milk ejection) reflex. Timing the sessions is less effective than monitoring milk ejections. Fast speed may trigger a milk ejection but then should be slowed during high flow periods. Narrow-diameter flanges may pinch the nipple and may be detrimental. (Difficulty: 3; Discipline: Clinical Skills; Taxonomy: Plan)

11.88 **The answer is a.** The infant's epiglottis covers the trachea during swallowing, preventing milk from entering the airway. Between swallows, it prevents air from entering the esophagus. (Difficulty: 4; Discipline: Development; Taxonomy: Knowledge)

11.89 **The answer is c.** Pollard et al. found that babies who are regularly given pacifiers may forget how to suck their own fingers. Sucking may help trigger respiration in some babies and be protective against SIDS. Babies suck on pacifiers, their own fingers, mother's fingers, and mother's breasts during breastfeeding. The findings of this article cannot be generalized to "all babies" or breastfeeding babies. (Difficulty: 3; Discipline: Clinical Skills; Taxonomy: Evaluate)

11.90 **The answer is b.** The independent variable is manipulated by the experiment. The dependent variable is the result of the manipulation. The other three statements about experimental research designs are false. (Difficulty: 2; Discipline: Clinical Skills; Taxonomy: Knowledge)

11.91 **The answer is b.** It may be a breach of the Code of Professional Conduct if the speaker did not ask permission to use your material and does not properly attribute its source. IBCLCs are required to obtain permission from the original source of printed, visual, or other intellectual property. (Difficulty: 4; Discipline: Clinical Skills; Taxonomy: Collaboration)

11.92 **The answer is c.** LCs work in collaboration with clients' primary care providers. The IBCLC may provide information to the mother, work with her physician to identify medical conditions, and/or discuss alternative therapies with her primary care provider. (Difficulty: 4; Discipline: Clinical Skills; Taxonomy: Collaboration)

11.93 **The answer is d.** The International Code Article 7.4 states that "samples of infant formula or other products within the scope of this Code, or of equipment or utensils for their preparation or use, should not be provided to health workers except when necessary for the purpose of professional evaluation or research at the institutional level." Choices a, b, and c are permitted. (Difficulty: 3; Discipline: Clinical Skills; Taxonomy: Knowledge)

11.94 **The answer is b.** LC practice is based on scientific principles, current research, and published guidelines. The first step is to provide clinical evidence supporting or refuting this practice and discuss the evidence with your colleague. Choice a would be appropriate later, if choices b and c are do not result in a change of practice. Choice d is inappropriate. (Difficulty: 4; Discipline: Clinical Skills; Taxonomy: Collaboration)

11.95 **The answer is a.** Making or downloading one copy of a copyrighted work for personal use is considered "fair use." Making multiple copies without permission from the copyright holder violates copyright laws. Pictures and images posted on Internet sites are protected by international copyright laws. You may use legitimately purchased images in your presentations with proper attribution, but further distributing these images without specific permission, as in printed handouts, is not considered fair use. (Difficulty: 3; Discipline: Clinical Skills; Taxonomy: Knowledge)

11.96 **The answer is d.** Aerobic bacteria require oxygen and are more potentially harmful than anaerobic bacteria, which do not require oxygen. The mucous membranes are the most common route for infections of the newborn. (Difficulty: 4; Discipline: Pathology; Taxonomy: Knowledge)

11.97 **The answer is b.** SIgA plays a powerful role in preventing neonatal septicemia. Choices c and d also provide some protection against neonatal septicemia. (Difficulty: 4; Discipline: Development; Taxonomy: Knowledge)

11.98 **The answer is b.** Breastfeeding at least 7 months reduces risk of urinary tract infections for up to 2 years, because of SIgA and lactoferrin in milk and human milk's anti-inflammatory and anti-infective properties. The difference seems to be more pronounced in girls because of genitourinary anatomy. (Difficulty: 5; Discipline: Pathology; Taxonomy: History)

11.99 **The answer is b.** Donor milk is dispensed by prescription only, especially in the United States. Regardless of the amount of milk available, its use is prioritized (ranked) according to severity of need by the recipient. (Difficulty: 3; Discipline: Clinical Skills; Taxonomy: Collaboration)

11.100 **The answer is a.** Telling a client to take an herbal preparation for milk supply issues falls outside the legitimate scope of practice of IBCLCs. Role fidelity is one of the principles of biomedical ethics. Role fidelity means that individuals caring for patients/clients should practice within the scope of practice for which they are qualified. Operating outside one's scope of practice is a violation of an ethical principle that can lead to harm for the patient. (Difficulty: 2; Discipline: Clinical Skills; Taxonomy: Knowledge)

11.101 **The answer is d.** Feeding on demand, or "on cue," is Step 8 and applies to all babies, especially breastfeeding babies. It is also described as "Encourage unrestricted breast-feeding." Step 2 addresses staff training of at least 20 hours; feeding only breastmilk (Step 6) applies only to healthy term babies, Step 9 calls for avoidance of teats or pacifiers for breastfed babies. Step 9 does not specify which other devices may be used. (Difficulty: 5; Discipline: Clinical Skills; Taxonomy: Knowledge)

11.102 **The answer is c.** Overweight/obese women are more likely to have a lower prolactin response to suckling, which is a major factor negatively affecting breastfeeding. Repeat pregnancies, underweight, and age over 35 years are not documented risk factors per se, but could be indicators of other maternal problems that might affect lactation. (Difficulty: 3; Discipline: Pathology; Taxonomy: History)

11.103 **The answer is d.** A current, referenced text designed for lactation professionals is the most reliable of the sources. For example, the database LactMed from the National Library of Medicine, the American Academy of Pediatrics publication on transfer of drugs into human Milk, or Medications and Mothers milk by Hale are considered reputable sources of information. (Difficulty: 2; Discipline: Pharmacology; Taxonomy: Collaboration)

11.104 **The answer is c.** Choice c is a major tenet of the International Code, Article 5.1, and therefore the correct answer to this question. Choice a is verified by many studies. Choice d is true and a major reason why the World Health Organization publishes guidelines for safe preparation and use of powdered formulas. Cost of formula to the parents is not addressed in the International Code of Marketing of Breast-milk Substitutes. (Difficulty: 4; Discipline: Clinical Skills; Taxonomy: Collaboration)

11.105 **The answer is c.** No pacifier use is allowed. For the Lactational Amenorrhea Method (LAM) to work, all nutritive and non-nutritive sucking must be done at breast. (Difficulty: 4; Discipline: Physiology; Taxonomy: Knowledge)

11.106 **The answer is c.** Tactile sensation of the breast in the mouth ("mother in the mouth") is a critical part of imprinting and emotional and psychological development. The oral experience of breastfeeding is pleasurable and normal. The infant controls and molds the shape of the breast in its mouth. (Difficulty: 5; Discipline: Development; Taxonomy: Knowledge)

11.107 **The answer is b.** This rash on the baby's thigh is one manifestation of allergic responses (atopic disease). An LC may not make a diagnosis nor prescribe, so choices a and d are inappropriate responses. (Difficulty: 5; Discipline: Clinical Skills; Taxonomy: Plan)

11.108 **The answer is d.** CNS development is highly linked to lactose in human milk. Choices a and c are also accurate. Lactose aids absorption of calcium and iron. (Difficulty: 4; Discipline: Development; Taxonomy: Knowledge)

11.109 **The answer is d.** Cow's milk (bovine) formulas are safer than the other options listed. Soy products contain no lactose and are not recommended for general use. Powdered formulas are never sterile and may be contaminated with pathogenic bacteria. Goat's milk is deficient in folic acid and other nutrients needed by human infants. (Difficulty: 4; Discipline: Pharmacology; Taxonomy: Knowledge)

11.110 **The answer is d.** Human milk varies in color with mother's diet, medications, and other factors. Colored milk has never been shown to be detrimental or harmful to babies. No testing needs to be done, and no dietary changes are needed. (Difficulty: 3; Discipline: Pathology; Taxonomy: Plan)

11.111 **The answer is a.** Lactoferrin binds to iron, which starves pathogenic bacteria of the iron needed to proliferate. (Difficulty: 5; Discipline: Development; Taxonomy: Knowledge)

11.112 **The answer is d.** The white blanched area is a vasospasm of the nipple, usually triggered by cold air or trauma, also known as Raynaud phenomenon. Keeping the nipple warm especially immediately after the baby finishes nursing should help avoid triggering this painful circulatory condition. (Difficulty: 3; Discipline: Clinical Skills; Taxonomy: Plan)

11.113 **The answer is d.** Three or more key symptoms are found in 70% of diagnosed candidal infection of the nipples. According to Morrill's research, key symptoms strongly correlated to candidal infections are burning pain, stabbing pain, nonstabbing pain, shiny skin, and flaky skin. Other symptoms can also occur. (Difficulty: 5; Discipline: Pathology; Taxonomy: Evaluate)

11.114 **The answer is a.** The intent-to-treat design allocates research participants to groups according to a planned intervention. Whether the mothers actually breastfeed is not considered in the group assignment. (Difficulty: 4; Discipline: Clinical Skills; Taxonomy: Knowledge)

11.115 **The answer is b.** The number of milk ejections strongly correlates to the amount of milk consumed by the infant at a feed. Multiple milk ejections are common. (Difficulty: 2; Discipline: Development; Taxonomy: Knowledge)

11.116 **The answer is a.** Twenty-four-hour rooming-in for all babies is Step 7. Infant formula may be administered to a breastfed baby if a medical reason is documented. Very few conditions of the mother or baby are considered acceptable medical reasons for supplementation. (Difficulty: 4; Discipline: Clinical Skills; Taxonomy: Knowledge)

11.117 **The answer is b.** The independent variables in this study were the feeding devices (tubes, cups). Because these were not analogous, their effectiveness cannot be compared to the location of the feeding, which is the dependent variable. Choice a is a less serious flaw. (Difficulty: 3; Discipline: Clinical Skills; Taxonomy: Evaluate)

11.118 **The answer is b.** Products and equipment used or distributed by an LC must be covered by the product liability insurance of the manufacturer. Altered syringes would not be covered by product liability insurance and would put the LC at greatest liability. (Difficulty: 5; Discipline: Clinical Skills; Taxonomy: Document)

11.119 **The answer is a.** Human alpha-lactalbumin (HAMLET) in laboratory experiments was found to inactivate at least 40 forms of tumors. Beta-lactoglobulin is not found in human milk. Lactoferrin and gangliocides are also important immunofactors in human milk. (Difficulty: 4; Discipline: Development; Taxonomy: Evaluate)

11.120 **The answer is b.** Maternal IDDM increases the risk of infections in general, including breast infections. (Difficulty: 2; Discipline: Pathology; Taxonomy: Knowledge)

11.121 **The answer is d.** This choice has high levels of dietary calcium. Choices b and c are good nutrients but are not high in calcium. Rice and potatoes are low in calcium. (Difficulty: 4; Discipline: Development; Taxonomy: Knowledge)

11.122 **The answer is a.** This nipple is short and flat with a barely visible wound on the superior surface. The baby was tongue-tied. The combination of a flat nipple and a baby with poor tongue mobility caused the abrasion. (Difficulty: 3; Discipline: Development; Taxonomy: Document)

11.123 **The answer is a.** The mammary ridge forms at 4–5 weeks' gestation. (Difficulty: 3; Discipline: Development; Taxonomy: Knowledge)

11.124 **The answer is d.** One half-life is the time it takes for half of the drug to be metabolized. In the first half-life, 20 mg would be metabolized leaving 20 mg. After the second half-life, half of the remaining 20 mg would be metabolized, leaving 10 mg. After the third half-life, 5 mg would be left. After 4 half-lives, 2.5 mg of the drug would remain. (Difficulty: 4; Discipline: Pharmacology; Taxonomy: Knowledge)

11.125 **The answer is b.** The release of cholecystokinin causes satiety and relaxation. (Difficulty: 2; Discipline: Development; Taxonomy: Knowledge)

11.126 **The answer is b.** The median score is the middle score, which may or may not also be the mean (average) or mode (most frequent) score. (Difficulty: 3; Discipline: Clinical Skills; Taxonomy: Knowledge)

11.127 **The answer is c.** Case reports are often the first level of research of a new phenomenon. Observational studies and qualitative surveys are also appropriate initial studies. A clinical trial is a very rigorous approach and rarely undertaken early in an investigation of a phenomenon or treatment. (Difficulty: 4; Discipline: Clinical Skills; Taxonomy: Collaboration)

11.128 **The answer is b.** False-negative (Type II) errors occur when a real difference exists, but a flaw in the design or other aspect of the research does not identify the real difference. Inadequate sample size is one cause of Type II errors. Choice a is a Type I error, and a control group is necessary for any comparative analysis of groups. (Difficulty: 3; Discipline: Clinical Skills; Taxonomy: Knowledge)

11.129 **The answer is d.** Pasteurized donor milk does not transmit the HIV virus. Pasteurization kills the HIV virus and other pathogens that may be present in milk. The other options are common to both pasteurized donor milk and mothers' own milk. (Difficulty: 5; Discipline: Clinical Skills; Taxonomy: Knowledge)

11.130 **The answer is a.** A is the more common sequence: depression can lead to breastfeeding cessation. Supporting mothers who are depressed is critical. Many will tell them that they should wean in order to recover from depression. It is important to find out what the mother wants to do. If she wants to continue breastfeeding through depression, support her. It will help with her depression and help her feel connected to her baby. You may be the only one supporting her decision. (Difficulty: 3; Discipline: Psychology; Taxonomy: Goals)

11.131 **The answer is c.** The alveoli contain secretory cells that produce milk. (Difficulty: 3; Discipline: Development; Taxonomy: Knowledge)

11.132 **The answer is a.** Studying experiences of an event is a qualitative research method. The other responses are quantitative designs: b is descriptive, c is correlational, and d is experimental research. (Difficulty: 4; Discipline: Clinical Skills; Taxonomy: Knowledge)

11.133 **The answer is c.** The most appropriate principle is to use the least intervention for the shortest time. Discuss options with the mother, and obtain her consent before proceeding. Avoid devices that fall within the scope of the International Code of Marketing of Breast-milk Substitutes. (Difficulty: 3; Discipline: Techniques; Taxonomy: Plan)

11.134 **The answer is c.** In premature babies, a thin silicone nipple shield was found to increase transfer of milk. Old thick or rigid designs blocked milk flow. A shield is fairly easy to keep clean and should be cleaned thoroughly after each use. However, the risk of contamination by pathogens is still present. (Difficulty: 5; Discipline: Clinical Skills; Taxonomy: Plan)

11.135 **The answer is a.** Screening every mother and baby is most appropriate and avoids over- and under-supplementing of those with documented needs for supplements. After screening everyone and supplementing those with a need, also discussing risk of sunscreens is appropriate. (Difficulty: 5; Discipline: Clinical Skills; Taxonomy: Collaboration)

11.136 **The answer is a.** The timing of gut closure and developmental readiness for complementary foods is one example of mutual interdependency. Mother's milk helps build baby's immune system. Environmental chemicals that may appear in mother's milk have no documented effect on the baby or its immune system. (Difficulty: 4; Discipline: Development; Taxonomy: Knowledge)

11.137 **The answer is b.** Milk ducts sometimes terminate on the areola, causing milk to be released during the milk-ejection reflex. This is a normal breast configuration. (Difficulty: 3; Discipline: Knowledge; Taxonomy: Knowledge)

11.138 **The answer is d.** LCs' scope of practice does not include diagnosis, treatment of infections, dispensing of medications, or wound / infection care. The purulent bacterial infection pictured should be referred to the mother's primary care provider for evaluation and treatment. Breastfeeding should continue, because the baby has already been exposed and could even be the source of the infection. (Difficulty: 4; Discipline: Clinical Skills; Taxonomy: Collaboration)

11.139 **The answer is c.** The nipple stretches to twice its resting length (100%) during normal breastfeeding. (Difficulty: 3; Discipline: Development; Taxonomy: Knowledge)

11.140 **The answer is c.** The orbicularis oris is a circular sphincter-like muscle that circles the mouth and closes the lips around an object in the mouth. Masseter muscles close the jaw, temporal muscles also close the jaw and are visible during sucking, and the internal and external pterygoids move the jaw sideways, as in grating the teeth. (Difficulty: 5; Discipline: Development; Taxonomy: History)

11.141 **The answer is c.** Drugs that are highly absorbable via oral ingestion more easily transfer to breastmilk. The other properties reduce the amount that may get to the baby. (Difficulty: 2; Discipline: Pharmacology; Taxonomy: Knowledge)

11.142 **The answer is d.** A birth injury is the most likely reason because it is likely to be painful for the baby. Placing the sore side higher than the normal side may reduce pain, resulting in the baby's strong preference for the more comfortable position. Breasts differ in configuration and flow, and one side may be much easier for the baby to manage in the early weeks. Undetected breast cancer (choice c) is very unlikely this early postbirth. (Difficulty: 4; Discipline: Pathology; Taxonomy: History)

11.143 **The answer is d.** Caffeine is highly fat soluble and therefore easily transfers to milk. (Difficulty: 5; Discipline: Pharmacology; Taxonomy: Goals)

11.144 **The answer is c.** After 5 half-lives have passed, approximately 98% of the drug or isotope has been eliminated. Each drug or isotope has a specific half-life. (Difficulty: 3; Discipline: Pharmacology; Taxonomy: Knowledge)

11.145 **The answer is b.** Baby B's rate of weight gain was the fastest, as represented by the steeply increasing angle of slope of the graph. None of the other conclusions can be drawn from the data presented. (Difficulty: 3; Discipline: Clinical Skills; Taxonomy: Evaluate)

11.146 **The answer is d.** Mothers' dietary practices have very little effect on lactation. Following good dietary practices is important for the breastfeeding mother's general health, yet has little relevance to milk volume or composition. (Difficulty: 5; Discipline: Development; Taxonomy: Collaboration)

11.147 **The answer is a.** The baby can and should continue to feed on the affected side. If the incision was close to the nipple, hand expressing should be used to prevent milk stasis. The expressed milk can be given to the baby. Massage on or near the surgical site is not appropriate. Cold packs may feel comfortable but are ineffective in reducing milk stasis. (Difficulty: 4; Discipline: Techniques; Taxonomy: Plan)

11.148 **The answer is a.** Human milk whey: casein ratio is about 80:20 in the early weeks. The casein portion binds calcium and scatters light and therefore appears white; the whey portion of soluble components is slightly blue. Cow's milk has a whey: casein ratio of about 20:80, which means the high portion of casein causes the white opaque color of cow's milk. (Difficulty: 2; Discipline: Development; Taxonomy: Knowledge)

11.149 **The answer is d.** A large proportion (~70%) of the glandular tissue is located within a 30-mm radius of the nipple, according to recent ultrasound studies. (Difficulty: 5; Discipline: Development; Taxonomy: Knowledge)

11.150 **The answer is d.** Mothers talking to other mothers has been shown to be an effective strategy for supporting breastfeeding since at least the 1920s. (Difficulty: 5; Discipline: Psychology; Taxonomy: Knowledge)

11.151 **The answer is b.** The risk for premenopausal breast cancer is higher for women who do not breastfeed/lactate after pregnancy. There is a relationship between not breastfeeding and choices c and d. As of this writing, no relationship between breastfeeding and the risk of cervical cancer has been investigated. (Difficulty: 4; Discipline: Clinical Skills; Taxonomy: Knowledge)

11.152 **The answer is c.** The definition of breastfeeding is so broad as to fail to differentiate between the cohorts. Choice a is incorrect because there is no way to determine if the sample size is adequate without further statistical analysis. Choice b is incorrect because the standard deviation alone is not meaningful. (Difficulty: 2; Discipline: Clinical Skills; Taxonomy: Evaluate)

11.153 **The answer is c.** The infant gut takes up to 2 weeks to recover from damage caused by a reaction to a single bottle of artificial baby milk. (Difficulty: 4; Discipline: Pathology; Taxonomy: Knowledge)

11.154 **The answer is a.** A standard deviation of 0.6 is smaller than a standard deviation of 1.2. Therefore, the breastfeeding mothers had cholesterol levels that were closer together than the non-breastfeeding mothers. Choices c and d are incorrect because the standard deviation alone is not a comparison of data between cohorts. (Difficulty: 2; Discipline: Clinical Skills; Taxonomy: Evaluate)

11.155 **The answer is c.** Allowing the baby to finish the first breast first allows the baby's appetite to best determine the balance of nutrients he obtains during a feed. Enforcing other patterns may result in less-than-optimal intake of nutrients and calories. (Difficulty: 5; Discipline: Techniques; Taxonomy: Plan)

11.156 **The answer is b.** Operational definitions, or how the authors define the term "breastfeeding," are critical. (Difficulty: 3; Discipline: Clinical Skills; Taxonomy: Evaluate)

11.157 **The answer is b.** Placing the fingers at the edge of the areola is the best place to begin assessing a nipple–areola complex for inversion. (Difficulty: 5; Discipline: Techniques; Taxonomy: Assessment)

11.158 **The answer is b.** Current ultrasound research on healthy normal lactating breasts reveals an average of 9 ducts (range 4–18) terminating on the nipple. (Difficulty: 4; Discipline: Development; Taxonomy: Knowledge)

11.159 **The answer is a.** Your first action should be to listen to the history of this situation, carefully documenting what the mother tells you and what you observe. Choices b and d might be appropriate. Choice c is not within the scope of practice of an IBCLC. This mother had surgery for a breast abscess the day before. (Difficulty: 4; Discipline: Clinical Skills; Taxonomy: Document)

11.160 **The answer is c.** With very rare exceptions, breastfeeding should continue if the mother is ill at the time of birth or if she becomes ill during breastfeeding. (Difficulty: 3; Discipline: Pathology; Taxonomy: Plan)

11.161 **The answer is d.** Only the IBCLC credential is considered legally valid in the United States. Internationally, IBCLC is the recognized credential for professional LCs. (Difficulty: 4; Discipline: Clinical Skills; Taxonomy: Knowledge)

11.162 **The answer is d.** This mother needs immediate medical evaluation. Any breast lesion that does not quickly respond to common treatment for common problems during breastfeeding could have an ominous cause. This lesion is nipple cancer (Paget's disease). (Difficulty: 2; Discipline: Clinical Skills; Taxonomy: Collaboration)

11.163 **The answer is c.** When there is no prior knowledge of a potential conflict of interest, the most ethical course of action is to disclose the source of conflict and how you have avoided the conflict of interest. Researching the funding for an event before accepting the invitation would have been better. (Difficulty: 3; Discipline: Clinical Skills; Taxonomy: Collaboration)

11.164 **The answer is b.** Tube-feeding devices were originally designed for situations where the baby has a good suck, and mother provides food via the tube while building up her milk supply. (Difficulty: 4; Discipline: Clinical Skills; Taxonomy: Plan)

11.165 **The answer is c.** Polycystic ovary syndrome is a leading cause of infertility due to higher levels of androgens and disrupts other reproductive hormones as well. Depression is not known to affect induced lactation. Mild anemia is unlikely to affect lactation, and can likely be corrected with dietary supplements. Hypertension is not currently known to affect lactation, natural or induced. (Difficulty: 4; Discipline: Physiology; Taxonomy: Assessment)

11.166 **The answer is b.** Cow's milk is the most common food allergen in children, responsible for multiple allergic symptoms. Soy is almost as common an allergen. Cabbage and rice are uncommon allergens in most populations. (Difficulty: 3; Discipline: Pathology; Taxonomy: History)

11.167 **The answer is a.** The lymphatic system always drains from the breast tissue; it does not supply components of milk manufacture. Choices b and c are also correct, since these are sometimes relevant. (Difficulty: 4; Discipline: Development; Taxonomy: Knowledge)

11.168 **The answer is d.** Exposure to foreign proteins, in this case manufactured formula made from cow's milk or soy protein, before gut closure can permanently sensitize that child's immune system to many other allergens. When subjects and controls are both exposed to the intervention, results are confounded and therefore unreliable. (Difficulty: 4; Discipline: Clinical Skills; Taxonomy: Evaluate)

11.169 **The answer is b.** An effective asymmetrical latch by the baby would place more of the breast underneath the nipple in the baby's mouth, assuming the baby in this situation typically nurses in a head-up (upright) position. Yellow crusts are unlikely to be related to infant saliva. Typical visual signs of *Candida* are different from the appearance of this breast. Color of the areola is irrelevant. This mother was told that her nipple problem was due to "friction" from the baby's mouth, yet the problem resolved when she applied an antibiotic cream. (Difficulty: 3; Discipline: Pathology; Taxonomy: Knowledge)

11.170 **The answer is a.** Feeding-tube devices were designed to provide food to an adopted baby when the mother was not producing adequate milk. Choices b and d are appropriate uses. Tube-feeding devices do not correct a dysfunctional sucking pattern. (Difficulty: 4; Discipline: Clinical Skills; Taxonomy: Plan)

11.171 **The answer is a.** IBCLC (International Board Certified LC) is the only globally recognized credential for LCs. (Difficulty: 3; Discipline: Clinical Skills; Taxonomy: Knowledge)

11.172 **The answer is c.** The symptoms most likely indicate infectious mastitis. She needs medical evaluation and treatment with an antibiotic, bedrest, and continued breastfeeding and/or increasing milk drainage from the affected breast. She would greatly benefit from help with her baby. (Difficulty: 5; Discipline: Pathology; Taxonomy: Assessment)

11.173 **The answer is b.** Sedation or drowsiness is the most likely infant reaction to an anticonvulsant drug taken during breastfeeding. Other signs include poor suck, poor weight gain, or jaundice; all should be reported to the child's physician. The other signs listed are not likely to be related to anticonvulsant therapy. (Difficulty: 3; Discipline: Pharmacology; Taxonomy: Collaboration)

11.174 **The answer is c.** An incision around the perimeter of the areola that is deep enough to remove underlying tissue is likely to sever the fourth intercostal nerve, thereby diminishing oxytocin and prolactin response. Choice a is incorrect because it is possible to estimate the milk supply based on the known factors. Choice b is incorrect because it is likely there will be diminished milk. Choice d is incorrect because the factors listed are critical to determining her milk supply. (Difficulty: 5; Discipline: Pathology; Taxonomy: History)

11.175 **The answer is a.** Quasi-experimental studies are more likely to show that the explanation really did cause the outcome; therefore, these designs have the highest internal validity. (Difficulty: 3; Discipline: Clinical Skills; Taxonomy: Knowledge)

11.176 **The answer is c.** World Health Assembly Resolution WHA 49.15 (1996) urges governments "to ensure that the financial support for professionals working in infant and young child health does not create conflicts of interest, especially with regard to the WHO/UNICEF Baby Friendly Hospital Initiative." The other sources of funding are ethical. (Difficulty: 3; Discipline: Clinical Skills; Taxonomy: Collaboration)

11.177 **The answer is a.** The International Code is silent regarding breast pumps. However, feeding bottles (baby bottles) that are not used as collection containers attached to breast pumps fall within the scope of the International Code. (Difficulty: 2; Discipline: Clinical Skills; Taxonomy: Knowledge)

11.178 **The answer is c.** Lysozyme kills bacteria by disrupting cell walls. Mucins adhere to pathogens, preventing their attachment to mucous membranes. Fatty acids disrupt cell membranes of some viruses. Casein does not appear to be protective against inflammation or pathogens. (Difficulty: 4; Discipline: Development; Taxonomy: Knowledge)

11.179 **The answer is d.** Leukocytes, and other white cells and immune components, are absent in all manufactured milks. The other components are found in artificial feeding products. A few contain real lactose; the others have fructose and other carbohydrates. (Difficulty: 5; Discipline: Development; Taxonomy: Knowledge)

11.180 **The answer is c.** The LC can provide published references to the mother but cannot pronounce a drug as "safe" or "unsafe." Determining the safety of maternal medications is reserved for appropriately licensed health care providers. Choices b and d are appropriate for the LC. (Difficulty: 4; Discipline: Clinical Skills; Taxonomy: Collaboration)

11.181 **The answer is c.** Lipase present in human milk digests and breaks down the fatty acids and may change the taste and smell of stored milk. The stored milk is still safe and healthy for the baby. (Difficulty: 3; Discipline: Clinical Skills; Taxonomy: Knowledge)

11.182 **The answer is c.** The IBLCE Code of Professional Conduct (IBLCE CPC) at 3.2 says "Refrain from photographing, recording or taping (audio or video) a mother or her child for any purpose unless the mother has given advance written consent on her behalf and that of her child" (emphasis added). See also Core Curriculum for LC Practice, 3rd ed at p. 20. (Difficulty: 4; Discipline: Clinical Skills; Taxonomy: History)

11.183 **The answer is d.** This is a description that is factual and does not suggest uses for the product. Marketing is designed to get people to buy the product by suggesting uses, benefits, and desirability of the product. (Difficulty: 3; Discipline: Clinical Skills; Taxonomy: Evaluate)

11.184 **The answer is d.** Article 6.3 states "Facilities of health care systems should not be used for the display of products within the scope of the Code." Factual descriptions are allowed. A company can provide information on preparation or use of its own products, including the company logo. The Code applies to manufacturers and distributors of products that fall within the scope of the Code, not professionals. The Code permits health care workers to accept supplies at the institutional level for research and evaluation, but specifically prohibits these from being distributed to mothers. Resolution WHA49.15 (2008) on infant and young child nutrition "recognizes the need to ensure that the commitment and support for breastfeeding and optimal infant and young child nutrition are not undermined by conflicts of interest." (Difficulty: 5; Discipline: Clinical Skills; Taxonomy: Collaboration)

11.185 **The answer is c.** Feeding bottles and teats (nipples), infant formula, and foods marketed for babies less than 6 months old fall within the scope of the International Code of Marketing of Breast-milk Substitutes and subsequent World Health Assembly Resolutions. As of 2014, breast pumps are not addressed in the Code. Diapers and swaddling blankets do not fall within the scope of the Code. (Difficulty: 3; Discipline: Clinical Skills; Taxonomy: Collaboration)

11.186 **The answer is c.** The mother's secretory immune system provides targeted protection through the enteromammary and bronchomammary pathways. (Difficulty: 5; Discipline: Development; Taxonomy: Knowledge)

11.187 **The answer is c.** Nerves are known to regrow at an established rate. Ducts have been shown to regrow in response to hormonal stimulation The longer the time interval between the surgery and the event of lactation, the more extensive the reinnervation and recanalization will be. Choice a is incorrect because the time factor is dismissed. Choice b is incorrect because the hormonal response is not a significant factor between these two ages. Choice d is incorrect because the interval of time is an important factor in recanalization and reinnervation. (Difficulty: 5; Discipline: Pathology; Taxonomy: Evaluate)

11.188 **The answer is c.** . Breastfeeding, particularly exclusive breastfeeding, downregulates the mother's stress system, improves her sleep, and lowers her risk of depression. (Difficulty: 5; Discipline: Psychology; Taxonomy: History))

11.189 **The answer is b.** Peer-support or mother-support breastfeeding groups have the strongest evidence of effectiveness in supporting mothers to exclusively breastfeed for 6 months and maintain breastfeeding at least 2 years. Peer support is especially effective in low-income or minority populations. The other options may have value in helping her reach her goals as well. (Difficulty: 5; Discipline: Psychology; Taxonomy: Goals)

11.190 **The answer is d.** This is an accessory nipple on the woman's upper, inner thigh, which is an unusual location for an accessory nipple. This woman found the sensitivity of the skin paralleled her menstrual cycles. (Difficulty: 4; Discipline: Development; Taxonomy: Assessment)

11.191 **The answer is c.** Nutrition and immunological therapy for premature infants is the most common historical use of banked donor milk. The other uses of donor milk may occur, depending on availability of donors. (Difficulty: 5; Discipline: Development; Taxonomy: Knowledge)

11.192 **The answer is d.** Prolonged milk stasis is the most common and most important contributing factor to a breast abscess. The other choices could have played a role in the milk stasis. (Difficulty: 5; Discipline: Pathology; Taxonomy: History)

11.193 **The answer is a.** For a maternal medication to affect the baby, it must pass into milk and be ingested by the baby. Drugs that are not absorbed from the GI tract are very low risk because the baby's GI tract would not absorb the drug even if it's in the milk. (Difficulty: 5; Discipline: Pharmacology; Taxonomy: Knowledge)

11.194 **The answer is c.** Fathers easily bond with their exclusively breastfed babies. Educating fathers and other relatives improves breastfeeding rates. (Difficulty: 3; Discipline: Psychology; Taxonomy: History)

11.195 **The answer is a.** The probability of a chance occurrence is usually established at 1.0. The smaller the probability value, the least likely it is that the event happened by chance. (Difficulty: 3; Discipline: Clinical Skills; Taxonomy: Knowledge)

11.196 **The answer is d.** Distributing products covered by the scope of the Code to all pregnant women is unethical and violates the International Code of Marketing of Breastmilk Substitutes. Feeding bottles are within the scope of the Code. Marketing of any product covered by the Code in ways that undermine direct breastfeeding is a violation of the Code and unethical. (Difficulty: 5; Discipline: Clinical Skills; Taxonomy: Document)

11.197 **The answer is c.** Whether or not she is breastfeeding, a new mother with MS is likely to experience an increase in acute episodes during the postbirth period. Often, breastfeeding is wrongly blamed for this phenomenon. (Difficulty: 4; Discipline: Clinical Skills; Taxonomy: Knowledge)

11.198 **The answer is a.** Without milk removal, they will quickly atrophy and the milk will be reabsorbed. Choice b is incorrect because the introduction of external bacteria is not possible when the duct has been severed and hematogenous infection is unlikely. Choice c is unlikely. Choice d is incorrect because a baby suckling well will drain most glands in the breast. (Difficulty: 4; Discipline: Pathology; Taxonomy: Assessment)

11.199 **The answer is a.** The axillary nodes collect most of the lymph fluid; the intermammary and subclavicular nodes collect some lymph from the breast. The mesenteric nodes are in the abdomen. (Difficulty: 4; Discipline: Development; Taxonomy: Knowledge)

11.200 **The answer is a.** Non-human proteins are the key trigger in allergic disease. Choices b and c are both additional factors in allergic disease. Choice d is incorrect: white cells in milk do not directly attack dietary allergens. (Difficulty: 4; Discipline: Development; Taxonomy: Knowledge)

11.201 **The answer is c.** Under Principle 1.3 of the IBLCE CPC the mother should be fully informed about all her care options. The IBCLC Scope of Practice does not permit an IBCLC to "prescribe" even over-the-counter products. The mother should consult with her health care provider and can bring with her information she has learned from the IBCLC. (Difficulty: 4; Discipline: Clinical Skills; Taxonomy: Goals)

11.202 **The answer is b.** The degree of breast fullness/emptiness is the most important regulator of milk production in the short term. Components of milk retained in the alveoli provide chemical feedback to the cells. The highest rate of production occurs when the breasts are emptiest. (Difficulty: 4; Discipline: Development; Taxonomy: Knowledge)

11.203 **The answer is c.** The breastfeeding dyad is a unique biological and psychological entity. (Difficulty: 5; Discipline: Psychology; Taxonomy: Knowledge)

11.204 **The answer is a.** Accurate documentation merely describes what is visually apparent. Choice b is subjective, and choices c and d are not accurate because determination of sufficient or insufficient glandular tissue for lactation cannot be determined by visual examination alone. (Difficulty: 3; Discipline: Clinical Skills; Taxonomy: Document)

11.205 **The answer is c.** Implementing the BFHI has strong evidence of improving initiation, duration, and exclusivity of breastfeeding. All of the other answers are also backed by evidence. (Difficulty: 5; Discipline: Clinical Skills; Taxonomy: Collaboration)

11.206 **The answer is c.** Docosahexaenoic acid is a long-chain fatty acid that is found in the fatty portion of milk,. The others are found in the whey fraction. (Difficulty: 2; Discipline: Development; Taxonomy: Knowledge)

11.207 **The answer is b.** Living cells including macrophages are killed by freezing. The other components are not significantly affected by freezing. (Difficulty: 2; Discipline: Clinical Skills; Taxonomy: Knowledge)

11.208 **The answer is c.** Fenugreek is believed to enhance milk production, although research does not confirm its safety or effectiveness, and the placebo effect may explain its results. Fluid intake to thirst is sufficient to maintain milk production. Electrolyte-replacing fluids are probably harmless. Beer was once thought to be a galactagogue, but the alcohol in beer may actually decrease milk production. Sage is believed to reduce milk production, although its effect has not been thoroughly evaluated. Before any ingested strategy is attempted, better breastfeeding management should be ensured. (Difficulty: 3; Discipline: Pharmacology; Taxonomy: Collaboration)

11.209 **The answer is d.** An open cup is safest, especially in emergency situations. Closed systems (teats/nipples, tubes, syringes) are harder to clean and can disrupt the baby's oral behaviors at breast. (Difficulty: 5; Discipline: Clinical Skills; Taxonomy: Plan)

11.210 **The answer is a.** The Innocenti Declaration was adopted in 1990 and signed by representatives of many nations. It was modified and reconfirmed in November 2005. The other documents also support breastfeeding. The action steps of the Innocenti Declaration are more specific. (Difficulty: 4; Discipline: Clinical Skills; Taxonomy: Knowledge)

11.211 **The answer is d.** The LC supports the breastfeeding relationship, including helping the mother to explore all her options in any given situation. Choices a and b could be included in the conversation. (Difficulty: 4; Discipline: Psychology; Taxonomy: Goals)

11.212 **The answer is c.** Prolactin is produced in high levels at all stages of lactation and has an anti-stress effect on mother. Estrogen and progesterone levels are low in ongoing lactation, and placental lactogen is absent after the delivery of the placenta. (Difficulty: 3; Discipline: Development; Taxonomy: Knowledge)

11.213 **The answer is b.** Breastfeeding reduces risk of leukemia by 20% to 30%, depending on duration and exclusivity of breastfeeding. (Difficulty: 5; Discipline: Clinical Skills; Taxonomy: Knowledge)

11.214 **The answer is d.** Lumpectomy is the type of breast surgery most likely to preserve lactation function. The mother should be followed closely for 2 weeks after giving birth if she has had any breast surgery. (Difficulty: 3; Discipline: Clinical Skills; Taxonomy: History)

11.215 **The answer is c.** The LC does not need a referral from a physician before assisting a baby with cleft palate to breastfeed. She should always work closely and collaboratively with the baby's physician(s) before and after any surgery for repair of the cleft. (Difficulty: 2; Discipline: Clinical Skills; Taxonomy: Collaboration)

11.216 **The answer is a.** Exclusive breastfeeding means that the baby satisfies all nutrition and sucking at his mother's breast. Adding supplemental vitamins is not exclusive breastfeeding, nor is adding other fluids or pacifiers. (Difficulty: 5; Discipline: Clinical Skills; Taxonomy: History)

11.217 **The answer is a.** Communicating relevant information to primary care provider(s) is required of LCs. (Difficulty: 3; Discipline: Clinical Skills; Taxonomy: Collaboration)

11.218 **The answer is c.** Fat-soluble vitamin intake is related to fat levels in milk, which vary with several factors. Protein, minerals, and lactose do not vary with infant feeding patterns. (Difficulty: 2; Discipline: Development; Taxonomy: History)

11.219 The answer is a. A nipple shield has been shown to be useful for some premature babies with weak suck, which is supported by research. Although nipple shield use is poorly researched, some professionals suggest their use for the other situations listed. (Difficulty: 5; Discipline: Techniques; Taxonomy: PlanJC9696019-R1-026-11A)

11.220 The answer is c. Drugs with high milk:plasma (blood) ratio readily transfer into milk and may even accumulate in milk. The active ingredient in cannabis (marijuana) is THC, which can accumulate in milk. As of 2015, the Academy of Breastfeeding Medicine recommends that mothers who use cannabis be strongly counseled to avoid using cannabis during pregnancy and breastfeeding. Long-term studies are needed. The other choices are drug properties that inhibit drug transfer into milk. (Difficulty: 2; Discipline: Pharmacology; Taxonomy: Collaboration)

11.221 The answer is a. Citing published medical guidelines on medications is the most ethical and appropriate first response. Her baby may get diarrhea or thrush from her treatment, which might be the next piece of information to share with her. Increasing family foods is irrelevant in this situation. (Difficulty: 3; Discipline: Pharmacology; Taxonomy: Collaboration)

11.222 The answer is c. Article 5 of the International Code prohibits advertising of products within the scope of the Code, including infant formula, to the general public. Choice a is scientifically true and supports the aim of the Code but is not specifically mentioned in the Articles of the Code. Choices b and d are false. (Difficulty: 3; Discipline: Clinical Skills; Taxonomy: Knowledge)

11.223 The answer is a. Consent must be obtained before touching the mother or baby or taking photographs. Unwanted touching could be considered battery. Written consent is preferred over verbal. The other actions are appropriate after obtaining consent from the mother. (Difficulty: 2; Discipline: Clinical Skills; Taxonomy: History)

11.224 The answer is d. Education provided by sources with a conflict of interest is inappropriate and is likely to be inaccurate and unhelpful. Formula, bottles, and teats are products that fall within the International Code. (Difficulty: 2; Discipline: Clinical Skills; Taxonomy: Assessment)

11.225 The answer is a. Cultures that sexualize the breast are often the most resistant to women using their breasts to feed their infants anywhere and everywhere. (Difficulty: 5; Discipline: Psychology; Taxonomy: Evaluate)

11.226 The answer is d. Maternity protection has a profound effect on breastfeeding rates, which has been documented since the 1900s. Family violence has not yet been linked to breastfeeding at the policy level. One study suggests that violence in the home is a barrier to women breastfeeding. (Difficulty: 3; Discipline: Clinical Skills; Taxonomy: Clinical Skills)

11.227 The answer is b. Manufacturers omitted chloride in a mistaken effort to impact adult cardiac disease by changing infant intake of salt. Chloride is an essential nutrient for human brain development. (Difficulty: 5; Discipline: Development; Taxonomy: History)

11.228 The answer is c. Position papers are official documents of the organization, and they carry much influence within the profession and to the public. (Difficulty: 4; Discipline: Clinical Skills; Taxonomy: Document)

11.229 **The answer is a.** The most important goal for any lactation professional is to support the mother in reaching her own goals for breastfeeding. (Difficulty: 2; Discipline: Clinical Skills; Taxonomy: Goals)

11.230 **The answer is b.** Peer support is the most effective strategy in virtually all populations that have been studied to date. The other strategies may help in addition to peer or mother-to-mother support. (Difficulty: 5; Discipline: Clinical Skills; Taxonomy: Goals)

11.231 **The answer is c.** In a Baby-Friendly Hospital, infant formula may be administered to a breastfed baby only if a medical reason is documented. This is a typical and appropriate scene on a maternity unit in a Baby-Friendly Hospital. (Difficulty: 3; Discipline: Clinical Skills; Taxonomy: Knowledge)

11.232 **The answer is c.** The current Academy of Breastfeeding recommendation for a breastfed baby undergoing general anesthesia is to withhold breastfeeding and breastmilk for 4 hours. The most serious consequence of nonfasting is pulmonary aspiration, and even breastmilk can be problematic. The Academy of Breastfeeding Medicine protocol is an evidence-based guidance document carefully researched by experts in both pediatric anesthesia and breastfeeding. (Difficulty: 5; Discipline: Pharmacology; Taxonomy: Collaboration)

11.233 **The answer is b.** Viral fragments trigger baby's immune response. Viral fragments in milk do not appear to actually transmit disease from mother to infant. (Difficulty: 4; Discipline: Development; Taxonomy: Knowledge)

11.234 **The answer is c.** Implementing the International Code is an operational target of the Innocenti Declaration. Implementing BFHI and forming a national committee and national coordinator are not operational targets of the Innocenti Declaration but are important health policies. The fourth provision of the 1990 Innocenti Declaration protects the breastfeeding rights of working women, not their right to breastfeed in public. (Difficulty: 4; Discipline: Clinical Skills; Taxonomy: Collaboration)

11.235 **The answer is b.** BFHI's Step 9 is "Give no teats or pacifiers to breastfed babies," so Step 2 staff training must include non-teat feeding methods. Cup-feeding is the safest and recommended technique for feeding babies who cannot breastfeed, and staff should be able to teach and assist all mothers in this skill. Choice c is also true but of lesser overall importance than option b. Choice a is incorrect, and choice d is irrelevant because BFHI applies to all settings. (Difficulty: 4; Discipline: Clinical Skills; Taxonomy: Plan)

11.236 **The answer is c.** Because not enough milk is a chief cause of breastfeeding failure, any educational material should contain information about how to make plenty of milk. Choices a and d are good information but less important than milk production. Comparing breastfeeding with artificial feeding suggests their equivalence, which is neither accurate nor helpful information. (Difficulty: 4; Discipline: Clinical Skills; Taxonomy: Evaluate)

11.237 **The answer is a.** Involving all pertinent staff, planning sufficient education is the most important step and providing substantial evidence of the safety and effectiveness of the new policy are also successful strategies for changing policies. Forcing new policies on staff (choice d) is likely to result in open and covert resistance. (Difficulty: 4; Discipline: Clinical Skills; Taxonomy: Collaboration)

11.238 **The answer is b.** Taking a history is always the first step in documenting a client encounter. An LC could then conduct choices a and d, although diagnosis is outside the scope of practice. Choice c is incorrect because providing medications is not within the current scope of practice of the LC. (Difficulty: 4; Discipline: Clinical Skills; Taxonomy: Plan)

11.239 **The answer is b.** The International Code specifies that information on artificial feeding provided to health workers should be scientific and accurate. Detailed accurate information on product composition, provided to health workers, is appropriate marketing of products within the scope of the Code. (Difficulty: 2; Discipline: Clinical Skills; Taxonomy: Collaboration)

11.240 **The answer is b.** Confounding variables are factors that could influence the outcome of research that were not described or eliminated by the research design. (Difficulty: 3; Discipline: Clinical Skills; Taxonomy: Knowledge)

11.241 **The answer is d.** Forming a team is the first step in developing evidence-based policies of any sort. Developing a policy is an interactive and educational process that requires input from all affected parties. (Difficulty: 4; Discipline: Clinical Skills; Taxonomy: Collaboration)

11.242 **The answer is a.** This technique is most likely used to massage open a plugged nipple pore (bleb); anecdotal stories suggest it might be helpful for choices a and d. It is ineffective for expressing milk because it occludes milk ducts. (Difficulty: 4; Discipline: Techniques; Taxonomy: Plan)

11.243 **The answer is c.** If a well-defined hard area remains after appropriate mastitis treatment, it could be an abscess. The LC should refer the mother to a physician for thorough evaluation and treatment. The LC should remain in contact with the mother's providers and be prepared to support the mother and provide referenced resources for the providers if requested. Choice a is always appropriate but will not resolve an abscess. Choice b is inappropriate and possibly dangerous. Choice d is inappropriate; breastfeeding can continue on the affected breast in most situations. (Difficulty: 3; Discipline: Clinical Skills; Taxonomy: Collaboration)

11.244 **The answer is a.** SIgA is the main antibody appearing on mucous membranes and the gastrointestinal tract. SIgA binds microbes and blocks them from entering tissues; therefore, the immune system in tissues is not triggered. IgM and IgG neutralize toxins, but trigger an inflammatory reaction. IgE is elevated during allergic reactions. (Difficulty: 4; Discipline: Pathology; Taxonomy: Knowledge)

11.245 **The answer is b.** A clear description of your observation is most appropriate. Choice a is less clear; choice c is offering a diagnosis, and choice d includes the mother's subjective feelings ("painful"). (Difficulty: 5; Discipline: Clinical Skills; Taxonomy: Document)

11.246 **The answer is a.** Closely supervised breastfeeding may help her. The key is close supervision to protect her and her baby. (Difficulty: 2; Discipline: Psychology; Taxonomy: Collaboration)

11.247 **The answer is d.** The U.S. Centers for Disease Control does not does not list human breast milk as a body fluid for which most healthcare personnel should use special handling precautions, except in high-exposure situations such as donor milk banking. (Difficulty: 5; Discipline: Clinical Skills; Taxonomy: Collaboration)

11.248 **The answer is b.** Breastfeeding mothers in emergency situations benefit most from private areas where they can tend and feed their babies. Re-lactation support should also be built in to policies of the emergency services as a secondary form of support. Ready-to-feed formula may be a safer but unrealistic choice for formula-fed babies, and powdered formula is the least desirable option, even if it is prepared with clean bottled water. (Difficulty: 5; Discipline: Clinical Skills; Taxonomy: Collaboration)

11.249 **The answer is c.** Caffeine is the most likely to affect the baby because it is a central nervous system stimulant and highly lipid soluble. Insulin is poorly absorbed orally; digoxin acts on muscle tissue and passes poorly into milk; warfarin has a large molecular weight and does not pass into milk. (Difficulty: 2; Discipline: Pharmacology; Taxonomy: Knowledge)

11.250 **The answer is b.** Reduction mammoplasty frequently results in nipple/areolar nerve impairment. Many mothers experience an initially high milk supply that diminishes at about 2 to 3 weeks. A continuation of monitoring output and weight is necessary to assess the milk supply in case of this reduction. Choices a, c, and d are appropriate but less important than b. (Difficulty: 5; Discipline: Pathology; Taxonomy: History)

11.251 **The answer is b.** B-lymphocytes produce targeted antibodies that quickly appear in milk. (Difficulty: 4; Discipline: Development; Taxonomy: Knowledge)

11.252 **The answer is d.** A research article published in a peer-reviewed professional journal is a primary reference. Choice a is a review, which is a secondary reference. Choice b is a chapter in a book, which is a secondary or tertiary source. Choice c is a book, interpreting other sources in its recommendations. (Difficulty: 4; Discipline: Clinical Skills; Taxonomy: Evaluate)

11.253 **The answer is b.** Step 2 of the BFHI is training all staff on the BFHI steps and breastfeeding management, including feeding on cue. During the training, old ideas can be explored and clarified, and references provided. Documentation and policies should be based on evidence and are more accepted after training. Disciplinary measures should not be the first policies developed. (Difficulty: 4; Discipline: Clinical Skills; Taxonomy: Collaboration)

11.254 **The answer is c.** Flange diameter that allows the mother's nipple to move freely will avoid compressing milk ducts and thus restricting milk flow. Choices a and b are important as well. All parts of the pump that touch the milk should be cleaned according to the manufacturer's instructions. (Difficulty: 4; Discipline: Clinical Skills; Taxonomy: Evaluate)

11.255 **The answer is c.** About 1% of most medications administered to a lactating woman actually reaches her breastfed baby. There are exceptions, based on drug properties, dosage, age of the baby, and other factors. (Difficulty: 3; Discipline: Pharmacology; Taxonomy: Knowledge)

11.256 **The answer is b.** The lymph system has been the most studied because of its role in breast cancer. In the lactating breast, lymph maintains fluid homeostasis and is involved in early postbirth edema, which can have negative consequences on breastfeeding. (Difficulty: 2; Discipline: Development; Taxonomy: Knowledge)

11.257 **The answer is b.** Documentation is required and should be an accurate description of what is viewed by the LC. In this photograph, there is no indication of infection, and LCs do not diagnose infectious conditions. In choice B, "normal" is a subjective word, and there is no indication of what "normal" is for this woman. Choice d offers a judgment and prediction, and is inappropriate. (Difficulty: 4; Discipline: Clinical Skills; Taxonomy: Document)

11.258 **The answer is d.** Ultrasound research confirms that milk ducts are easily compressed, do not display "typical" sinuses, and are superficial to the breast surface. (Difficulty: 4; Discipline: Development; Taxonomy: Knowledge)

11.259 **The answer is b.** As of this writing (December 2015), recertification is required every 5 years, by either reexamination or accumulating CERPs. Recertification by reexamination is required at least every 10 years. (Difficulty: 3; Discipline: Clinical Skills; Taxonomy: Document)

11.260 **The answer is c.** Manufacturers are experimenting with the addition of nucleotides to increase the protective properties of their products. However, even with nucleotides added, the manufactured products fall far short of human milk's protective properties. (Difficulty: 2; Discipline: Development; Taxonomy: Collaboration)

11.261 **The answer is d.** Most breastfeeding mothers can follow the eating and fluid intake patterns of an average woman in a developed country. Fluid intake is unrelated to milk volume; excess calories are unnecessary, and B vitamins are found in many animal-based foods. (Difficulty: 4; Discipline: Development; Taxonomy: Evaluate)

11.262 **The answer is a.** When a procedure requires anesthesia, the mother should withhold breastfeeding at least 4 hours prior to anesthesia. Clear fluids can be given up to 2 hours before the procedure, the baby can breastfeed immediately after the procedure, and formula must be withheld 6 to 8 hours before anesthesia. (Difficulty: 4; Discipline: Pharmacology; Taxonomy: Collaboration)

11.263 **The answer is d.** Lipid solubility facilitates transfer of drugs into mother's milk. The other factors inhibit drug transfer to milk. (Difficulty: 5; Discipline: Pharmacology; Taxonomy: Knowledge)

11.264 **The answer is a.** SIgA is a primary antibody on the mucous membranes, which is where respiratory and gastrointestinal infections begin. SIgA binds microbes and blocks them from entering tissues. SIgA may be targeted to a specific pathogen but does not directly kill bacteria. It has an anti-inflammatory effect and activates the infant's immune system. (Difficulty: 2; Discipline: Development; Taxonomy: Knowledge)

11.265 **The answer is d.** Screening of donors is universal. Pasteurization is common but not universal in all nations. Screening for environmental contaminants is not routinely performed, although occasional case-by-case screening for a particular substance has been done. (Difficulty: 4; Discipline: Development; Taxonomy: Knowledge)

11.266 **The answer is d.** A systematic review is the strongest level of research evidence. The next strongest of the listed research methods is choice b, a randomized trial. A cohort study is the weakest of those three. The MCN article is qualitative research, while the others are quantitative methods. (Difficulty: 4; Discipline: Clinical Skills; Taxonomy: Evaluate)

11.267 **The answer is b.** Keeping the dyad together is the most supportive action. (Difficulty: 4; Discipline: Psychology; Taxonomy: Plan)

11.268 **The answer is d.** "Correlation does not prove causation"—it only states that there is a relationship. The true relationship could be that breastfeeding fosters use of breast pumps, rather than breast pumps foster breastfeeding. (Difficulty: 2; Discipline: Clinical Skills; Taxonomy: Evaluate)

11.269 **The answer is b.** Water-soluble vitamins such as B_6 and B_{12} in milk are strongly dependent on maternal dietary intake. These nutrients are essential to the baby. (Difficulty: 2; Discipline: Development; Taxonomy: Goals)

11.270 **The answer is d.** Most donor human milk is used for feeding premature babies and those with severe allergies. The others are also appropriate uses for donor milk, but lower priority than treating vulnerable infants. (Difficulty: 5; Discipline: Development; Taxonomy: Knowledge)

11.271 **The answer is a.** Effective milk transfer is the primary function of a pump. Pumps should have at least one setting operating at about the same number of cycles per minute as the baby would feed: 40 to 60 times per minute. (Difficulty: 4; Discipline: Clinical Skills; Taxonomy: Plan)

11.272 **The answer is d.** Live nursing mothers are the best teachers, especially for low-income, young, and low-education mothers. The other strategies can also be effective. (Difficulty: 5; Discipline: Clinical Skills; Taxonomy: Collaboration)

11.273 **The answer is a.** Any statement that favorably compares the product to breastfeeding is considered idealizing and violates the International Code of Marketing of Breast-milk Substitutes. Choices b, c, and d are factual statements. Breast pumps (choice d) are not covered by the International Code. (Difficulty: 2; Discipline: Clinical Skills; Taxonomy: Knowledge)

11.274 **The answer is d.** Iron in human milk is highly bioavailable. Exclusively breastfed babies are very unlikely to become anemic for at least 6 to 9 months. (Difficulty: 2; Discipline: Development; Taxonomy: Assessment)

11.275 **The answer is a.** The fourth intercostal nerve innervates the nipple and areola. Damage to this nerve can result in loss of sensation at the nipple and resultant lack of nerve feedback for lactation. (Difficulty: 4; Discipline: Development; Taxonomy: Knowledge)

11.276 **The answer is d.** The excess risk of gastrointestinal infections for formula-fed babies is far greater than the other risks. The other diseases are also more prevalent in formula-fed children. (Difficulty: 5; Discipline: Pathology; Taxonomy: History)

11.277 **The answer is b.** Babies consume about two-thirds of the available milk in a breast during any given feeding. (Difficulty: 3; Discipline: Development; Taxonomy: Assessment)

11.278 **The answer is d.** The ILO Convention provides job protection after maternity leave. It provides for 14 weeks' maternity leave and nursing breaks during the day. Although on-site child care is beneficial to all parents, especially breastfeeding mothers, the ILO convention of 2000 does not specifically address on-site child care. (Difficulty: 3; Discipline: Clinical Skills; Taxonomy: Collaboration)

11.279 **The answer is c.** Barrier methods are most compatible with breastfeeding because no hormones are involved. There are numerous anecdotal reports of progestin-only contraceptives interfering with lactation. Combined pills contain estrogen, which can significantly reduce milk supply. Emergency contraception (levonorgestrel) requires mothers to avoid breastfeeding for 8 to 24 hours after the dose. "Preven" (another emergency contraceptive) should be avoided because it contains both estrogen and progestin. (Difficulty: 3; Discipline: Physiology; Taxonomy: Goals)

11.280 **The answer is b.** LCs are expected to avoid situations that would put them into an ethical conflict of interest. Refusal to eat the "sponsored" food is appropriate. Avoiding the issue simply supports the conflict of interest. Although refusing to participate in the rest of the meeting would strongly raise the issue to everyone at the meeting, that action may not be the best for that particular situation. Choice d is inappropriate and violates the Code of Ethics for LCs. (Difficulty: 3; Discipline: Clinical Skills; Taxonomy: Plan)

11.281 **The answer is c.** IBCLC Clinical Competencies and IBLCE Scope of Practice say IBCLCs can perform comprehensive feeding assessments and oral examinations, and they can provide evidence-based information and support about any aspect of breastfeeding. Choice b is a good response after explaining normal and abnormal tongue function. Choice d might be a later or supplemental strategy. (Difficulty: 4; Discipline: Clinical Skills; Taxonomy: Goals)

11.282 **The answer is d.** LCs do not determine the safety of prescribed medications. It is within the IBCLC's scope of practice to provide references and written information to parents and providers of care. (Difficulty: 2; Discipline: Clinical Skills; Taxonomy: Knowledge)

11.283 **The answer is b.** Mothers who breastfeed often want to "tell the world," which is a strong theme of empowerment. (Difficulty: 3; Discipline: Psychology; Taxonomy: Evaluate)

11.284 **The answer is c.** Original research (primary references) is the most important type of source to include in a literature review. Texts and review articles may help you locate primary references on a subject. Lectures also may direct you to primary references. (Difficulty: 4; Discipline: Clinical Skills; Taxonomy: Evaluate)

11.285 **The answer is c.** SIgA is highest in the first 25 hours, with levels up to 15 to 40 times higher than at any other stage of lactation. This immunoglobulin protects the vulnerable newborn even in contaminated environments. (Difficulty: 3; Discipline: Development; Taxonomy: Knowledge)

11.286 **The answer is a.** Providing "free" samples of infant formula to mothers is a violation of the International Code. (Difficulty: 4; Discipline: Clinical Skills; Taxonomy: Assessment)

11.287 **The answer is d.** Minerals in human milk are stable to pasteurization and freezing. Many immune components are stable to heat treatment. White cells are destroyed by pasteurization and freezing. Lipids are stable to pasteurization but may break down into free fatty acids during freezing and thawing. (Difficulty: 4; Discipline: Assessment; Taxonomy: Knowledge)

11.288 **The answer is b.** Randomized controlled trials are considered the most rigorous evidence for a phenomenon. (Difficulty: 3; Discipline: Clinical Skills; Taxonomy: Knowledge)

11.289 **The answer is b.** In this mother's case, the baby had a shallow latch, which was quickly and easily corrected. This is the most common cause of this type of wound. Choices a and c are possible. Biting during nursing (choice d) is not likely to cause a wound in this position; it is more likely to cause a wound at the nipple–areola juncture. (Difficulty: 4; Discipline: Pathology; Taxonomy: Assessment)

11.290 **The answer is b.** Lipids are the most variable of the components listed. The proportion of fat in milk increases as the breast empties, and there is a slight variation in fatty acid profiles with maternal diet. The others are very stable across women, over the course of a day, and over the duration of breastfeeding. (Difficulty: 3; Discipline: Development; Taxonomy: Knowledge)

11.291 **The answer is b.** The proportion of fat in milk increases as the breast empties, so the proportion of fat from one breast is highest when the baby has fed several times from that breast. (Difficulty: 4; Discipline: Development; Taxonomy: Knowledge)

11.292 **The answer is c.** Mothers are reliable witnesses and reporters of their baby's condition. Sudden disinterest in breastfeeding may indicate a significant problem in the baby. (Difficulty: 3; Discipline: Clinical Skills; Taxonomy: History)

11.293 **The answer is c.** Herbs can pass into milk and exert an effect on the baby. Giving pharmaceutical advice is not within the scope of practice of the LC. The LC can provide the mother with published information about nonpharmacological remedies for minor health problems. (Difficulty: 2; Discipline: Clinical Skills; Taxonomy: Collaboration)

11.294 **The answer is b.** Macrophages and possibly neutrophils and T-lymphocytes actively kill microbes by phagocytosis. (Difficulty: 4; Discipline: Clinical Skills; Taxonomy: Knowledge)

11.295 **The answer is b.** Growth factors are most concentrated in colostrum and early milk. (Difficulty: 5; Discipline: Development; Taxonomy: Knowledge)

11.296 **The answer is a.** Support from her male partner is the most important of the options listed, although any support will increase the likelihood of her continuing to breast-feed. (Difficulty: 4; Discipline: Psychology; Taxonomy: Goals)

11.297 **The answer is b.** Beta-lactoglobulin is not even present in human milk and is the most likely to cause allergic reactions in babies. Alpha-lactalbumin is not found in bovine milk. Lactose and lactoferrin are found in both milks. (Difficulty: 4; Discipline: Pathology; Taxonomy: Evaluate)

11.298 **The answer is d.** Lipid solubility facilitates transfer of drugs into mother's milk. The other factors inhibit drug transfer to milk. (Difficulty: 4; Discipline: Pharmacology; Taxonomy: Knowledge)

11.299 **The answer is d.** Feeding bottles and teats fall within the scope of the Code under Article 2. Pacifiers do not fall under the Code because milk does not flow through them, but they are covered under Baby Friendly Hospital Initiative Step 9. Pumps and storage bags are not covered. (Difficulty: 4; Discipline: Clinical Skills; Taxonomy: Knowledge)

11.300 **The answer is a.** Whey:casein ratio changes over time from 90:10 in early lactation to ~60:40 as the baby approaches 6 months. Stools normally change from very loose and frequent to firmer and less frequent over time. (Difficulty: 5; Discipline: Development; Taxonomy: Knowledge)

11.301 **The answer is a.** Unsolicited donations of formula in emergency situations can undermine breastfeeding and worsen the health of all babies. UNICEF and the Emergency Nutrition Network recommend that unsolicited donations be locked up until the legitimate need can be determined. Safe preparation in emergencies is difficult to impossible. (Difficulty: 4; Discipline: Clinical Skills; Taxonomy: Collaboration)

11.302 **The answer is c.** Sucrose is not found in human milk but is often the carbohydrate used to manufacture infant formula. The other carbohydrates play an important role in infant growth and immune function. (Difficulty: 3; Discipline: Development; Taxonomy: History)

11.303 **The answer is d.** Specific antibodies to maternally acquired bacterial and viral illnesses are produced in mother's body and quickly appear in milk. Other immune properties in milk are active against a wide spectrum of pathogens. (Difficulty: 3; Discipline: Pathology; Taxonomy: Collaboration)

11.304 **The answer is c.** The string-like structure connecting the tongue to the floor of the mouth is the lingual frenulum (or frenum). The labial frenulum is on the upper (maxillary) gum ridge. The incisive papilla are behind the upper gum ridge, and mucous membrane covers most of the inside of the baby's mouth. (Difficulty: 4; Discipline: Development; Taxonomy: Assessment)

11.305 **The answer is b.** Most countries provide paid maternity leave for new mothers, which is the most supportive strategy to facilitate meeting global breastfeeding recommendations. All of the other choices are appropriate and helpful. (Difficulty: 5; Discipline: Psychology; Taxonomy: Collaboration)

11.306 **The answer is b.** The pale-colored lumps on the areola are Montgomery's tubercles (Montgomery's glands) and are completely normal. (Difficulty: 2; Discipline: Development; Taxonomy: Goals)

11.307 **The answer is d.** The active substance in *Cannabis* (marijuana) has a high milk:plasma ratio (8) and therefore is present in milk for a long time—it also has a long half-life (25 to 57 hours). The other substances are found at lower levels in the milk, yet still have an effect on the infant. (Difficulty: 5; Discipline: Pharmacology; Taxonomy: Collaboration)

11.308 **The answer is c.** The hypoglossal nerve (cranial nerve XII) is the primary motor nerve of the tongue. The other nerves listed are involved in suck–swallow–breathe but play a lesser role in tongue movement. (Difficulty: 5; Discipline: Development; Taxonomy: History)

11.309 **The answer is a.** This mother's nipple size is in the normal range. The puckering around the areola is probably because the air is cool. (Difficulty: 2; Discipline: Development; Taxonomy: Assessment)

11.310 **The answer is b.** Pumps are useful when the mother and baby need to be separated. Only if direct breastfeeding is not possible should pumping be suggested. A mother with a history of sexual abuse should first be encouraged to breastfeed. The other reasons for pumping are appropriate. (Difficulty: 4; Discipline: Clinical Skills; Taxonomy: Plan)

11.311 **The answer is b.** This nipple is flat. There is no distinct "shank" between the areola and nipple "bud" or tip. (Difficulty: 4; Discipline: Clinical Skills; Taxonomy: Document)

11.312 **The answer is a.** Atopic dermatitis is the most likely condition because it is locally contained and has sudden onset. The other conditions are possible and the LC should be collaborating with her medical care provider for a thorough diagnosis. Fungal infections on the lactating breast are typically not localized to one small area. (Difficulty: 4; Discipline: Pathology; Taxonomy: History)

11.313 **The answer is c.** Viruses and bacteria are eliminated by pasteurization. Many protective and nutritive elements are retained. (Difficulty: 5; Discipline: Development; Taxonomy: Document)

11.314 **The answer is d.** The question lists the foods from least priority to highest according to WHO recommendations. (Difficulty: 4; Discipline: Development; Taxonomy: Document)

11.315 **The answer is a.** Increased carrying when the baby is not fussy as well as when he is fussy reduces total crying per day. (Difficulty: 2; Discipline: Psychology; Taxonomy: Goals)

11.316 **The answer is d.** Teats have significant drawbacks in virtually every situation. Teats fall within the scope of the International Code of Marketing of Breastmilk Substitutes and should be considered only rarely and for therapeutic purposes. (Difficulty: 5; Discipline: Clinical Skills; Taxonomy: Plan)

11.317 **The answer is d.** Open cups or spoons are safe, especially in emergencies and disasters, and do not disrupt the baby's sucking response. (Difficulty: 4; Discipline: Clinical Skills; Taxonomy: Collaboration)

11.318 **The answer is b.** The highest risk of disease in children who were never breastfed is hospitalization for lower respiratory tract diseases (257% higher). Obesity is 32% higher, diarrhea and vomiting are 178% higher, and asthma is 67% higher in children who have never breastfed. (Difficulty: 5; Discipline: Clinical Skills; Taxonomy: Knowledge)

11.319 **The answer is c.** The lumps are Montgomery's tubercles (Montgomery glands) and are entirely normal. (Difficulty: 3; Discipline: Development; Taxonomy: Document)

11.320 **The answer is c.** This is "peau d'orange" or orange-peel texture of the skin is associated with breast cancer, overstretched skin, edema, hair follicle stimulation, and other conditions. Breast cancer should be ruled out by a qualified medical provider. The other answers would be appropriate after ruling out a dangerous condition. (Difficulty: 5; Discipline: Clinical Skills; Taxonomy: Collaboration)

11.321 **The answer is d.** The rolling action presses milk out of the milk ducts sinuses toward the nipple. Little milk is stored in the ducts, but of the techniques listed, this is likely the most effective method for hand expressing. (Difficulty: 3; Discipline: Techniques; Taxonomy: Plan)

11.322 **The answer is b.** A theoretical framework helps establish a systematic point of view and starting/reference point for professional activities. (Difficulty: 2; Discipline: Clinical Skills; Taxonomy: Knowledge)

11.323 **The answer is d.** Breastfeeding has a calming, stress-reducing effect on mothers. Breastfeeding may reduce risk of postpartum depression. Breastfeeding mothers miss work less often. Many mothers find breastfeeding emotionally fulfilling. (Difficulty: 3; Discipline: Psychology; Taxonomy: Collaboration)

11.324 **The answer is a.** The Baby Friendly Hospital Initiative (BFHI) is designed to protect breastfed babies from practices and policies that disrupt or interfere with breastfeeding. The 2009 Expanded and Integrated BFHI includes safe preparation of formula for the nonbreastfeeding baby. (Difficulty: 4; Discipline: Clinical Skills; Taxonomy: History)

11.325 **The answer is b.** Immune factors form a "layer" in milk that is the first to appear in the colostral phase and the last to disappear during weaning. Some factors even increase over time; some are stable to heating or freezing, and many develop after birth and change throughout the course of lactation. (Difficulty: 4; Discipline: Development; Taxonomy: Document)

11.326 **The answer is c.** Kangaroo care, or skin-to-skin contact, stabilizes infant temperature, reduces infant pain, and increases infant oxygen saturation. However, the temperature stabilization is most important because the mother's body provides greater thermal homeostasis than electric warmers and other humans. It is especially beneficial for premature infants. There is no increased risk for infant suffocation in this position. (Difficulty: 4; Discipline: Psychology; Taxonomy: Knowledge)

11.327 **The answer is c.** Domperidone (Motilium), metoclopramide (Reglan, Maxolon), and cimetidine (Tagamet) are sometimes used to increase milk production. Of these, domperidone and metoclopramide have been studied most for effectiveness and safety. Beer raises prolactin levels when tested in men, but babies do not like the flavor of alcohol in milk and breastfeed less when milk alcohol levels are elevated. (Difficulty: 3; Discipline: Pharmacology; Taxonomy: Collaboration)

11.328 **The answer is b.** PCOS is implicated in low and marginal milk production in some women. (Difficulty: 3; Discipline: Physiology; Taxonomy: Knowledge)

11.329 **The answer is a.** High lipid solubility would increase drug transfer into milk. The other factors would inhibit passage into milk. (Difficulty: 2; Discipline: Pharmacology; Taxonomy: Collaboration)

11.330 **The answer is c.** It is appropriate to discuss the potential side effects on milk supply with the mothers. The ethical principle in this case is the patients' rights to autonomy over their health care choices. (Difficulty: 5; Discipline: Clinical Skills; Taxonomy: Collaboration)

11.331 **The answer is a.** Bromocriptine (Parlodel, Bromolactin, Kripton, Bromohexal) has been used to suppress lactation. (Difficulty: 2; Discipline: Pharmacology; Taxonomy: Knowledge)

11.332 **The answer is b.** The tongue usually extends past the lower gum ridge (alveolar ridge) and is cupped around the breast. Occasionally, it will extend past the lower lip. (Difficulty: 4; Discipline: Development; Taxonomy: Assessment)

11.333 **The answer is a.** Omega-3 fatty acids DHA and AA are especially important in development of the central nervous system and are found in abundance in human milk. (Difficulty: 3; Discipline: Development; Taxonomy: Evaluate)

11.334 **The answer is a.** Rooting and sucking are key reflexes for infant feeding. (Difficulty: 5; Discipline: Development; Taxonomy: Knowledge)

11.335 **The answer is a.** Down syndrome is most likely to show this pattern of growth. The 2006 World Health Organization's Child Growth Standards (http://www.who.int/childgrowth/en/) are based on breastfed babies in six geographic regions of the world. (Difficulty: 3; Discipline: Clinical Skills; Taxonomy: Evaluate)

11.336 **The answer is b.** An oral structural defect is the most likely explanation for pain during nursing of two siblings who are not twins. The younger baby had a mild tongue-tie; after that was released, nursing was comfortable for the mother. Choices a and c are unlikely to cause breast or nipple pain, and there is no reason to think that her milk production is inadequate in any way. (Difficulty: 2; Discipline: Physiology; Taxonomy: Knowledge)

11.337 **The answer is a.** The question in the survey was prefaced by a positive statement about the value of breastfeeding. This type of a research flaw is called a "leading question." Choices b and c cannot be concluded from the information provided. Choice d might be true, but the flawed question would invalidate the results anyway. (Difficulty: 3; Discipline: Clinical Skills; Taxonomy: Knowledge)

CHAPTER 12

Case Reports with Practice Questions

Each case is an actual situation with some names and details changed to protect the clients' confidentiality. Several pertinent questions are associated with each case. The answers and explanations follow the questions for each case.

Case 1

A 4 week-old baby was adopted when 3 days old. The baby's birth mother was using heroin in her first trimester followed by methadone maintenance for the duration of her pregnancy. The baby was born by cesarean section at 39 weeks' gestation after a short labor. The adopting mother reports a history of mild depression and infertility; she is inducing lactation with the aid of domperidone and herbal supplements. The baby has been formula-fed from birth. The adopting mother's goal is "to have the baby nurse at breast."

Questions for Case 1

1. Which of the following newborn behaviors is MOST LIKELY related to newborn drug withdrawal from maternal opiate use during pregnancy?
   a. tremors and hyperactive reflexes
   b. coordinated suck–swallow–breathe
   c. lethargy for several hours after birth
   d. low muscle tone around the jaw and mouth

2. What is the FIRST action that an adopting mother should take to start transitioning her baby to nursing at breast?
   a. Try feeding the formula using a tube-feeding device at breast.
   b. Hold the baby in a nursing position near the breast during feeds.
   c. Replace the standard nipple(teat) with a slow-flow design.
   d. Wait until the baby is very hungry before attempting at breast.

3. An adopting mother is exploring maternal factors that may influence her ability to induce lactation. Which of the following factors or conditions is MOST LIKELY to reduce her chances of inducing lactation?
   a. clinical depression
   b. mild anemia
   c. polycystic ovary syndrome
   d. hypertension

4. Which hormone involved in lactogenesis is absent and cannot be provided artificially when a mother is inducing lactation and has never been pregnant?
   a. estrogen
   b. progesterone
   c. prolactin
   d. placental lactogen

5. A mother is inducing lactation for her adopted baby. After 4 weeks of effort, she reports pumping both breasts simultaneously about 4 times a day with a consumer-grade electric breast pump, getting about 1 oz per breast each time. Which strategy would be MOST LIKELY to increase her milk production?
   a. Change to pumping sequentially (not simultaneously).
   b. Use a hospital-grade (multiuser) pump instead of a consumer (single-user) pump.
   c. Increase the number of pumping sessions per day to at least 8.
   d. Use a larger-diameter flange on the collection container.

Answers for Case 1

1. **The answer is a.** Tremors and hyperactive reflexes are typical of newborn abstinence syndrome, which can significantly affect the infant's ability to feed. (Difficulty: 3; Discipline: Pathology; Taxonomy: Assessment; 1–2 Days)

2. **The answer is b.** The first goal is to encourage the baby to view the breast as the source of food, so holding the baby in nursing position with the baby's cheek touching the mother's bare breast is the best first strategy. Tube-feeding devices may be an option after the baby can latch and attempt to feed at breast, if the mother's milk production is low. Replacing the standard nipple with a slow-flow one is still not breastfeeding. Hungry babies are in no mood to change feeding methods easily, so attempting to directly breastfeed when the baby is not excessively hungry is more effective. (Difficulty: 4; Discipline: Techniques; Taxonomy: Goals; 15–28 Days)

3. **The answer is c.** Polycystic ovary syndrome is a leading cause of infertility due to higher levels of androgens and disrupts other reproductive hormones as well. Depression is not known to affect induced lactation. Mild anemia is unlikely to affect lactation, and can likely be corrected with dietary supplements. Hypertension is not currently known to affect lactation, natural or induced. (Difficulty: 4; Discipline: Physiology; Taxonomy: Assessment; General Principles)

4. **The answer is d.** Placental lactogen is the most important lactogenic hormone, deriving from the placenta. In induced lactation, it cannot be provided artificially. The other key lactogenic hormones can be provided with medications. (Difficulty: 3; Discipline: Physiology; Taxonomy: History; Prenatal)

5. **The answer is c.** Adding additional sessions is the most likely strategy to increase production. Sequential pumping is less effective than simultaneous pumping for most women, because simultaneous pumping takes advantage of the let-down reflex in both breasts. Any pump with sufficient pressures and appropriate rhythms would be effective, not whether the pump is designed for multiple or single users. A larger-diameter flange might be helpful if the flange diameter is inhibiting movement of the breast/nipple in the flange. (Difficulty: 4; Discipline: Techniques; Taxonomy: Plan; 15–28 Days)

Case 2

You are employed by a maternity hospital which is working toward Baby-Friendly designation. Part of that journey is reviewing options for obtaining, storing, and distributing commercially published materials for patient education, sources for staff education, infant formula (both standard and specialty-use), breast pumps, feeding bottles, nipples (teats), pacifiers, swaddling blankets, baby clothing including hats, diapers, etc. Up until now, the hospital has been receiving free or low-cost supplies of many of these products. The hospital also gives some of these supplies to new mothers at discharge.

Questions for Case 2

1. Which product falls within the scope of the International Code of Marketing of Breast-milk Substitutes?
   a. swaddling blankets
   b. breast pumps
   c. feeding bottles
   d. diapers

2. At a well-baby clinic affiliated with a Baby-Friendly Hospital, a mother of an exclusively breastfed 6-week-old baby asks whether she should introduce a pacifier to her baby. Your BEST response is:
   a. Breastfeeding is well-established, so introducing a pacifier will help protect against SIDS.
   b. Pacifiers will help your baby learn to self-soothe and fall asleep alone.
   c. Pacifiers are never recommended for breastfed babies.
   d. Pacifiers increase your baby's risk of ear infections (otitis media).

3. Your hospital is working toward Baby-Friendly designation but is currently giving out "discharge bags" donated by a formula company. Why does this violate the International Code of Marketing of Breast-milk Substitutes?
   a. Mothers are more likely to start early formula use if they get a free sample.
   b. Brand-name formula is more expensive than generic (store) brand products.
   c. The International Code prohibits distributing free samples to new mothers.
   d. The samples contain powdered formula, which is never sterile and possibly contaminated.

4. Which action is prohibited by the International Code of Marketing of Breast-milk Substitutes and subsequent World Health Assembly resolutions?
   a. factual descriptions of a product that falls within the scope of the Code
   b. company logo on instructions for using that company's breastmilk substitute
   c. a health care worker at a large institution accepting supplies for research and evaluation within their institution from a company
   d. using equipment or education materials sponsored or produced by companies when teaching mothers about infant feeding

5. Which of the following is a description, not a marketing statement, and thus meets the criteria of the International Code of Marketing of Breast-milk Substitutes and subsequent World Health Assembly resolutions?
   a. Brand AA's Stage One foods for babies 4 months and older introduce single-ingredient pureed fruits and vegetables.
   b. Breast milk is the first choice for your infant's growth and development. But if you choose formula, Brand BB provides organic infant formulas that contain all the nutrients your baby needs.
   c. Brand CC's bottle is the perfect product for babies of all ages, and this makes it easy for them to learn how to drink.
   d. Brand DD milk storage containers are compatible with most breast pumps, dishwasher-safe, leak-proof, and made of food-grade polypropylene.

6. Training expenses for Step 2 are sometimes a barrier for some facilities working toward Baby-Friendly designation. Which of these sources of funding is UNETHICAL?
   a. hospital or private charitable foundations with humanitarian missions
   b. government-funded grants, stipends, or budget-line allocations
   c. formula company–sponsored training courses
   d. religious institutions affiliated with the hospital

Answers for Case 2

1. **The answer is c.** Feeding bottles and teats (nipples), infant formula and foods marketed for babies less than 6 months old fall within the scope of the International Code of Marketing of Breast-milk Substitutes and subsequent World Health Assembly Resolutions. As of 2014, breast pumps are not addressed in the International Code. Diapers and swaddling blankets do not fall within the scope of the International Code. (Difficulty: 3; Discipline: Clinical Skills; Taxonomy: Collaboration; General Principles)

2. **The answer is d.** Pacifiers increase the risk of ear infections. Many studies have reported that pacifiers interfere with exclusive breastfeeding, especially if started before breastfeeding is well established. In rigorous research, pacifiers have not been shown to protect against SIDS. The Baby-Friendly Initiative Step 9 states: "Give no teats or pacifiers to breastfed babies." (Difficulty: 5; Discipline: Clinical Skills; Taxonomy: Goals; 1–3 Months)

3. **The answer is c.** Choice c is a major tenet of the International Code—Article 5.1 and therefore the correct answer to this question. Choice a is verified by many studies. Choice d is true and a major reason why the World Health Organization publishes guidelines for safe preparation and use of powdered formulas. Cost of formula to the parents is not addressed in the International Code of Marketing of Breast-milk Substitutes. (Difficulty: 4; Discipline: Clinical Skills; Taxonomy: Collaboration; General Principles)

4. **The answer is d.** Article 6.3 states: "Facilities of health care systems should not be used for the display of products within the scope of the Code." Factual descriptions are allowed. A company can provide information on preparation or use of their own products, including the company logo. The Code applies to manufacturers and distributors of products that fall within the scope of the Code, not professionals. The Code permits health care workers to accept supplies at the institutional level for research and evaluation, but specifically prohibits these from being distributed to mothers. Resolution WHA49.15 (2008) on infant and young child nutrition "recognizes the need to ensure that the commitment and support for breastfeeding and optimal infant and young child nutrition are not undermined by conflicts of interest." (Difficulty: 5; Discipline: Clinical Skills; Taxonomy: Collaboration; General Principles)

5. **The answer is d.** This is a description which is factual and does not suggest uses for the product. Marketing is designed to get people to buy the product by suggesting uses, benefits, and desirability of the product. (Difficulty: 3; Discipline: Clinical Skills; Taxonomy: Evaluation; General Principles)

6. **The answer is c.** WHA 49.15 (1996) urges governments "to ensure that the financial support for professionals working in infant and young child health does not create conflicts of interest, especially with regard to the WHO/UNICEF Baby Friendly Hospital Initiative. The other sources of funding are ethical. (Difficulty: 3; Discipline: Clinical Skills; Taxonomy: Collaboration; General Principles)

Case 3

The lactation consultant (LC) made a home visit to a mother with a 3-week-old baby. The mother has a master's degree in biology and works at a local university; the baby's father works for the government. The baby, who was born at 37 weeks' gestation, is barely back to birth weight, although when at the breast his feeding patterns are appropriate. The mother says her son sleeps for about 1 hour at a stretch, on and off during the day and night and wants to nurse every time he wakes. He does have periods of being awake and content as long as he is in her arms.

The LC asked her where the baby was sleeping. The mother said the nurse at the hospital told her never bring the baby in her bed, so she had been sleeping on the living room couch with the baby since she got home. She does have a crib for her baby in a separate bedroom. She has attempted to put him to sleep "alone, on his back, in the crib," as she has been advised, but finds he wakes up within a few minutes and cries. She is exhausted trying to get him to sleep alone. The parents are considering using a "sleep training" scheme so she can get more rest.

Questions for Case 3

1. What is a normal duration of a sleep cycle for a 3-week-old exclusively breastfed infant?
   a. from 3 to 4 hours between feeds, around the clock
   b. about an hour, with some longer and shorter periods
   c. irregularly during the day and 5 to 6 hours at night
   d. 2-hour naps during the day, plus a longer stretch at night

2. What is the MOST LIKELY evidence-based sleep pattern for a breastfeeding mother in the early weeks postpartum?
   a. awake during the daylight hours, then 8 hours of uninterrupted sleep
   b. sleeps longer when her baby is in the same room in a crib
   c. sleeps longer and deeper when her baby is formula-fed by someone else
   d. sleeps longer and has better-quality sleep when bedsharing with her nursing baby

3. Which is the MOST LIKELY outcome from "sleep training" regimens that allow a baby to "cry it out" to "teach them to sleep alone?
   a. parents get a full night's uninterrupted sleep within 3 days
   b. baby relaxes into a restful sleep when put to bed alone
   c. baby's nighttime cortisol levels remain elevated even when the baby appears to be asleep
   d. mother's daytime milk production adjusts to fewer nursings at night

4. In which of these sleep environments is the baby at increased risk for SIDS (sudden infant death syndrome)?
    a. unattended, away from adult noises and contact
    b. sleeping on the same surface as an adult
    c. lying supine in a firm, flat, clean crib
    d. sleeping next to a drunk or drugged adult

5. Which situation puts the infant at LOWEST risk of smothering?
    a. baby alone, placed supine on a soft adult mattress
    b. adult sleeping with baby on a sofa (couch)
    c. nursing mother sleeping with her baby on a firm adult mattress
    d. swaddled infant alone, supine, in a crib

6. Which suggestion MOST SUPPORTS continued exclusive breastfeeding for the mother of a 3-week-old baby who complains that her baby will not sleep alone?
    a. Give your baby some formula so he will sleep more soundly.
    b. Baby-proof your bed, then lie with your baby's face near your breast. You'll both fall asleep easily.
    c. Nurse your baby to sleep, then slowly ease him into his own crib near where you sleep.
    d. If you let him cry for a short time, he'll learn to put himself to sleep.

Answers for Case 3

1. **The answer is b.** Newborn sleep patterns are irregular, and short periods of sleep are typical. Babies do not sleep for long stretches for several months. By 3 months, some have begun to consolidate short sleep stretches into longer ones occasionally. (Difficulty: 4; Discipline: Development; Taxonomy: Assessment; 15–28 Days)

2. **The answer is d.** Research studies report that a breastfeeding mother who shares a safe bed with her baby has the best nocturnal sleep of every group of new parents tested. All postpartum women tend to have fragmented sleep regardless of how they feed their babies. (Difficulty: 4; Discipline: Development; Taxonomy: Assessment; 15–28 Days)

3. **The answer is c.** Sleep training schemes create sustained, elevated cortisol levels in infants and young children. Elevated cortisol levels are known to have long-term negative consequences because babies are more sensitive to stress in the early years. Parents might or might not sleep better. Babies physiologically cannot "put themselves to sleep" in the early weeks and months. Mother's milk production hinges on frequent removal of milk, including during the night; long stretches of milk stasis suppress production. (Difficulty: 5; Discipline: Development; Taxonomy: Evaluation; 1–3 Months)

4. **The answer is a.** Babies who sleep unattended—in a separate room, away from adult noises and activities, are at increased risk of SIDS. Choice b carries no independent risk. Supine sleeping appears to be a low-risk situation related to SIDS, if the baby is in proximity to responsible adults. Sleeping next to an impaired adult puts babies at risk of smothering, not SIDS. Exclusively breastfed babies have the lowest rates of SIDS and all-cause infant mortality. (Difficulty: 4; Discipline: Psychology; Taxonomy: Goals; 1–3 Months)

5. **The answer is c.** When a non-smoking, sober, breastfeeding mother sleeps next to her baby on a safe surface, the risk of smothering is extremely low to negligible. Babies left unattended on soft mattresses are at risk of rolling prone and smothering or becoming entrapped. Sofas are a high-risk situation for anyone sleeping with a baby, especially if the baby is on the inside (next to the back cushions). A swaddled baby alone in a crib is at increased risk of SIDS and smothering. (Difficulty: 4; Discipline: Psychology; Taxonomy: Evaluation; 1–3 Months)

6. **The answer is b.** Breastfeeding mothers instinctively sleep with their baby in a unique, protective posture. Exclusively breastfeeding mothers who sleep with their babies on a safe surface get the most sleep of all postbirth parents. Formula may suppress arousal, is a significant risk factor for many reasons, and interferes with exclusive breastfeeding. Crying is stressful for babies, with significant long-term negative consequences. (Difficulty: 4; Discipline: Psychology/Physiology; Taxonomy: Goals; 15–28 Days)

Case 4

You are consulting with the mother of a 10-day-old baby. Mother has severely injured nipples, and unceasing pain throughout the feed. You observe scabs across both nipple faces; the mother says they open and even bleed during a feed. Placing the mother in a reclined position, with the baby lying skin-to-skin, prone, on the mother's chest/torso, allowed for baby-led self-attachment. The mother describes this as the most comfortable latch she has experienced. Nonetheless, the baby has a difficult time maintaining latch, using a shallow gape and gripping with his lips, which causes a callus or blister to appear on his top lip, at the midline. After the feed, you do a visual and digital examination of the baby's mouth, and feel a short, tight lingual frenulum that pulls the tongue tip into a "heart" shape when extended.

Questions for Case 4

1. You want to document how a mother's nipples are healing under your care plan by taking a photograph at today's appointment. What permission is required?
   a. The mother's verbal consent, during the consult, is sufficient.
   b. No permission is required; photographs allow you to chart clinical progress.
   c. Written permission from the mother is required, prior to your taking the photograph.
   d. Written permission from the mother is required, at the conclusion of the consult.

2. A client mother's nipples are healing slowly but surely. She wants to send you cellphone photographs she has taken each day, showing the progress. She will transmit them via her cellphone directly to your cellphone. The best way to protect her privacy is to:
   a. explain that cell phone photograph transmission is not secure.
   b. delete the photograph from your phone after you look at it.
   c. refuse to accept the photographs because the mother took them, and you have no way of verifying the photograph is of her.
   d. delete them from your phone after adding the image to your password-protected secure charting system.

3. You are aware of research that reports that chronic wounds can heal with topical use of manuka honey, which is (U.S.) FDA approved for its inherent antibacterial properties. To avoid ethical concerns about discussion of the product as part of a mother's care plan for her cracked, you should:
   a. carry the product with you, to show how it is properly applied. Leave the sample with your client.
   b. tell the mother about how the product works, and ask her to discuss with her primary health care provider whether it is appropriate for her use given her medical history.
   c. discuss a variety of topical products that the mother might use to speed nipple healing, and ask her to consult with her primary health care provider first about which one to use.
   d. ask the mother if she has any allergy to honey first.

4. You suspect the mother and baby's breastfeeding situation will rapidly improve if the baby has the lingual frenulum revised or surgically released. To best meet your ethical obligations, you should:
   a. inform the mother of your diagnosis of ankyloglossia.
   b. provide several options of health care providers who can examine for and diagnose ankyloglossia.
   c. explain how the baby's tongue is used during normal feeding, and the impact of any anatomic restrictions.
   d. discuss use of breast compression during feeds to maximize flow and intake.

Answers for Case 4

1. **The answer is c.** The IBLCE Code of Professional Conduct (IBLCE CPC) at 3.2 says "Refrain from photographing, recording or taping (audio or video) a mother or her child for any purpose unless the mother has given advance written consent on her behalf and that of her child" (emphasis added). See also *Core Curriculum for Lactation Consultant Practice,* 3rd ed. at p. 20. (Difficulty: 4; Discipline: Clinical Skills; Taxonomy: History; General Principles)

2. **The answer is d.** See 3.1 of IBLCE CPC, regarding preserving confidentiality. The duty of prior written permission for photographs is when the IBCLC takes the picture, not the mother. But the IBCLC has an overall duty of care to preserve confidentiality if the mother decides to take and send a picture. (Difficulty: 4; Discipline: Clinical Skills; Taxonomy: History; General Principles)

3. **The answer is c.** Under Principle 1.3 of the IBLCE CPC the mother should be fully informed about all her care options. The IBCLC Scope of Practice does not permit an IBCLC to "prescribe" even over-the-counter products. The mother should consult with her health care provider and can bring with her information she has learned from the IBCLC. (Difficulty: 4; Discipline: Clinical Skills; Taxonomy: Goals; General Principles)

4. **The answer is c.** IBCLC Clinical Competencies and IBLCE Scope of Practice say IBCLCs can perform comprehensive feeding assessments and oral examinations, and they can provide evidence-based information and support about any aspect of breastfeeding. Choice b is a good response after explaining normal and abnormal tongue function. Choice d might be a later or supplemental strategy. (Difficulty: 4; Discipline: Clinical Skills; Taxonomy: Goals; General Principles)

Case 5

The mother of a 14-month-old girl ask you to testify at her divorce custody/visitation hearing. The child has multiple food and environmental allergies, some life-threatening; the child's physician has testified to the importance of this child continuing to breastfeed for at least 2 years or longer. The father of this child is opposed to continued breastfeeding and has accused the mother of forcing the child to breastfeed in order to avoid letting the child stay with him for multiple-day and overnight visits. The legal system in their location does not differentiate between the needs of a breastfed child and any other child, nor between the mother's or father's ability to care for a child under the age of 2 years.

Questions for Case 5

1. Which milk component is HIGHER at 14 months postbirth than in the early weeks?
   a. zinc
   b. lactose
   c. lysozyme
   d. alpha-lactalbumin

2. A mother is challenged to provide reasons that her 14-month-old child wants to nurse several times a day and night. The child is also eating a wide variety of family foods. The MOST LIKELY reason for the child to want to nurse into the second year or longer is:
   a. the child is seeking the immune protection found only in her mother's milk
   b. insufficient caloric levels in the family foods offered
   c. oral aversion to solid or lumpy foods
   d. emotional closeness and comfort

3. A mother is being accused of child abuse because her child is still nursing at 14 months and shares mother's bed all night every night. What is the MOST LIKELY long-term outcome of all-night bedsharing with sustained breastfeeding?
   a. enhanced self-esteem and confidence in the child
   b. delayed progression to independent sleeping for the child
   c. increased risk of maternal abuse of the child, including incest
   d. higher risk of dental caries in the child

4. How is the nursing mother–baby relationship in the second year of breastfeeding different from any other mother–baby or parent–baby relationship?
   a. The nursing mother's heart rate and respiratory rate continue to influence her child.
   b. A nursing toddler sleeps with her mother in a unique way, thus reducing risk for sleep-related death.
   c. Immune components in mother's own milk offer unique protection to the infant until at least age 3.
   d. Continued nursing suggests an overly dependent child or overcontrolling mother.

5. The mother of a 14-month-old wants suggestions for optimizing nutrition from complementary foods. Of the following foods, which would you recommend as MOST LIKELY to fill the nutritional gap between what breastfeeding provides and the child's needs?
   a. whole grains for their B vitamins
   b. animal products, especially red meat for iron
   c. fish or shellfish for the lipids
   d. green leafy vegetables for the fiber

Answers for Case 5

1. **The answer is c.** Lysozyme increases in milk over time, providing immune protection for the breast and the nursing child. Zinc decreases over time; lactose remains stable, and proteins including alpha-lactalbumin are relatively stable over time. (Difficulty: 3; Discipline: Development; Taxonomy: History; > 12 Months)

2. **The answer is d.** Children who continue nursing past infancy are meeting their needs for warmth, security, emotional closeness, comfort, and more. Nursing into the second year and beyond provides some important calories to the child and important immune protection. (Difficulty: 3; Discipline: Development; Taxonomy: Collaboration; > 12 Months)

3. **The answer is a.** Children whose needs for dependency and nursing are met willingly all day and night by their mother and parents show normal, desirable outcomes in all parameters. None of the other choices are supported by research. (Difficulty: 3; Discipline: Psychology; Taxonomy: Goals; > 12 Months)

4. **The answer is c.** Immune components unique to human milk protect the child until the child's immune system is fully mature at around 3 years of age. Heart and respiratory rate synchronicity occur primarily during the early days and weeks. While it is true that nursing babies and their mothers have different sleep habits than other adults, there is no evidence of elevated risk related to bedsharing after about 4 months. The last choice is false. (Difficulty: 4; Discipline: Psychology; Taxonomy: Evaluation; > 12 Months)

5. **The answer is b.** Complementary foods that best fill the nutritional gap between breastmilk and the needs of a 12- to 24-month-old child should be nutritionally dense and high in protein, iron, and/or zinc. A variety of other foods will provide a balanced set of nutrients. B vitamins are also found in animal products. Omega-3 fats in fish are also found in human milk. Young children need less fiber than adults, although green leafy vegetables are good sources of other nutrients. (Difficulty: 5; Discipline: Development; Taxonomy: Goals; > 12 Months)

Case 6

The parents of a 1-day-old baby, born at home, call your private practice for help, saying that nursing is painful for the mother, and her nipples are flat/bent after each feed. The baby urinated on the first day but has not yet passed a meconium stool. Their previous child was tongue-tied (short/tight lingual frenulum), which was successfully treated within a week after birth. The baby nurses for over 45 minutes, falls asleep for a few minutes, and then wakes again crying frantically. The baby has not yet been examined by a physician or skilled health care provider.

Questions for Case 6

1. The parents of a 1-day-old baby born at home without a skilled birth attendant want your help with painful breastfeeding. Your BEST response should be:
   a. I will help only after you've had your baby examined by a physician or skilled professional.
   b. I can talk with you by telephone a few times, off the record.
   c. I charge a fee for home or office visits and can see you later today.
   d. I cannot help, because I am required to work only under a physician's supervision.

2. A mother says that her baby latched on well at first, but now her nipple is painful and "looks flat." Your FIRST action should be:
   a. Carefully observe the baby's behavior at breast during a feed.
   b. Have the mother pull the baby's legs in closer.
   c. Make sure both upper and lower lips are flanged (rolled) outward.
   d. Remove the baby from her breast and re-start the feed.

3. After the baby releases the breast after a 20-minute feed, there is a crease across the nipple tip and the nipple appears flattened. The MOST LIKELY cause of this is:
   a. normal suck
   b. shallow latch
   c. baby's head is turned away
   d. torticollis in the baby

4. After repositioning a 2-day-old baby so he latches more deeply, the mother says her nipples are still creased and painful after a feed. The MOST LIKELY infant-related cause of this continued nipple pain is:
   a. small for gestational age
   b. tongue and inner cheeks have a white coating
   c. labial frenulum is long and elastic
   d. lingual frenulum is attached at the lower gum ridge

5. During a home visit on the second postbirth day, you learn that a baby has not yet passed a meconium stool. Your FIRST action should be:
   a. Assess the baby's skin turgor and reflexes, documenting your findings.
   b. Inform the baby's primary care provider of your findings.
   c. Reassure the parents that delayed passing of meconium is normal.
   d. Show the parents how to safely feed infant formula.

6. Which infant sleep pattern is MOST LIKELY during the first 2 days after birth? The mother received no drugs or pharmacological pain relief during labor, and the healthy term infant was placed in skin-to-skin contact with mother immediately, without suctioning or separation for any reason.
   a. 60 to 90 minutes of sleep at irregular intervals
   b. absence of REM sleep during daylight hours
   c. 5 to 6 hours of slow-wave sleep during darkness
   d. predictable periods of sleep if alone in a crib

7. On the second postbirth day, an otherwise healthy term baby nurses for 45 minutes, sleeps briefly, then wakes with frantic crying. What is the MOST LIKELY explanation for this pattern?
   a. normal pattern for day 2
   b. small for gestational age
   c. head injury during birth
   d. shallow latch at breast

Answers for Case 6

1. **The answer is c.** An LC can ethically provide postpartum consults in a client's home or in an office, providing the fees are discussed first. The other choices are not appropriate. All client consults, by phone or in person, or electronically, must be documented, and the LC must be in contact with the family's care provider(s). (Difficulty: 5; Discipline: Clinical Skills; Taxonomy: Collaboration; 1–2 Days)

2. **The answer is a.** The LC should observe a full feed before suggesting any changes. The other actions or suggestions might be appropriate, depending on what is observed. (Difficulty: 5; Discipline: Techniques; Taxonomy: Assess; 1–2 Days)

3. **The answer is b.** Shallow latch is the most likely reason that the mother's nipple is flattened after a feed with a crease across the nipple tip. Position of the baby and torticollis are possible explanations to explore after the depth of attachment is corrected. Normal suck should not crease, flatten or damage the mother's nipple. (Difficulty: 4; Discipline: Pathology; Taxonomy: Evaluate; 1–2 Days)

4. **The answer is d.** A short and/or tight lingual frenulum, or one that is attached near the lower gum ridge and/or tongue tip, is the most likely infant condition listed to cause persistent nipple pain. Small gestational age is not likely related to nipple pain. The white coating is likely oral *Candida* infection, which can be painful but unlikely to cause nipple distortion. The upper lip (labial) frenulum as described is normal. (Difficulty: 3; Discipline: Pathology; Taxonomy: Evaluate; 1–2 Days)

5. **The answer is b.** IBLCE's Code of Professional Conduct states that an LC is required to "Inform an appropriate person or authority if it appears that the health or safety of a client or a colleague is at risk." LC scope of practice alone does not include a medical assessment of the baby. Meconium should have been passed on day 1. Safe formula feeding may become necessary if other strategies are ineffective. (Difficulty: 4; Discipline: Clinical Skills; Taxonomy: Collaboration; 1–2 Days)

6. **The answer is a.** Newborn sleep cycles are approximately 60 to 90 minutes in irregular patterns throughout the first few months. REM sleep and slow-wave sleep are part of sleep cycling. Babies cannot sleep long periods until at least 6 months of age. Solitary sleep results in less sleep for the infant and parents. (Difficulty: 2; Discipline: Development; Taxonomy: Evaluation; 1–2 Days)

7. **The answer is d.** Shallow latch and/or weak suck is the most likely explanation for this pattern in a healthy term infant. A normal pattern is in the range of 10 to 30 minutes of effective sucking, followed by a longer sleep stretch. Frantic crying suggests hunger from inadequate milk transfer during the feed. While b and c are possible, d is the most likely explanation for this infant's behavior. (Difficulty: 4; Discipline: Development; Taxonomy: Evaluation; 1–2 Days)

Case 7

A mother was collecting milk with an electric breast pump for her baby born at 28 weeks' gestation. The baby developed necrotizing enterocolitis (NEC) and died yesterday. She is now painfully engorged, deeply grieving, and desperate for help. There is a donor milk bank in your area that accepts bereavement milk.

Questions for Case 7

1. You have been working with a mother whose baby was born at 28 weeks of gestation. Today you learn that her baby has died. The FIRST thing you should say to her is:
   a. It's OK to stop pumping your milk now.
   b. Oh, NO, what a shock! And just when you thought she was improving.
   c. I can help you gradually reduce your milk production comfortably.
   d. What was your baby's name?

2. A mother stopped pumping milk for her premature baby 48 hours ago, and now her breasts are painfully full of milk, Your FIRST action to reduce her discomfort should be:
   a. Suggest she stand in a warm shower to trigger a let-down response.
   b. Put cold cloths on her breasts to reduce inflammation.
   c. Help her massage and express some milk.
   d. Apply a breast binder to suppress lactation.

3. Of the following factors, which is the MOST LIKELY reason that a premature baby developed necrotizing enterocolitis (NEC)?
   a. The baby received only pumped human milk.
   b. The baby received a supplement derived from soy protein.
   c. Digested formula can destroy the baby's white cells.
   d. Exclusive breastfeeding cannot protect an infant from NEC.

4. What is the MOST LIKELY use of pasteurized milk donated by mothers whose baby died?
   a. Support adults with IgA deficiencies or are receiving solid-organ transplants
   b. Research on milk properties, storage, or other factors
   c. Dispensed to sick or premature babies on prescription
   d. Extract human stem cells for research purposes

5. Which of the following recommendations would be MOST HELPFUL for a mother who is reducing milk production after her premature baby died?
   a. Pump or express only enough milk to soften your breasts when they become full.
   b. Bind your breasts tightly with a firm cloth or binder for at least a week.
   c. Restrict your fluid intake for the next 2 to 3 weeks.
   d. Ask your doctor to prescribe a medication containing estrogen and progesterone.

Answers for Case 7

1. **The answer is b.** In a highly emotional situation, the LC should acknowledge the mother's feelings first. Choice b is an example of an empathetic statement. Asking about the baby (d) might be a good second response. Clinical help or suggestions can be provided after feelings are acknowledged. (Difficulty: 5; Discipline: Clinical skills; Taxonomy: Goals; Prematurity)

2. **The answer is c.** The first strategy is always to help the mother with self-care skills. Gentle hand expression and massage should help the milk to start moving, and requires no equipment or devices. A warm shower may help trigger a let-down and is the next best suggestion. There is no indication of inflammation, so cold compresses are inappropriate at best. A breast binder is likely to increase pain and does not reduce short-term milk synthesis. (Difficulty: 4; Discipline: Techniques; Taxonomy: Goals; Prematurity)

3. **The answer is c.** Researchers Penn et al. reported that "Lipase digestion of formula, but not milk, caused significant death of neutrophils (ranging from 47% to 99% with formulas vs. 6% with milk) with similar results in endothelial and epithelial cells." Human milk nearly completely protects premature infants from NEC, whether the milk is pumped and fed, or the baby breastfeeds directly. Soy protein may also be a risk for NEC. (Difficulty: 3; Discipline: Pathology; Biochemistry; Taxonomy: Evaluate; Prematurity)

4. **The answer is b.** Bereavement milk is most likely to be used for research purposes. Occasionally it may be pasteurized and used for lower-risk babies or adults. Bereavement milk is usually not given to the most vulnerable newborns because the mothers were not screened before donating. (Difficulty: 5; Discipline: Nutrition; Taxonomy: Collaborate; Prenatal)

5. **The answer is a.** Removing some milk but not emptying the breasts will comfortably use the principle of autocrine control of lactation and gradually diminish milk secretion. Breast binding does not suppress lactation and can induce pathology. Fluid intake is unrelated to milk production, and restricting fluids can harm other aspects of mother's health. An estrogen-containing medication will likely suppress milk production, with or without progesterone, but may take several days to be effective. Meanwhile, the mother's milk stasis is painful for her and can trigger other pathology. (Difficulty: 3; Discipline: Techniques; Taxonomy: Goals; Prematurity)

Case 8

First email: "I am wondering if I will be able to breastfeed my second child if I was unable to breastfeed my first child. After my son was born he received colostrum, but my milk never came in. I never got engorged and after about 1.5 weeks of trying to breastfeed and pump I still never got any milk. I am just wondering if I should still try to breastfeed our daughter when she is born, or if the same thing will happen again. I REALLY want to breastfeed, but understand if I cannot. If you could help me on this situation I would greatly appreciate it. Again, I am just wondering if it is possible that my milk may not come in this second time around either."

LC's reply: The LC responded by email and offered to help the mother by phone.

Second email: "I do not have long distance on my phone, and my cellphone is out of the service area for the next 2 weeks. Otherwise I would be happy to call you.

I tried to breastfeed the first time, but we ended up having a C-section due to my high BP and his heart rate dropping . . . before the C-section I was put on magnesium–which I had to be on for a full 24 hours and it made me really sick. (vomiting, headache, etc.) then I had SEVERE reactions to pain meds and was only on extra-strength Tylenol™ (acetaminophen) for the pain, which did not help very much . . . so they would bring Brian into me to breastfeed, shove him in my face, grab and pull and tug until he latched on . . . he would latch for 20 minutes each breast . . . so I am not sure if it was because I was really stressed out with the pain, the vomiting, and it being my first baby and first breastfeeding experience. But I never actually got milk . . . never got engorged. I also have large breasts . . . which I know the size does not affect milk production or the ability to breastfeed, but thought I would let you know that fact. I have little sensation in my breasts when they are touched as well.

I can tell you this much, this time around I will have more control over my pain, as we have found a pain med that I do not get sick from and am opting for the C-section so that I do not risk the chance of being put on magnesium again. I will also have more control over the nurses just giving me my daughter and then asking them to leave and letting me do it myself . . . hoping that all of this will help me relax more and be able to breastfeed.

Again, I was just wondering if it will help or if I should buy bottles and get the formula of choice just in case. I am also sorry that I do not have the option of calling you at this moment."

Questions for Case 8

1. A mother pregnant for the second time asks, "Will I be able to breastfeed my second child if I was unable to breastfeed my first baby?" Which of the following should be your FIRST response to her?
   a. You are wise to be asking these questions now, during pregnancy.
   b. Yes, most second babies breastfeed better than first babies.
   c. The answer depends on the reason you had problems the first time.
   d. No, because your breasts have insufficient glandular tissue.

2. Which of the following maternal perinatal factors is MOST LIKELY to interfere with initiation of breastfeeding?
   a. cesarean surgery
   b. magnesium sulfate administered during labor
   c. intravenous hydration during labor
   d. history of failed breastfeeding in previous pregnancy

3. Which maternal prenatal factor is MOST LIKELY to compromise lactation?
   a. three previous closely spaced pregnancies
   b. maternal underweight
   c. maternal obesity
   d. mother older than 35 years

4. Which technique for helping a mother breastfeed has been found to be offensive to mothers?
   a. placing the baby skin-to-skin and allowing the baby to self-latch
   b. grasping the mother's breast and shoving it into the baby's mouth
   c. showing the mother how to support her breast from underneath
   d. showing a movie or video of several positions for breastfeeding

5. Which prenatal breast condition is MOST LIKELY to affect lactation?
   a. no leaking of colostrum by the third trimester
   b. flat nipples
   c. no change in pigment of the nipple and areola
   d. no change in breast size during pregnancy

6. Which medication given to a laboring woman is MOST LIKELY related to newborn sucking problems?
   a. magnesium sulfate
   b. fentanyl
   c. propofol
   d. penicillin

7. Which of the following conditions of labor is MOST LIKELY to delay the onset of lactogenesis II (copious milk production)?
   a. very rapid labor
   b. delivery before 37 weeks' gestation
   c. long, difficult labor
   d. vomiting during labor

8. A mother complains of incision pain following her cesarean birth and requests pain relief medication but is worried about the effect on her baby. Your FIRST response to her should be:
   a. You cannot have any drugs for pain relief while breastfeeding.
   b. Try using patterned breathing like you learned in childbirth classes.
   c. We'll monitor you and your baby closely after you've received pain medication
   d. Today is the worst—the pain should be less by tomorrow.

9. A pregnant woman is worried that her milk may not come in with her second baby. She said she never actually got milk after her first baby's birth, and never got engorged. Which of the following birth complications is MOST RELATED to delayed-onset lactogenesis?
   a. cesarean birth
   b. retained placental fragment
   c. premature birth
   d. episiotomy

10. Which hormone's rapid decline after childbirth triggers the onset of lactogenesis II (onset of copious milk production)?
    a. estrogen
    b. prolactin
    c. oxytocin
    d. progesterone

Answers for Case 8

1. **The answer is a.** Supporting the mother's decision to explore the reasons for her previous unsuccessful breastfeeding experience is the best first response, because that technique helps build her confidence. After an empathetic response, providing a problem-solving answer would be appropriate. (Difficulty: 4; Discipline: Clinical Skills; Taxonomy: Goals; Prenatal)

2. **The answer is a.** Cesarean surgery is associated with breastfeeding difficulties in several research studies, regardless of the reason for the cesarean. Magnesium sulfate is suspected of causing problems; likewise for IV hydration. A history of failed breastfeeding could be from numerous causes including infant factors. (Difficulty: 4; Discipline: Psychology; Taxonomy: Knowledge; Labor/birth)

3. **The answer is c.** Overweight/obese women are more likely to have a lower prolactin response to suckling, which is a major factor negatively affecting breastfeeding. Repeat pregnancies, underweight, or age over 35 years are not documented risk factors per se, but could be indicators of other maternal problems that might affect lactation. (Difficulty: 3; Discipline: Pathology; Taxonomy: History; General Principles)

4. **The answer is b.** Mothers do not like for staff members to grab their breasts or push the baby onto their breasts, and may be too intimidated to express their displeasure. Demonstrating with a doll or with a video may be more helpful. Option a, self-attachment, is usually very helpful and effective. Supporting the breast from underneath may compress some surface milk ducts. (Difficulty: 3; Discipline: Techniques; Taxonomy: Goals; Prenatal)

5. **The answer is d.** No change in breast size during pregnancy can indicate suppressed development of lactocytes (milk-making cells), appearing as breast hypoplasia. Secreted colostrum may not appear at the nipple until after birth when oxytocin levels are high. Nipple shape and protractility often change in pregnancy. Pigmentation changes of the nipple and areola have not been researched related to lactation. (Difficulty: 4; Discipline: Development; Taxonomy: History; Labor/birth)

6. **The answer is b.** Fentanyl is associated with breastfeeding problems, according to randomized controlled studies of high, low, and, and none. Propofol is rapidly metabolized and has not been researched for breastfeeding outcomes. (Difficulty: 3; Discipline: Pharmacology; Taxonomy: History; 1–2 Days)

7. **The answer is c.** Delayed lactogenesis (onset of copious milk production delayed past 72 hours) is most likely associated with long, difficult labor. Specific factors and interventions of long, difficult labors may also play a role. Rapid labor, premature delivery, and vomiting during labor are not known to be related to the timing of onset of lactogenesis II. (Difficulty: 3; Discipline: Pathology; Taxonomy: Knowledge; Labor/birth)

8. **The answer is c.** Pain medications for surgical deliveries are generally compatible with breastfeeding. The LC and nursing staff should monitor the mother and baby for poor or ineffective feeding, excessive drowsiness, or lethargy. (Difficulty: 2; Discipline: Pharmacology; Taxonomy: Goals; 1–2 Days)

9. **The answer is b.** A retained placental fragment is the most likely factor associated with delayed onset of lactogenesis. cesarean surgery may also delay onset of lactogenesis. (Difficulty: 3; Discipline: Pathology; Taxonomy: History; Prenatal)

10. **The answer is d.** Delivery of the placenta causes a sudden drop in levels of progesterone, triggering the onset of lactogenesis II. (Difficulty: 3; Discipline: Physiology; Taxonomy: Knowledge; 1–2 Days)

Case 9

The mother had well-controlled gestational diabetes and wanted a natural birth. At 37 weeks, labor was induced for high blood pressure.

She was admitted to the hospital and given intravenous administration of pitocin (synthetic oxytocin) for 3 days without onset of regular contractions. During that time she received only intravenous fluids and consumed no other food or drink. She did not sleep well because of the regular but ineffective contractions from the pitocin.

After 3 days, she was sent home for the weekend and returned Monday for another attempt at induction. Instead, she requested a cesarean delivery, which was refused three times.

Labor induction was again attempted with IV pitocin, but her uterus ruptured. She was rushed to the operating room, where cesarean surgery was immediately performed. The surgery took several hours, during which she received >30 units of blood.

Her baby was taken to the intensive care unit for a week. She requested a hospital-grade breast pump but was refused. She requested that her baby be given donor human milk, which was available on prescription at the Donor Milk Bank in the same city instead of infant formula, but that request was refused as well.

The hospital has been openly resistant to implementing the Baby-Friendly Hospital Initiative. The mother has contacted an attorney for possible legal action against the hospital and its staff.

Questions for Case 9

1. A pregnant woman has gestational diabetes. She can reduce her risk of developing type 2 diabetes if she breastfeeds for how long?
   a. at least 3 months
   b. at least 6 months
   c. at least 12 months
   d. breastfeeding does not change the risk

2. A mother's labor is being induced at 37 weeks because of high blood pressure. What is the MOST LIKELY consequence to her baby's ability to breastfeed?
   a. No problem; babies have mature sucking responses at 37 weeks of gestation.
   b. The baby's oral muscles are too weak to suck normally.
   c. The baby may have short sucking bursts.
   d. The drugs used for labor induction affect baby's coordination.

3. A mother required multiple units of blood by transfusion during a difficult birth. By postbirth day 7, her milk has not yet "come in." What is the MOST LIKELY cause of her delayed lactogenesis?
   a. long, difficult labor
   b. Sheehan syndrome
   c. separation from her baby
   d. she did not start expressing or pumping soon enough

4. Which milk expression method(s) would be your FIRST recommendation for a mother whose 37-week gestation baby is hospitalized in a neonatal intensive care unit?
   a. Hand-express, starting at 24 hours after birth.
   b. Hand-express within 1–2 hours, then add a hospital-grade pump.
   c. Double-pump with an adjustable-speed hospital-grade pump.
   d. Single-pump with a wide-diameter, flexible-flange pump.

5. Which is the MOST COMMON use for donor human milk worldwide?
   a. term babies whose mothers cannot breastfeed
   b. adopted babies
   c. premature babies
   d. babies of mothers who are infected with HIV

6. Which components of human milk are MOST STABLE to pasteurization and freezing?
   a. proteins
   b. lipids
   c. cellular components
   d. minerals

7. A pregnant woman is worried about giving birth prematurely because of hypertension. Which strategy is MOST LIKELY to prevent or reduce risk of pregnancy-related hypertension?
   a. well-balanced diet with sufficient protein
   b. high-carbohydrate diet
   c. drinking at least 2 L of milk every day
   d. prenatal vitamin supplements

Answers for Case 9

1. **The answer is a.** For pregnant women with gestational diabetes, breastfeeding at least 3 months reduces the risk of developing type 2 diabetes. (Difficulty: 4; Discipline: Pathology; Taxonomy: Knowledge; Prenatal)

2. **The answer is c.** At 37 weeks of gestation, many babies' suck patterns are less organized than at full term even though some babies will breastfeed effectively. Oral muscle strength should be sufficient for breastfeeding by 37 weeks. Drugs for induction have not been researched for effect on baby's suck coordination. (Difficulty: 4; Discipline: Psychology; Taxonomy: Assessment; Prematurity)

3. **The answer is b.** Sheehan syndrome is the most likely reason for her delayed lactogenesis and may affect her lactation permanently. Severe blood loss related to birth can cause necrosis of all or part of the pituitary gland, which produces prolactin needed for lactogenesis. Long, difficult labor may also delay lactogenesis. Separation from her baby and delay in milk expression can also hinder onset of lactation. (Difficulty: 5; Discipline: Pathology; Taxonomy: History; Labor/birth)

4. **The answer is b.** Expressing or pumping within 1–2 hours combined with pumping with a hospital-grade pump would be the most likely strategy to maximize milk collection and production. Delaying expression for 24 hours can compromise lactation. A double pump with adjustable speed may be helpful combined with hand expression. Single-pumping is more time-consuming and does not utilize milk ejection as well as other strategies. (Difficulty: 4; Discipline: Techniques; Taxonomy: Plan; Prematurity)

5. **The answer is c.** Premature and sick babies are the most common recipients of donor milk. Depending on the local situation and available donated milk, other recipients can include the other choices and more. (Difficulty: 3; Discipline: Clinical Skills; Taxonomy: Knowledge; Prematurity)

6. **The answer is d.** Minerals in human milk are stable to pasteurization and freezing. Many immune components are stable to heat treatment. White cells are destroyed by pasteurization and freezing. Lipids are stable to pasteurization but may break down into free fatty acids during freezing and thawing. (Difficulty: 4; Discipline: Development; Taxonomy: Knowledge; General Principles)

7. **The answer is a.** A well-balanced, nutritious diet with sufficient protein may prevent or reduce risk of pregnancy-related hypertension. The other dietary strategies are unlikely to be effective. (Difficulty: 3; Discipline: Development; Taxonomy: Collaboration; Prenatal)

Case 10

First email: I have a beautiful 2-week-old baby girl. Although in my heart I really wanted to breastfeed my daughter . . . it has not worked out. We have never been able to have a latch (mainly because I have flat nipples). We tried using a shield but she still was not getting enough and I would still have to pump after.

Basically since she's been born I have been exclusively pumping and it is just too much. I've had a public health nurse/LC over to my home a few times and 3 days ago we decided it would be best to switch her to formula. So with that said I am now trying to have my milk dry up and I have not had any success.

I am following the guidelines on your website. Pumping when I'm full and emptying just to feel comfortable. I used to pump for 15 minutes every 3 hours to feed my baby and now I am pumping only 7 or 8 minutes every 4 hours. But I am still producing more milk. Today I pumped 4 oz in like 6 minutes! I started crying. Just 3 days ago it took me 15 minutes to pump 3 oz . . .

I also had mastitis during the first week, so I am afraid of going too long without pumping in case I have a relapse.

I just do not know what to do anymore and I feel like the milk will just never dry up. I am tired of being chained to a pump and not being able to go out freely.

Please, if there is anything you can do to help me I would be so grateful.

LC's email reply: At 2 weeks, your breasts are still adjusting. If you tell me where you live (city, state), I will find someone near you who can help you.

Questions for Case 10

1. The mother of a 2-week-old baby asks for help drying up her milk, saying, "I do not know what to do anymore–I feel like the milk will just never dry up." Your FIRST response to her should be:
   a. You sound desperate! At 2 weeks, your breasts are still adjusting to making milk.
   b. What did you expect when you decided to stop breastfeeding?
   c. Have you tried using a breast binder?
   d. Your milk will eventually dry up if you stop all that pumping.

2. Which strategy would be MOST EFFECTIVE for a mother who is producing far more milk than her healthy, term 2-week-old daughter needs?
   a. Breastfeed on cue (8 to 12 or more times a day) while milk production adjusts.
   b. Drink 1 cup of sage tea three times a day to reduce milk production.
   c. Wear a supportive bra and apply cold packs if overfull.
   d. Offer only one breast per feed, and express the other breast.

3. Which factor is MOST IMPORTANT in regulating the short-term rate of milk production?
   a. mother's intake of fluids
   b. degree of breast fullness
   c. maternal serum prolactin level
   d. age of baby

4. A mother trying to dry up her milk quickly develops mastitis when her baby is 10 days old. Which is the MOST LIKELY predisposing factor?
   a. flat nipples that retain bacteria in skin folds.
   b. bacterial contamination of her absorbent bra pads
   c. recurring milk stasis
   d. inadequate cleaning of breast pump parts

5. After trying to wean her baby to formula unsuccessfully, a mother of a 2-week-old baby requests help in re-starting breastfeeding. She had trouble with latching in the early days, says her nipples are flat, and has been feeding pumped milk in a bottle with silicone teat. Your FIRST action should be:
   a. Teach her suck-training techniques.
   b. Show her how to use a nipple-pulling device to extend her nipples.
   c. Have her place the bottle teat over her own nipple for a few feeds.
   d. Place the baby skin-to-skin on mother's body and support attempts at self-attachment

6. A mother is adamant about not wanting to breastfeed or provide her pumped milk, nor obtain donor human milk. She asks which manufactured formula would be next safest for her baby. Your BEST suggestion is:
   a. soy-based liquid
   b. goat's milk
   c. cow's-milk–based powdered
   d. cow's milk–based liquid

7. A mother is trying to reduce milk production through pumping, and found that pumping for 15 minutes every 3 hours was producing excess milk. Which strategy would be MOST LIKELY to reduce total amount pumped per day?
   a. Pump at the highest comfortable pressure.
   b. Use a large-diameter flange.
   c. Pump only past one let-down (milk-ejection reflex).
   d. Pump more often so the breasts do not have time to fill.

Answers for Case 10

1. **The answer is a.** Your first response should be a validation of her concern and a factual statement related to her situation. Blaming her for stopping is inappropriate; breast binders do not hasten weaning and may increase pain; and sudden cessation of pumping may result in more breast pathology. (Difficulty: 2; Discipline: Clinical Skills; Taxonomy: Goals; 3–14 Days)

2. **The answer is a.** Lactating breasts will calibrate and adjust to the baby's needs by around 6 weeks. There is no indication of discomfort, so remedies for engorgement are inappropriate. Herbal products to reduce production are poorly researched; suppression of production so early in lactation is inappropriate. Patterns of breast usage are unrelated to total milk volume produced. (Difficulty: 3; Discipline: Techniques; Taxonomy: Plan; 3–14 Days)

3. **The answer is b.** The degree of breast fullness/emptiness is the most important regulator of milk production in the short term. Components of milk retained in the alveoli provide chemical feedback to the cells. The highest rate of production occurs when the breasts are emptiest. (Difficulty: 4; Discipline: Development; Taxonomy: Knowledge; General Principles)

4. **The answer is c.** Milk stasis is the most likely predisposing factor in developing mastitis. Once milk stasis occurs, then commonly occurring bacteria can multiply. (Difficulty: 4; Discipline: Pathology; Taxonomy: History; 3–14 Days)

5. **The answer is d.** Placing the baby skin-to-skin on mother's chest often leads to infant self-attachment by triggering the infant's instincts. After 2 weeks, any early minor suck problems should have resolved. Babies with normal suck can latch on to many different nipple configurations, and the pumping would likely have improved her nipple elasticity. (Difficulty: 5; Discipline: Techniques; Taxonomy: Plan; 3–14 Days)

6. **The answer is d.** Cow's milk (bovine) formulas are safer than the other options listed. Soy products contain no lactose and are not recommended for general use. Powdered formulas are never sterile and may be contaminated with pathogenic bacteria. Goat's milk is deficient in folic acid and other nutrients needed by human infants. (Difficulty: 4; Discipline: Pharmacology; Taxonomy: Knowledge; General Principles)

7. **The answer is c.** Milk is released in a bolus-type pattern during milk ejections. Limiting total pumping time to only one let-down would result in less total milk collected. The other three options would increase the rate of production and/or amount collected. (Difficulty: 3; Discipline: Clinical Skills; Taxonomy: Plan; 3–14 Days)

Case 11

My client is being treated for Lyme disease with a several-month prescription of doxycycline. Her doctor told her to stop breastfeeding her 10-month-old because of tooth staining. I searched the LactNet archives and saw a post on Lyme disease, so I thought I would ask you about it. I read Hale's book *Medications and Mothers' Milk*, and will share that with her.

I do not understand why we have to use doxy when there are several other combos mentioned. One thing is that Rocephin is IV, so oral is preferable to IV. But why not amoxicillin? I knew that Lyme is a very debilitating disease that is underrecognized and takes a long time to recover from if not treated well in the beginning stage. I know several folks who have been treated for it.

This is the first time I've looked into breastfeeding and medications for Lyme, and I appreciate that all out warfare has been proclaimed, but I hate to lose breastfeeding in there. This client had put off her treatment a few weeks ago because she did not want to quit breastfeeding, and today she told me the rest of the story, and that now and again she cannot resist nursing—which looks okay, according to Hale.

We have an infectious-disease doctor here who does not care what Hale says; he will not prescribe doxycycline if a woman if breastfeeding due to the bone issue. Maybe she only has a couple weeks left of medications to go and could review all the information with her pediatrician.

Questions for Case 11

1. The mother of a healthy 10-month-old must take tetracycline for 2 weeks and asks about possible effects on her baby. Your FIRST response should be:
   a. Tetracycline is considered compatible with breastfeeding by the American Academy of Pediatrics.
   b. Your baby will likely have diarrhea for the duration of your treatment.
   c. Ask your doctor for an antifungal for your nipples to prevent thrush.
   d. Offer more family foods to your baby while you are taking this medicine.

2. A mother has postponed treatment for Lyme disease for fear of the effects of long-term doxycycline on her breastfed 10-month-old baby. Your FIRST response should be:
   a. Go ahead and take the medicine. Formula would be worse than any outcome from the medication.
   b. You've breastfed long enough for all the benefits to have reached your baby.
   c. You sound ambivalent about these options. Can we explore the risks of the disease and treatment in more detail?
   d. Lyme is a terrible disease and your treatment outweighs any benefit of continuing to breastfeed your baby.

3. You are asked to help develop treatment policies that support breastfeeding for maternal infectious diseases in a family/general medical practice office. Which statement is MOST ACCURATE concerning risk to the breastfed baby of maternal infectious diseases?
   a. Most maternal infections are passed to the baby through her milk; therefore, immediate weaning is advised.
   b. Antibiotics for maternal infections are likely to cause severe problems in the breastfed baby.
   c. Babies can continue to breastfeed during maternal bacterial infections, but not viral infections.
   d. Mother's immune system makes specific antibodies to infections acquired during breastfeeding, so breastfeeding should continue.

4. What is the MOST LIKELY nursing-related behavior pattern of a 10-month-old baby?
   a. Baby willingly goes to sleep alone in a crib.
   b. Prefers lumpy or mashed food from jars to common foods eaten by the family.
   c. Baby is usually negotiable about where and when to breastfeed.
   d. Baby is very social; goes quickly and readily to strangers.

5. Which of the following is the MOST APPROPRIATE complementary food for a 10-month-old breastfed baby?
   a. baked potato without salt
   b. strips of lightly cooked pork
   c. orange and grapefruit segments
   d. steamed broccoli and carrots

6. A breastfeeding mother was bitten by a tick and is being treated for Lyme disease and is worried about transmitting the disease to her baby. Which action is MOST LIKELY to protect her baby from becoming infected?
    a. Stop breastfeeding immediately.
    b. Increase family foods and decrease breastfeeding.
    c. Continue breastfeeding and take prescribed antibiotics.
    d. Continue breastfeeding and increase intake of vitamin C.

Answers for Case 11

1. **The answer is a.** Citing published medical guidelines on medications is the most ethical and appropriate first response. Her baby may get diarrhea or thrush from her treatment, which might be the next piece of information to share with her. Increasing family foods is irrelevant in this situation. (Difficulty: 3; Discipline: Pharmacology; Taxonomy: Collaboration; General Principles)

2. **The answer is c.** An empathetic statement is your best FIRST response. This situation is a true dilemma because Lyme is a serious disease, and doxycycline during breastfeeding can have long-term effects on babies. A thorough exploration of risks of both the disease and its treatments in collaboration with her primary care providers is an important role of the LC. (Difficulty: 4; Discipline: Clinical Skills; Taxonomy: Goals; 7–12 Months)

3. **The answer is d.** Specific antibodies to maternally acquired bacterial and viral illnesses are produced in mother's body and quickly appear in milk. Other immune properties in milk are active against a wide spectrum of pathogens. (Difficulty: 3; Discipline: Pathology; Taxonomy: Collaboration; General Principles)

4. **The answer is c.** By 10 months, most breastfed toddlers are somewhat negotiable about location and timing. Their need to breastfeed is more flexible than in the first 6 months. They often breastfeed to sleep, enjoy many family foods, and may be cautious or even frightened when approached by strangers. (Difficulty: 3; Discipline: Development; Taxonomy: Plan; 7–12 Months)

5. **The answer is b.** Nutrient-dense and iron-rich foods are the most important complementary foods for the breastfed child between 6 and 12 months. The other foods are lower in nutrient value, although still important in the child's overall diet. (Difficulty: 5; Discipline: Development; Taxonomy: Knowledge; 7–12 Months)

6. **The answer is c.** The many immune components in breastmilk have been shown to be protective against the spirochete that causes Lyme. Virtually all antibiotics used to treat Lyme are compatible with breastfeeding, according to several sources. (Difficulty: 3; Discipline: Pathology; Taxonomy: Collaboration; 7–12 Months)

Case 12

"I talked to you briefly about my daughter who spit up a lot while I was breastfeeding and thought that she was simply overeating or suffered with reflux (GERD) as that was what the doctor told me. You had suggested that she may have a milk allergy. If it is a milk allergy what other symptoms would she have? Also if I were to get an allergy test done on her would the milk allergy show up?

If you could send me some information regarding the milk allergy issue and what steps I should take that would be greatly appreciated.

I am very concerned about not letting her have milk, as it would be a challenge to replace the vitamin D and calcium that is provided by milk and milk products. Also she loves all dairy products, and they are the main part of her diet. She and is a very hard child to feed."

Questions for Case 12

1. A 16-month-old breastfeeding child has severe eczema on her face. She breastfeeds several times a day and at night, and loves dairy products which are the main part of her diet. Your FIRST suggestion should be:
   a. Cut down on her intake of dairy products to less than two servings a day.
   b. Ask your pediatrician for a suitable lotion or cream for the eczema.
   c. Does she rub her face on her pillow or stuffed toys?
   d. Has anyone discussed the possibility of your daughter having a dairy allergy?

2. The mother of a 16-month-old partly breastfed child is concerned that he started spitting up frequently and has had an itchy rash on his face ever since starting day care. His lunch meal is provided by the day care center. Which is the MOST LIKELY cause of his new spitting up and rash?
   a. age of the child
   b. gastroenteritis
   c. anxiety at being separated from his mother
   d. allergy to a food he is eating at day care

3. A mother asks about sources of vitamin D for her 16-month-old breastfeeding child. Your FIRST recommendation should be:
   a. Continue breastfeeding; you and he should get direct sunlight about 30 minutes a week.
   b. Give him two to three servings of dark green leafy vegetables every day.
   c. An egg yolk every day will provide enough vitamin D.
   d. Start replacing breastfeeding with vitamin D–fortified cow's milk.

4. Which of the following foods is the BEST source of calcium for a partly breastfeeding 16-month-old who cannot tolerate dairy products?
   a. sesame seed paste
   b. fresh oranges
   c. spinach
   d. oatmeal cereal

5. A 16-month-old partly breastfed child has been diagnosed with food allergies. Which of the following is the MOST LIKELY allergy trigger?
   a. rice
   b. cow's milk
   c. soy
   d. cabbage

6. A mother is being pressured to wean her 16-month-old child and wants to know why continued breastfeeding is encouraged. Your FIRST response to her should be:
   a. They have a point. Breastfeeding past 12 months has little value.
   b. It's fine to continue for another few months.
   c. Would you like suggestions on discreet breastfeeding in public?
   d. Your milk continues to provide important immunity and nutrition to your child.

7. A mother living in a far northern latitude with limited sunlight several months a year asks about vitamin D supplements for her 5-month-old exclusively breastfed baby. Your BEST suggestion is:
   a. Mix some cod liver oil into pumped breastmilk and give it to your baby.
   b. Set up several sun lamps inside your home in the darkest months.
   c. Consider taking a supplement of 6400 IU daily yourself
   d. Supplement your baby with 4 oz of vitamin D–fortified formula daily.

8. You work in a public health department that is developing a vitamin D policy for pregnant women, breastfeeding mothers, and infants. Your BEST recommendation based on global research is:
   a. Screen all mothers and babies, and supplement those who are at risk or have low levels.
   b. Supplement all pregnant women, breastfeeding mothers, and breastfed babies.
   c. Warn all mothers to avoid using sunscreen on babies under 6 months old.
   d. Provide vitamin D supplements to dark-skinned mothers and babies.

9. Which prenatal or birth practice is MOST LIKELY to result in higher iron stores for the exclusively breastfed infant's first 6 months?
   a. Mother takes prenatal iron supplements.
   b. Delay clamping of the umbilical cord until pulsing stops.
   c. Mother eats foods high in iron for the first 6 months.
   d. Supplement the baby with iron-fortified formula.

Answers for Case 12

1. **The answer is d.** Eczema on the face is a common symptom of food allergies, especially allergy to cow's-milk protein. Cutting down on dairy will probably not help, because any amount of dairy protein may trigger a reaction. (Difficulty: 3; Discipline: Pathology; Taxonomy: History; >12 Months)

2. **The answer is d.** Food allergy is the most likely cause of his dermatologic and gastrointestinal symptoms of allergy. The mother should investigate what foods he is being given. Gastroenteritis would not simultaneously produce a face rash. Neither his age nor any anxiety would explain both symptoms. (Difficulty: 3; Discipline: Pathology; Taxonomy: History; >12 Months)

3. **The answer is a.** Levels of vitamin D in mother's milk are related to the mother's own vitamin D stores. A half-hour of direct sunlight assures adequate levels of D in many locations. If direct sunlight is not available, supplements of D for the mother should be considered. Leafy vegetables for the child may help; so will egg yolk. Weaning to formula is not appropriate. (Difficulty: 3; Discipline: Pathology; Taxonomy: Plan; General Principles)

4. **The answer is a.** Of the foods listed, sesame seeds ground into a paste are highest in calcium. Oxalic acid in spinach binds calcium, making spinach a poor source. Oranges and oatmeal are appropriate foods for a child this age, but not especially high in calcium. (Difficulty: 4; Discipline: Development; Taxonomy: Knowledge; >12 Months)

5. **The answer is b.** Cow's milk is the most common food allergen in children, responsible for multiple allergic symptoms. Soy is almost as common an allergen. Cabbage and rice are uncommon allergens in most populations. (Difficulty: 3; Discipline: Pathology; Taxonomy: History; General Principles)

6. **The answer is d.** Breastfeeding well into the second year and beyond provides important immunological components and nutrition to the child. There is no documented age beyond which breastfeeding has no value. (Difficulty: 2; Discipline: Psychology; Taxonomy: Goals; >12 Months)

7. **The answer is c.** Supplementing the breastfeeding mother with high doses of vitamin D (6400 IU) will raise the levels of D in her milk. Testing the child is appropriate before any direct supplements to the child are given. Local recommendations may differ; research on adequate levels of vitamin D continues to challenge our understanding of the importance of vitamin D for many health conditions. (Difficulty: 3; Discipline: Pathology; Taxonomy: Plan; 4–6 Months)

8. **The answer is a.** Screening every mother and baby is most appropriate and avoids over- and under-supplementing of those with documented needs for supplements. After screening everyone and supplementing those with a need, also discussing risk of sunscreens is appropriate. (Difficulty: 5; Discipline: Clinical Skills; Taxonomy: Collaboration; General Principles)

9. **The answer is b.** Delayed clamping of the umbilical cord until it stops pulsing assures that the infant receives the normal amount of placental blood. Anemic pregnant or breastfeeding women should increase iron intake for their own health. Supplementation with iron-fortified formula increases risk to the infant and is inappropriate. (Difficulty: 4; Discipline: Psychology; Taxonomy: Collaboration; Labor/birth)

Case 13

The mother and baby came to our lactation clinic for follow when the baby was 4 days old. Mother was limiting feeds to 10 minutes per side per advice of the floor nurse "because if the baby nurses longer than that, he's just using you as a pacifier and you'll get sore." The baby was up 29 g from discharge weight: weight was 6 lb 11 oz at birth and 6 lb 5 oz at release.

The baby's bilirubin was 10 mg/dL on second day and is now down to 9. 4 mg/dL Our clinic LC gave the mother correct info; the mother latched the baby in football (underarm) position successfully; the baby nursed >20 minutes and came off in "milk coma."

The mother had delivered by cesarean section. The staff nurse gave the mother a breast pump but did not show her how to use it; it has never been taken out of its box. The baby was already nursing well at breast. The staff called the lactation clinic in a panic to set up a visit because the patient was leaving the hospital, and her baby was not nursing appropriately.

The mother is obese—or rather, very large. A staff nurse could not tell if the mother was latching her baby on correctly.

When we saw her in clinic, the mother was in tears and overwhelmed with relief that baby had gained weight and bilirubin level was down. We're frustrated because this sort of thing happens on a weekly basis.

Questions for Case 13

1. You are helping a mother at her first postpartum visit on day 4. She has been limiting her baby's feeds to 10 minutes per breast because a hospital nurse told her "if he nurses longer than that, he's only using you as a pacifier and you'll get sore." Your FIRST statement to her should be:
   a. See what he can do with nursing at breast at his own pace.
   b. That advice was wrong—long feeds do not cause nipple pain.
   c. The baby gets most of your milk in the first 10 minutes.
   d. How are your breasts feeling today?

2. You are working to implement the Baby-Friendly Hospital Initiative in your facility. Scheduled feeds are often recommended for outdated and incorrect reasons. Your FIRST strategy should be:
   a. Design charting forms with at least 8 to 12 spaces to record number of feeds per day.
   b. During Step 2 training, explore and correct all the reasons that are given for scheduling feeds.
   c. Develop disciplinary measures for staff who continue to advise scheduled feeds.
   d. Meet with the prenatal class teachers and provide accurate patient handouts.

3. A staff nurse called the LC to help assess an obese mother breastfeeding her baby on day 2. Which indicator would be the MOST REASSURING indicator of effective feeding?
   a. Baby stays attached at least 10 minutes.
   b. Rooting and swallowing are observed.
   c. Baby's ear, shoulder, and hips are aligned.
   d. The mother reports gentle tugging on her breast.

4. An obese mother's baby weighed 6 lb 12 oz (3.07 kg) at birth; 6 lb 4 oz (2.83 kg) at discharge on day 2, and 6 lb 14 oz (3.12 kg) on a day 4 checkup. She is relieved, because obesity may have which effect on lactation:
   a. reduced prolactin response to sucking
   b. overactive let-down response that overwhelms the baby
   c. suppressed milk synthesis because of excess lipid tissue in the breast
   d. overproduction because of excess blood glucose

5. You are called to help an obese mother with breastfeeding on the second postbirth day. Her baby has not yet breastfed effectively despite several attempts. Your FIRST action should be:
   a. Put a rolled-up towel under the mother's breast.
   b. Compress her nipple and areola to make a breast "sandwich."
   c. Demonstrate deep latch with a breast model and doll.
   d. Have her sit upright with pillows under her arms.

6. You are helping a frightened, overwhelmed mother on day 4 with her first baby. She has been calling everyone she knows to get advice on what to expect in the early days of breastfeeding, and has heard confusing stories. You observe that she responds to her baby's cues and the baby nurses effectively for about 20 minutes before falling asleep and releasing her breast spontaneously. Your FIRST response should be:
   a. Now that's what I call a textbook example of a great breastfeed!
   b. Does she usually take only one breast like she just did?
   c. Are you getting enough help at home?
   d. Your baby looks better today than when you were discharged.

Answers for Case 13

1. **The answer is a.** Feeding the baby is the first action to take, and feeding on cue for length and frequency is the first issue to address. B is incorrect because feed length and nipple pain are not correlated. Although c is somewhat correct, that response does not take the baby's ability to feed into consideration. Addressing her breast comfort would be one of the next issues to address. (Difficulty: 4; Discipline: Clinical Skills; Taxonomy: Goals; 3–14 Days)

2. **The answer is b.** Step 2 of the BFHI is training all staff on the BFHI steps and breastfeeding management, including feeding on cue. During the training, old ideas can be explored and clarified, and references provided. Documentation and policies should be based on evidence, and are more accepted after training. Disciplinary measures should not be the first policies developed. (Difficulty: 4; Discipline: Clinical Skills; Taxonomy: Collaboration; General Principles)

3. **The answer is b.** Rooting and observed swallowing are reliable indicators that the baby is effectively breastfeeding during the first 4 days. Length of feeds can vary and still be effective. Alignment can vary. The mother's sensation is not a reliable indicator of a good feed. (Difficulty: 3; Discipline: Techniques; Taxonomy: Assessment; 3–14 Days)

4. **The answer is a.** Obesity is associated with reduced prolactin response to suckling in the early days of lactation. Prolactin response to suckling is more important for milk production in the first postbirth week than it is later in lactation. (Difficulty: 2; Discipline: Physiology; Taxonomy: Goals; 1–2 Days)

5. **The answer is c.** Deep attachment is key to comfortable, effective breastfeeding. Demonstrating with a model and a doll empowers the mother and develops her own skill in holding and positioning her baby effectively. The other techniques may be helpful if the next attempt at latching is unsuccessful. (Difficulty: 5; Discipline: Techniques; Taxonomy: Plan; 1–2 Days)

6. **The answer is a.** Supporting the mother with a positive, enthusiastic statement about her skills or ability is very confirming, especially for uncertain mothers. The other questions address clinical progress and might be appropriate after praising and reinforcing the mother's breastfeeding-related behavior. (Difficulty: 5; Discipline: Clinical Skills; Taxonomy: Goals; 3–14 Days)

Case 14

We worked with a mother whose baby reversed progress in growth when switched to formula at 6 months. The baby was healthy and thriving at 6 months. The mother read advertisements for formula with added DHA and AA, and switched her baby to formula. The baby stopped growing and had repeated illnesses. She contacted our office for help with re-lactating at 16 months.

No new teeth have appeared since 6 months when she switched the baby to formula. The baby now is irritable, and has bowel problems and sleep problems. The mother had read the formula company's advertisements claiming better cognitive development. Prior to switching to formula, the baby had been a happy thriving baby.

Questions for Case 14

1. You are helping a mother re-lactate after her baby became quite ill when she weaned the baby to formula at 6 months. Which of the following is the MOST LIKELY reason her baby suddenly had more illness?
   a. She prepared the formula with contaminated water from her backyard well.
   b. Withdrawal of the immune components in human milk left the baby with little defense against pathogens.
   c. The baby was exposed to more environmental pathogens as he became more mobile.
   d. The chemicals in the bottle and teat reacted with the formula to produce illness.

2. A mother saw a television advertisement for infant formula with added long-chain fatty acids, claiming the product would "result in early mental development scores." Why is this ad a violation of the International Code of Marketing of Breast-milk Substitutes?
   a. No manufactured product made from animal milk can replicate human milk.
   b. Long-chain fatty acids are not associated with early mental development.
   c. The International Code forbids advertising of products covered by the Code to the general public.
   d. The International Code requires television stations to give equal air time to breastfeeding promotion.

3. A mother stopped breastfeeding at 6 months, but her baby could not tolerate formula and she is requesting your help with re-starting to breastfeed. What is the FIRST suggestion you would make?
   a. We can talk to your doctor about prescribing medications to resume your milk production.
   b. Start by putting your baby close to your breast, skin-to-skin, several times a day, to see how he responds.
   c. Pump with a hospital-grade breast pump with double collection kit at least 8 times a day.
   d. It's too late now—once breastfeeding is stopped, it cannot be resumed.

4. A mother weaned her baby at 6 months and is now trying to re-establish breastfeeding at 16 months. Which components of milk are the "last to go" during weaning and involution?
   a. carbohydrates
   b. white cells
   c. enzymes
   d. immunoglobulins

5. What is the MOST IMPORTANT reason for continuing to breastfeed into the second year of life and beyond?
   a. immune protection tailored to the child's environment
   b. nutrition and trace minerals
   c. muscular development of the jaw and mouth
   d. emotional attachment between mother and child

6. The parents of a breastfeeding 16-month-old are divorcing, and the father is arguing that breastfeeding is a control mechanism by the mother. As an expert witness for the mother, your BEST response should be:
   a. The mother does not control the child in a breastfeeding relationship; rather, the child breastfeeds and the mother responds.
   b. The mother could pump her milk for her child; she does not have to breastfeed directly at this age.
   c. Overnight separation from the mother at this age will not damage their breastfeeding relationship.
   d. Mothers do have strong control over the breastfeeding relationship, which can be overbearing.

7. You are contacted by a mother who was exposed to influenza at work. Her child is 15 months old, sleeps with her, and breastfeeds several times a day and at night. Your BEST recommendation to her would be:
   a. You should wear a face mask when breastfeeding to protect your child.
   b. Your baby has already been exposed to your illness, so keep breastfeeding so he gets some antibodies.
   c. Pump your milk while you are sick, and have someone else give it to your child by cup.
   d. Your milk can transmit the flu virus, so pump and heat-treat the milk before feeding it to your child.

8. A breastfeeding mother resumes menstruation for the first time when her child is 16 months old. Which statement is MOST ACCURATE concerning her fertility at this time?
   a. Breastfeeding at this age offers no protection against pregnancy.
   b. You may experience several menstrual cycles before ovulation begins again.
   c. Ovulation usually precedes the first menstrual cycle in breastfeeding women.
   d. Taking a hormonal contraceptive will have no effect on lactation at this stage.

Answers for Case 14

1. **The answer is b.** Human milk contains many protective components, and the baby's immune system is still immature at 6 months. Choices a and c could have contributed to the child's illness. Chemicals in bottles and teats are being investigated for potential harmful effects. (Difficulty: 4; Discipline: Pathology; Taxonomy: Knowledge; 4–6 Months)
2. **The answer is c.** Article 5 of the International Code prohibits advertising of products within the scope of the Code, including infant formula, to the general public. Choice a is scientifically true and supports the aim of the International Code but is not specifically mentioned in the Articles of the Code. Choices b and d are false. (Difficulty: 3; Discipline: Clinical Skills; Taxonomy: Knowledge; General Principles)
3. **The answer is b.** Getting the baby re-interested in the breast is the first step in resuming breastfeeding after it was stopped. If the baby will latch and attempt breastfeeding, then the other suggestions are more likely to be successful. Choice d is incorrect. (Difficulty: 4; Discipline: Techniques; Taxonomy: Goals; 7–12 Months)

4. **The answer is d.** Immunoglobulins are a primary component of colostrum, the first secretion of the lactocytes during pregnancy; the same components essentially form an "immune layer" throughout lactation. As weaning and involution progress, lactose is the first component to diminish. (Difficulty: 4; Discipline: Development; Taxonomy: Knowledge; >12 Months)

5. **The answer is a.** The immune properties of human milk cannot be duplicated by any other source, and the protection against disease from breastmilk is irreplaceable. The other choices are also important reasons to continue breastfeeding as long as the child and mother desire. (Difficulty: 5; Discipline: Psychology; Taxonomy: Knowledge; >12 Months)

6. **The answer is a.** When children have outgrown the need to breastfeed, they stop. Mothers cannot make their children breastfeed at any age. Pumped milk is not the same as breastfeeding, and overnight separations before the child is ready to separate can be damaging to the mother–baby relationship. Choice d is false. (Difficulty: 4; Discipline: Psychology; Taxonomy: Collaboration; >12 Months)

7. **The answer is b.** For most maternal illnesses including viruses, the child has already been exposed and mother's body is already making antibodies specific to the infectious pathogen. Choice a is rarely necessary; c is appropriate only if the mother is too sick to care for her child. Choice d is incorrect. (Difficulty: 4; Discipline: Pathology; Taxonomy: Plan; >12 Months)

8. **The answer is b.** When a breastfeeding mother resumes menstruation after birth, even more than 12 months later, she may have several nonovulatory cycles before ovulating. The Lactational Amenorrhea Method is most effective when the baby is less than 6 months old. Choices a and c are incorrect. Estrogen-containing contraceptives affect lactation at all stages. (Difficulty: 2; Discipline: Physiology; Taxonomy: Knowledge; >12 Months)

Case 15

"I have been taking phenobarbital (Carbamazepine) for at least 6 years now and it has controlled my seizures (I've had seizures for almost 20 yrs.) I was previously told with both my other children NOT to breastfeed due to the phenobarbital. Therefore, they were both formula fed.

However, recently the neurologist I now see said, yes, breastfeeding is fine. I spoke with an LC who referenced Hale's book and said that it's safer to breastfeed with taking the medication than it is to be pregnant and taking it. I am completely confused and trying to figure out who to believe. I could deliver in as few as 3 weeks as my others came at 35 weeks, so I do not have a lot of time to figure it out.

Could you please tell me what you know about the safety for the baby with breastfeeding while I'm taking phenobarbital? I would have breastfed my other two children, except all the doctors I saw at that time, neurologists, maternal fetal medicine specialists, pediatricians, etc. said not to.

I'm now feeling confused as to what's best for my baby, and who to listen to. If I could find more info that supports breastfeeding while taking phenobarbital I would feel more comfortable. Also, switching to another seizure medicine would not be a good option, as this medication has worked for me, and I've used many, so I want to stay with one that is working.

Any help will be GREATLY appreciated!"

Questions for Case 15

1. A pregnant woman taking phenobarbital for several years asks about the safety of this medication when breastfeeding. Where would find the BEST source of information on drug compatibility with breastfeeding?
   a. a neighborhood pharmacist
   b. the drug package insert
   c. her obstetrician or midwife
   d. published current breastfeeding text

2. A woman who took taking phenobarbital (Carbamazepine) during pregnancy to control seizures wants to exclusively breastfeed. Which of the following infant signs is MOST LIKELY to be related to this drug transferring to her milk and should be reported to the primary care provider(s)?
   a. facial rash
   b. sedation or drowsiness
   c. vomiting or spitting up
   d. fussiness, excess crying

3. A mother with epilepsy wants to breastfeed her third baby, after formula-feeding her first two. Which aspect of breastfeeding should you spend MOST TIME discussing with her?
   a. increased infant alertness
   b. looser and more frequent stools
   c. more breast and nipple pain
   d. more frequent infant spitting up

4. A pregnant woman taking an antiseizure medication was advised to not breastfeed her first two children because of the medication. She is being encouraged to breastfeed this third child by her neurologist. What is the MOST SUPPORTIVE information you should share with her now?
   a. Your neurologist must know what he's talking about, so following his advice is wise.
   b. Your milk has many components that support brain growth, even if some medication is in the milk.
   c. You followed the best advice at the time with your other children, so do not feel guilty.
   d. Your milk's nutritional properties are not changed by the medication that might be present.

Answers for Case 15

1. **The answer is d.** A current, referenced text designed for lactation professionals is the most reliable of the above sources. For example, the database LactMed from the U.S. National Library of Medicine or Medications and Mothers Milk by Hale are considered reputable sources of information. (Difficulty: 2; Discipline: Pharmacology; Taxonomy: Collaboration; General Principles)
2. **The answer is b.** Sedation or drowsiness is the most likely infant reaction to an anticonvulsant drug taken during breastfeeding. Other signs include poor suck, poor weight gain, or jaundice; all should be reported to the child's physician. The other signs listed are not likely to be related to anticonvulsant therapy. (Difficulty: 3; Discipline: Pharmacology; Taxonomy: Collaboration; General Principles)

3. **The answer is a.** Breastfed infants are more alert and responsive compared to formula-fed babies due to the increased interaction with mother, composition of milk, and sucking at breast instead of a bottle. Formula-fed babies may sleep longer than breastfed babies, putting them at higher risk for SIDS. The stool composition may surprise her; breast and nipple pain should not occur. Breastfed babies are less likely to spit up than formula-fed babies. (Difficulty: 4; Discipline: Clinical Skills; Taxonomy: Goals; 3–14 Days)

4. **The answer is b.** Brain growth in infants is the most common concern when mother is taking any psychoactive medication, and antiseizure medications are considered compatible with breastfeeding. Choice a is incorrect because information was requested, not opinion. Choice c is inappropriate because implying feeling is not providing information. Choice d is accurate but less supportive than b. (Difficulty: 4; Discipline: Clinical Skills; Taxonomy: Collaboration; Prenatal)

Case 16

Is it possible for babies to be allergic to breastmilk? Our clinic just received a call message about a 3-month-old in one of our remote fly-in Aboriginal communities. His weight dropped from the 70th to the 10th percentile in weeks. He has spent several weeks in the children's hospital and is being followed by a specialist. They finally diagnosed him with an allergy to breastmilk, cow's milk, and soy.

I asked about whether they tried removing all dairy and soy from the mother's diet, and the nurse said that the situation was too urgent, as he was getting very sick. The doctor has prescribed Neocate for this baby, and he is now doing well and gaining weight. Is there any chance to resume breastfeeding if mom stops dairy and soy?

Questions for Case 16

1. A 3-month-old baby was hospitalized for sudden failure to thrive when his mother began giving supplements of formula. He was diagnosed with an allergy to breastmilk, cow's milk protein, and soy, and is being fed a bovine-based elemental formula. The mother wants to resume breastfeeding. Which is the MOST LIKELY cause of the baby's sudden growth problem?
   a. alpha-lactalbumin in the mother's milk
   b. beta-lactoglobulin in cow's-milk formula
   c. absence of lactose in soy formula
   d. nipple confusion from bottle supplements

2. The mother of a 3-month-old hospitalized for sudden failure to thrive asks for your help in resuming breastfeeding. The baby is allegedly allergic to breastmilk, cow's milk, and soy. In addition to increasing her milk production by pumping, the MOST IMPORTANT strategy for helping her is:
   a. Teach the mother why and how she should eliminate all bovine and soy protein from her own diet.
   b. Tell her to stop drinking whole cow's milk for a week.
   c. Provide her with a dietary supplement of calcium to replace cow's milk.
   d. Send a letter to her baby's care providers disputing the baby's allergy to breastmilk.

Answers for Case 16

1. **The answer is b.** Beta-lactoglobulin in cow's milk protein is a common allergen, and most likely to have caused this child's allergic reaction and failure to thrive. Soy is the second most common allergen. Babies are never allergic to mother's own milk or any of its natural components, but may react to foreign proteins that pass into milk. Nipple confusion is unlikely to begin at 3 months. (Difficulty: 2; Discipline: Pathology; Taxonomy: Evaluate; 1–3 Months)

2. **The answer is a.** Assuming the baby is truly allergic, eliminating cow's-milk protein and soy from the mother's diet is the most important strategy. Cow's-milk protein takes more than 1 week to be eliminated. LCs do not provide dietary supplements as part of their role. Although directly disputing a medical diagnosis is unethical, providing accurate information on allergen transfer into mother's milk to the mother and her providers is appropriate. (Difficulty: 4; Discipline: Pathology; Taxonomy: Goals; 1–3 Months)

Case 17

A true story: Kati Kim was snowbound in her car in a remote mountain area with her 4-year-old daughter and 7-month-old breastfed baby. Cellphone service was unavailable, and temperatures were below freezing. She and her husband James burned tires for warmth after the car ran out of fuel. After 7 days James left her and the children in the car and attempted to hike out and seek help. She kept both children alive until the rescue teams arrived 9 days later by breastfeeding both the baby and older child. James was found dead of exposure and hypothermia after hiking 16 miles to find help.

This occurred in southern Oregon (USA), Monday, Dec. 4, 2006. The mother and children were airlifted to Three Rivers Community Hospital in Grants Pass. The hospital earned designation as a Baby-Friendly Hospital in 1999 and has maintained its Designation through 2019.

Questions for Case 17

1. A mother, 4-year-old daughter, and 7-month-old baby were trapped in a snowbound car for 9 days. The mother breastfed both children after their small supply of food and liquids was exhausted. Which factor is MOST RELEVANT to milk production in this situation?
   a. The cold temperature slowed the children's' metabolism and caloric needs.
   b. Milk synthesis is mostly unrelated to maternal food or fluid intake.
   c. Water-soluble vitamins in her milk would be diminished by 9 days.
   d. The mother became malnourished and dehydrated by producing so much milk.

2. A mother, 4-year-old daughter, and 7-month-old baby were trapped in a snowbound car for 9 days. The mother breastfed both children after the small supply of food and liquids was exhausted. Which lactation-related hormone helped reduce stress in this mother?
   a. estrogen
   b. progesterone
   c. prolactin
   d. placental lactogen

3. A mother kept her 4-year-old daughter and 7-month-old baby alive by breastfeeding both children while snowbound in their car 9 days. Which component of breastmilk at this stage was HIGHER than at previous stages of lactation?
   a. lactoferrin
   b. secretory IgA
   c. bifidus factor
   d. lysozyme

Answers for Case 17

1. **The answer is b.** Maternal hydration and nutritional status is relevant to lactation capacity only if the mother is nearly in starvation herself. A well-nourished mother can produce large volumes of milk at little metabolic cost to herself, as in this true situation. (Difficulty: 3; Discipline: Development; Taxonomy: Knowledge; General Principles)
2. **The answer is c.** Prolactin is produced in high levels at all stages of lactation and has an antistress effect on the mother. Estrogen and progesterone levels are low in ongoing lactation, and placental lactogen is absent after the delivery of the placenta. (Difficulty: 3; Discipline: Development; Taxonomy: Knowledge; General Principles)
3. **The answer is d.** Lysozyme increases over the early months of lactation and is higher at 3 months than at 1 month. The other components vary less over time and are still important protective factors. (Difficulty: 5; Discipline: Development; Taxonomy: Knowledge; General Principles)

Case 18

The outpatient clinic received a call from a mother who is a 29-year-old teacher. Her first baby refuses to latch-on to the breast. He is 5 days old and appears yellow, and is neither voiding nor stooling regularly yet. She is painfully engorged, and all attempts to latch her baby onto the breast have failed miserably.

Questions for Case 18

1. A first-time mother and her 5-day-old infant called you for help. They live in a very remote area far from a health care facility. The baby is 5 days old, neither voiding or stooling regularly, and appears yellow. The mother's breasts are painfully engorged, and all attempts at latching the baby onto the breast have failed. Your FIRST action should be:
   a. Take her name and contact information and refer her to a home health care provider.
   b. Coach her on hand-expressing her milk over the phone.
   c. Ask her if she has a breast pump or any formula at home.
   d. Call the hospital where she gave birth and complain about lack of follow-up

2. A first-time mother and her 5-day-old infant called you for help. The baby is neither voiding or stooling regularly, and appears yellow. While the mother's breasts were engorged, all attempts at latching the baby onto the breast failed. She expressed 2 oz of milk total (60 mL). What is the NEXT action she should take?
   a. Pour the milk into a bottle and feed it with a wide-base nipple (teat).
   b. Place the baby skin-to-skin on her chest and see if he will self-attach.
   c. Use a small open cup to pour the pumped milk into the baby's mouth.
   d. Drip the pumped milk into the baby's mouth with a small dropper.

3. You are helping a mother exclusively breastfeed her 1-month-old child. Assuming the mother is responsive to her baby's cues, what is the MOST LIKELY feeding pattern to expect for this infant over the first 6 months?
   a. Feeding from both breasts every session, including at night
   b. Feeding from one breast each time he feeds
   c. Feeding from one or both breasts in no particular pattern
   d. Clusters of two to three feeds close together, then long stretches between

4. A 5-day-old baby has yellow-tinged skin and is not feeding well. After the baby's primary care provider has ruled out any pathology, the MOST IMPORTANT action would be:
   a. Give 1 oz (30 mL) of infant formula after each breastfeed for the next 24 hours.
   b. Place the unwrapped baby near a window with direct sunlight to reduce the level of bilirubin.
   c. Give the baby 1 oz (30 mL) of glucose water after feeds to flush out the bilirubin.
   d. Keep the mother and baby together and assure the baby has at least 8–12 effective feeds each day.

Answers for Case 18

1. **The answer is b.** Teaching hand-expression by phone is the fastest and usually the easiest way to solve two urgent issues: her breast engorgement and obtaining milk to feed her baby. (Difficulty: 2; Discipline: Techniques; Taxonomy: Assessment; 3–14 Days)

2. **The answer is b.** Direct breastfeeding is preferred over using a device to feed the baby, so an attempt at self-latching would be the next best strategy. If the attempt is unsuccessful, feeding the pumped milk with open cup is the next best option, allowing the baby to lap or sip the milk. A dropper may work, but can be tedious for all. A bottle with teat is the least desirable of these options. (Difficulty: 4; Discipline: Techniques; Taxonomy: Plan; 3–14 Days)

3. **The answer is c.** The most common 24-hour feeding pattern observed (57%) in a cohort of normal exclusively breastfed babies in Australia is feeding from one or both breasts in no particular pattern. The other patterns were also observed, although less frequently: 30% of babies studied never took both breasts; 13% always took both breasts, and some babies tended to cluster their feeds more than others. (Difficulty: 4; Discipline: Development; Taxonomy: Assessment; 3–14 Days)

4. **The answer is d.** Frequent effective breastfeeds are the best way to reduce bilirubin levels. If the baby is not feeding well, mother should hand-express and cup-feed her milk until the baby feeds better. Giving formula exposes the baby to a foreign protein. Direct sunlight may help if the baby is getting sufficient milk. Bilirubin is not water-soluble, so choice c is incorrect. (Difficulty: 4; Discipline: Pathology; Taxonomy: Collaboration; 3–14 Days)

Case 19

While out of town visiting relatives, a mother developed a high fever and a red, hot, swollen breast and went to a local emergency room. She was diagnosed with a breast abscess and referred to a surgeon. Today is the third day after surgery, and her breast is still swollen but she is otherwise healthy. Her baby is 6 weeks old, and she intends to breastfeed until he is at least a year old.

Questions for Case 19

1. You are helping a mother 3 days after a surgical procedure to drain a breast abscess. Her breast is firm, and milk is leaking from the incision, which is on the lateral side of the breast near her chest wall. What is the FIRST action she should take?
   a. Put the baby to breast on the affected side to relieve milk stasis.
   b. Express or pump milk from the affected breast and discard the milk.
   c. Massage the affected breast to push milk out of the incision and out of the nipple.
   d. Apply cold packs to the affected side and continue to feed on the other breast.

2. A mother had surgery to drain a breast abscess. What is the MOST IMPORTANT contributing factor for breast abscess?
   a. partial formula-feeding
   b. mother had influenza
   c. sore nipples
   d. prolonged milk stasis

3. A pregnant woman had surgery to drain a breast abscess during a previous lactation and asks about consequences to breastfeeding this time. Which aspect of the surgery are MOST LIKELY to negatively affect breastfeeding?
   a. the circumstances leading up to the abscess
   b. how long ago the surgery was performed
   c. location of the incision relative to milk ducts and nerves
   d. stage of lactation when the surgery was done

Answers for Case 19

1. **The answer is a.** The baby can and should continue to feed on the affected side. If the incision was close to the nipple, hand-expressing should be used to prevent milk stasis. The expressed milk can be given to the baby. Massage on or near the surgical site is not appropriate. Cold packs may feel comfortable but are ineffective in reducing milk stasis. (Difficulty: 4; Discipline: Techniques; Taxonomy: Plan; General Principles)
2. **The answer is d.** Prolonged milk stasis is the most common and most important contributing factor to a breast abscess. The other choices could have played a role in the milk stasis. (Difficulty: 5; Discipline: Pathology; Taxonomy: History; General Principles)
3. **The answer is c.** The location of the incision is most likely to affect lactation. Incisions that sever the 4th intercostal nerve or many milk ducts are more likely to negatively affect subsequent lactation than incisions elsewhere in the breast. (Difficulty: 3; Discipline: Development; Taxonomy: History; Prenatal)

Case 20

The baby in these photos is 5 days old. The mother has breastfed her other children.

Questions for Case 20

1. What is the FIRST thing you should say to the mother of this 5-day-old baby?

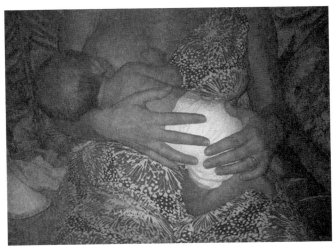

   a. Can you see your baby's lips when you hold him like that?
   b. How are your breasts feeling during and after each feed?
   c. Would you like suggestions on feeding more discretely?
   d. How is breastfeeding going for you and your baby today?

2. What should be your FIRST action in helping this baby breastfeed?

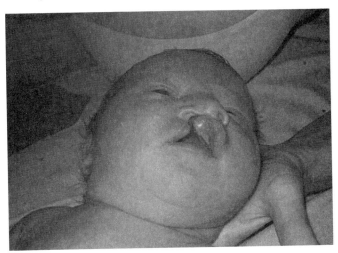

   a. Help mother position baby deeply at breast so her breast fills the baby's cleft lip.
   b. Help mother hand-express her milk to feed with an open cup.
   c. Provide an electric breast pump with double collection kit until the baby can latch.
   d. Give the mother a silicone nipple shield to create negative pressure in baby's mouth

3. What is the MOST LIKELY breastfeeding outcome for this baby?

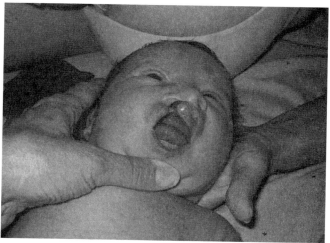

a. exclusive breastfeeding without assistive devices for 6 months
b. 30% chance mother will need to support her milk production and supplement with expressed milk
c. 50% chance of failure to thrive on breastmilk alone
d. baby will need a fitted obturator and multiple surgeries to breastfeed

Answers for Case 20

1. **The answer is d.** Asking an open-ended question about what's going right are the FIRST comments you should make. Once you've made positive rapport with a mother, then addressing any concerns that she has would be next. (Difficulty: 4; Discipline: Psychology; Taxonomy: Goals; 3–14 Days)

2. **The answer is a.** Direct breastfeeding is always the first choice. This baby was able to feed directly at breast because the mother's soft breast filled the cleft lip. The other strategies might be appropriate if direct breastfeeding was ineffective. (Difficulty: 5; Discipline: Techniques; Taxonomy: Goals; 1–2 Days)

3. **The answer is b.** Many babies with a unilateral cleft lip can breastfeed and grow normally without assistive devices. However, about one-third will not grow adequately on direct breastfeeding alone. Mother may need to pump or express to maintain milk production, and supplement the pumped milk with a cup. Breastmilk is especially important for babies with facial anomalies. (Difficulty: 4; Discipline: Pathology; Taxonomy: Collaboration; 3–14 Days)

Bibliography and Resources

There is no one single text or resource that covers the entire body of knowledge pertinent to breastfeeding and human lactation. The questions in this book were prepared from multiple sources and references.

Textbooks

Allain, A., & Chetley, A. (2010). Protecting Infant Health: A Health Workers' Guide to the International Code of Marketing of Breastmilk Substitutes (11th ed.). Penang: IBFAN/ICDC.

American Academy of Pediatrics (AAP). (2012). Guidelines for Perinatal Care (7th ed.). Elk Grove, IL: Author.

Apple, R. (1987). Mothers and Medicine. Madison, WI: University of Wisconsin Press.

Arnold, L. D. W. (2010). Human Milk in the NICU: Policy into Practice. Sudbury, MA: Jones & Bartlett.

Arvedson, J., & Brodsky, L. (1993). Pediatric Swallowing and Feeding: Assessment and Management. San Diego, CA: Singular Publishing Group.

Banyard, V. L., Edwards, V. J., & Kendall-Tackett, K. (2009). Trauma and Physical Health. New York: Routledge/Taylor & Francis.

Boshart, C. (2001). The Pacifier: Making the Decision. Temecula, CA: Speech Dynamics, Inc.

Brazelton, T. B., & Nugent, J. K. (1995). Neonatal Behavioral Assessment Scale (3rd ed.). New York: Cambridge University Press.

Brodribb, W. (Ed.) (2014). Breastfeeding Management (4th ed.). Melbourne, Australia: Australian Breastfeeding Association.

Brooks, E. C. (2013). Legal and Ethical Issues for the IBCLC. Burlington, MA: Jones and Bartlett Learning.

Buckley, S. J. (2005). Gentle Birth, Gentle Mothering. Brisbane, Australia: One Moon Press.

Bumgarner, N. J. (2000). Mothering Your Nursing Toddler (rev. ed.) Schaumburg, IL: La Leche League International.

Cadwell, K. (2002). Reclaiming Breastfeeding for the United States. Sudbury, MA: Jones & Bartlett.

Cadwell, K., & Turner-Maffei, C. (2009). Continuity of Care in Breastfeeding: Best Practices in the Maternity Setting. Sudbury, MA: Jones & Bartlett.

Cadwell, K., & Turner-Maffei, C. (2014). Breastfeeding A-Z: Terminology and Telephone Triage (2nd ed.). Sudbury, MA: Jones & Bartlett.

Cadwell, K., Turner-Maffei, C., O'Connor, B., Blair, A. C., Arnold, L. D. W., & Blair, E. M. (2006). Maternal and Infant Assessment for Breastfeeding and Human Lactation (2nd ed.). Sudbury, MA: Jones & Bartlett.

Carreiro, J. E. (2003). An Osteopathic Approach to Children. Philadelphia: Churchill Livingstone/ Elsevier.

Centers for Disease Control and Prevention. (2013). Strategies to Prevent Obesity and Other Chronic Diseases: The CDC Guide to Strategies to Support Breastfeeding Mothers and Babies. Atlanta: Department of Health and Human Services.

Christensson, K. (1994). Care of the Newborn Infant: Satisfying the Need for Comfort and Energy Conservation. Stockholm, Sweden: Karolinska Institutet.

Davis-Floyd, R. (1992). Birth as an American Rite of Passage. Los Angeles: University of California Press.

Enkin, M. W., Keirse, M., Renfrew, M. J., & Neilson, J. (2000). A Guide to Effective Care in Pregnancy and Childbirth (3rd ed.). Oxford: Oxford University Press.

Flower, H. (2003) Adventures in Tandem Nursing. Schaumburg IL: La Leche League international.

Francis, S., James, S., Schellenberg, P. J., & Lopez-Jones, N. (2002). The Milk of Human Kindness. London: Crossroads Books.

Genna, C. W. (2008). Supporting Sucking Skills in Breastfeeding Infants (2nd ed). Sudbury, MA: Jones & Bartlett.

Genna, C. W. (2013). Selecting and Using Breastfeeding Tools: Improving Care and Outcomes. Amarillo, TX: Hale Publishing.

Golden, J. (2001). A Social History of Wet Nursing in America. Columbus: Ohio State University Press.

Greenhalgh, T. (2014). How to Read a Paper: The Basics of Evidence-Based Medicine (5th ed.). Oxford: Wiley-Blackwell (BMJ Books).

Gromada, K. K. (2007). Mothering Multiples: Breastfeeding and Caring for Twins or More (3rd ed.). Schaumburg, IL: La Leche League International.

Hale, T. W., & Berens, P. D. (2010). Clinical Therapy in Breastfeeding Patients (3rd ed.). Amarillo, TX: Hale Publishing.

Hale, T. W., & Hartmann, P. E. (2007). Textbook of Human Lactation. Amarillo, TX: Hale Publishing.

Hale, T. W., & Ilett, K. F. (2002). Drug Therapy and Breastfeeding. New York: Parthenon Publishing Group.

Hale, T. W., & Rowe, H. E. (2014). Medications and Mothers' Milk (16th ed.). Amarillo, TX: Hale Publishing.

Hanson, L. A. (2004). Immunobiology of Human Milk: How Breastfeeding Protects Babies. Amarillo, TX: Hale Publishing.

Harper, B. (2005). Gentle Birth Choices. Portland, OR: Healing Arts Press.

Hausman, B. L. (2003). Mother's Milk: Breastfeeding Controversies in American Culture. New York: Routledge.

Hrdy, S. B. (1999). Mother Nature: A History of Mothers, Infants, and Natural Selection. New York: Pantheon Books.

Human Milk Banking Association of North America. (2011). Guidelines for the Establishment and Operation of a Donor Human Milk Bank. Ft. Worth, TX: Human Milk Banking Association of North America.

Institute of Medicine. (1991). Nutrition During Lactation. Washington, DC: National Academy of Sciences.

International Lactation Consultant Association. (2013). Core Curriculum for Lactation Consultant Practice (3rd ed.). Sudbury MA: Jones and Bartlett Learning.

Ivey, A. E., & Ivey, M. B. (2003) Intentional Interviewing and Counseling: Facilitating Client Development in a Multicultural Society (5th ed.). New York: Wadsworth.

Jensen, R. G. (1995). Handbook of Milk Composition. San Diego: Academic Press.

Kendall-Tackett, K. A. (2005). Depression in New Mothers: Causes, Consequences and Treatment Alternatives. Binghamton, NY: Haworth Press.

Kendall-Tackett, K. A. (2005). Handbook of Women, Stress and Trauma. New York: Brunner-Routledge/Taylor & Francis Group.

King, F. S. (1992). Helping Mothers to Breastfeed (revised ed.). Nairobi, Kenya: African Medical Research Foundation.

King, T, Brucker, M. C., Kriebs, J. M., Fahey, J. O., Kriebs, J. M., Gegor, C. L., & Varney, H. (2015). Varney's Midwifery (5th ed.). Sudbury, MA: Jones & Bartlett.

Klaus, M. H. (1993). Mothering the Mother. Jackson, TN: Perseus Books Group.

Klaus, M. H., & Kennell, J. (1982). Parent-Infant Bonding. St. Louis: C. V. Mosby.

Klaus, M. H., & Klaus, P. H. (1998). Your Amazing Newborn. Reading, MA: Perseus Books.

Koletzko, B., Michaelson, K. F., & Hernell, O. (2000). Short and Long Term Effects of Breastfeeding on Child Health. New York: Kluwer Academic/Plenum Publishers.

La Leche League International (2014). Sweet Sleep: Nighttime and Naptime Strategies for the Breastfeeding Family. (Wiessinger, D., West, D., Smith, L. J., & Pittman, T.) New York: Random House - Ballantine Books.

La Leche League International. (2010). The Womanly Art of Breastfeeding (D. Wiessinger, D. West, & T. Pittman, Eds.; 8th ed.). New York: Random House/Ballantine Books.

Lang, S. (2002). Breastfeeding Special Care Babies (2nd ed.). Edinburgh: Balliere Tindall/Harcourt Publishers.

Lauwers, J., & Swisher, A. (Eds.). (2016). Counseling the Nursing Mother: A Lactation Consultant's Guide (6th ed.). Sudbury, MA: Jones & Bartlett.

Lawrence, R. A., & Lawrence, R. M. (2016). Breastfeeding: A Guide for the Medical Profession (8th ed.). Philadelphia: Elsevier Mosby.

Lockwood, C. J., & Lemons, J. A. (Eds.). (2012). Guidelines for Perinatal Care (7th ed.). Elk Grove Village, IL: American Academy of Pediatrics.

Ludington-Hoe, S., & Golant, S. K. (1993). Kangaroo Care: The Best You Can Do to Help Your Preterm Infant. New York: Bantam Books.

Mannel, R., Martens, P. J., & Walker, M. (Eds.). (2013). Core Curriculum for Lactation Consultant Practice (3rd ed.). Sudbury, MA: Jones & Bartlett.

Mohrbacher, N. (2010). Breastfeeding Answers Made Simple. Amarillo, TX: Hale Publishing.

Montagu, A. (1986). Touching: The Human Significance of the Skin (3rd ed.). New York: Harper & Row.

Morris, S. E., & Klein, M. D. (2000). Pre-Feeding Skills: A Comprehensive Resource for Mealtime (2nd ed.). San Antonio, TX: Therapy Skill Builders.

Murray, S. F. (1996). Baby Friendly, Mother Friendly. London: Mosby.

Newton, N. (1955). Maternal Emotions. New York: Harper & Brothers.

Palmer, G. (2009). The Politics of Breastfeeding: When Breasts Are Bad for Business (3rd ed.). London: Pinter and Martin.

Sergueef, N. (2007). Cranial Osteopathy for Infants, Children and Adolescents. Philadelphia: Churchill Livingstone/Elsevier.

Simkin, P., & Ancheta, R. (2011). The Labor Progress Handbook (3rd ed.). Oxford: Blackwell Publishing.

Small, M. F. (1998). Our Babies, Ourselves: How Biology and Culture Shape the Way We Parent. New York: Anchor Books.

Smith, L. J. (2002). Coach's Notebook: Games and Strategies for Lactation Education. Sudbury, MA: Jones & Bartlett.

Smith, L. J. (2003). The Lactation Consultant in Private Practice: The ABCs of Getting Started. Sudbury, MA: Jones & Bartlett.

Smith, L. J., & Kroeger, M. (2010). Impact of Birthing Practices on Breastfeeding (2nd ed.). Sudbury, MA: Jones and Bartlett.

Stuart-Macadam, P., & Dettwyler, K. A. (1995). Breastfeeding: Biocultural Perspectives. New York: Aldine/Transaction Publishers.

Sunderland, M. (2006). The Science of Parenting. New York: DK Publishing.

Tappero, E., & ME, H. (1993). Physical Assessment of the Newborn. Petaluma: NICULink Book Publishers.

Trevathan, W. R., Smith, E. O., & McKenna, J. J. (1999). Evolutionary Medicine. New York: Oxford University Press.

Tuchman, D., & Walter, R. (1994). Disorders of Feeding and Swallowing in Infants and Children: Pathophysiology, Diagnosis and Treatment. San Diego, CA: Singular Publishing Group, Inc.

Upledger, J. (1983). Craniosacral Therapy. Seattle, WA: Eastland Press.

Upledger, J. E. (1996). A Brain Is Born. Berkeley, CA: North Atlantic Books.

US Department of Health and Human Services. (2011). The Surgeon General's Call to Action to Support Breastfeeding. Washington, DC: US Department of Health and Human Services, Office of the Surgeon General

Uvnas-Moberg, K. (2003). The Oxytocin Factor. Cambridge, MA: Da Capo Press/Perseus Books Group.

Van Esterik, P. (1989). Beyond the Breast-Bottle Controversy. New Brunswick, NJ: Rutgers University Press.

Van Esterik, P. (2002). Risks, Rights and Regulations: Communicating About Risks and Infant Feeding. Penang: World Alliance for Breastfeeding Action (WABA).

Walker, M. (2014). Breastfeeding Management for the Clinician: Using the Evidence (3rd ed.). Sudbury MA: Jones & Bartlett.

Wambach, K, & Riordan, J. (eds) (2016). Breastfeeding and Human Lactation (6th ed.). Sudbury, MA: Jones & Bartlett.

Ward, R. C. (2003). Foundations for Osteopathic Medicine (2nd ed.). Philadelphia: Lippincott Williams & Wilkins.

West, D., & Hirsch, E. M. (2008). Breastfeeding after Breast and Nipple Procedures: A Guide for Healthcare Professionals. Amarillo, TX: Hale Publishing.

West, D., & Marasco, L. (2009). Making More Milk. New York: McGraw-Hill.

Wight, N. E., Morton, J. A., & Kim, J. H. (2008). Best Medicine: Human Milk in the NICU. Amarillo, TX: Hale Publishing.

Wilson-Clay, B., & Hoover, K. (2013). The Breastfeeding Atlas (5th ed.). Manchaca, TX: LactNews.

Wolf, J. H. (2001). Don't Kill Your Baby. Columbus: The Ohio State University Press.

Wolf, L., & Glass, R. (1992). Feeding and Swallowing Disorders in Infancy: Assessment and Management. Tucson, AZ: Therapy Skill Builders/Communicator Skills Builders.

Young, E. W. D. (1989). Alpha and Omega: Ethics at the Frontiers of Life and Death. Reading, MA: Addison-Wesley Publishing Company.

Academy of Breastfeeding Medicine Clinical Protocols
http://www.bfmed.org/Resources/Protocols.aspx

ABM Clinical Protocol #1: Guidelines for Blood Glucose Monitoring and Treatment of Hypoglycemia in Term and Late-Preterm Neonates, Revised 2014. Wight, N., & Marinelli, K. A. (2014). *Breastfeeding Medicine, 9*(4), 173–179.

ABM Clinical Protocol #2: Guidelines for Hospital Discharge of the Breastfeeding Term Newborn and Mother: "The Going Home Protocol," Revised 2014. Evans, A., Marinelli, K. A., & Taylor, J. S. (2014). *Breastfeeding Medicine, 9*(1), 3–8.

ABM Clinical Protocol #3: Hospital Guidelines for the Use of Supplementary Feedings in the Healthy Term Breastfed Neonate. Academy of Breastfeeding Medicine. (ABM). (2009). *Breastfeeding Medicine, 4*(3), 175–182.

ABM Clinical Protocol #4: Mastitis, Revised March 2014. Amir, L. H. (2014). *Breastfeeding Medicine, 9*, 239–243.

ABM Clinical Protocol #5: Peripartum Breastfeeding Management for the Healthy Mother and Infant at Term, Revision 2013. Holmes, A. V., McLeod, A. Y., & Bunik, M. (2013). *Breastfeeding Medicine, 8*(6), 469–473.

ABM Clinical Protocol #6: Guideline on Co-Sleeping and Breastfeeding (revision). Academy of Breastfeeding Medicine (ABM). (2008). *Breastfeeding Medicine, 3*(1), 38–43.

ABM Clinical Protocol #7: Model Breastfeeding Policy (revision). (2010). *Breastfeeding Medicine, 5*(4), 173–177.

ABM Clinical Protocol #8: Human Milk Storage Information for Home Use for Full-Term Infants (original protocol March 2004; revision 1 March 2010). (2010). *Breastfeeding Medicine, 5*(3), 127–130.

ABM Clinical Protocol #9: Use of Galactogogues in Initiating or Augmenting the Rate of Maternal Milk Secretion (First Revision January 2011). Academy of Breastfeeding Medicine (2011). *Breastfeeding Medicine, 6*(1), 41–49.

ABM Clinical Protocol #10: Breastfeeding the Late Preterm Infant (34 0/7 to 36 6/7 Weeks Gestation) (first revision June 2011). Academy of Breastfeeding Medicine. (2011). *Breastfeeding Medicine, 6*(3), 151–156.

ABM Clinical Protocol #11: Guidelines for the Evaluation and Management of Neonatal Ankyloglossia and Its Complications in the Breastfeeding Dyad. Academy of Breastfeeding Medicine (ABM). (2004). New Rochelle, NY: Author.

ABM Clinical Protocol #12: Transitioning the Breastfeeding-/Breastmilk-Fed Premature Infant From the Neonatal Intensive Care Unit to Home. Academy of Breastfeeding Medicine (ABM). (2004). New Rochelle, NY: Author.

ABM Clinical Protocol #13: Contraception During Breastfeeding, Revised 2015. Berens, P., & Labbok, M. (2014). *Breastfeeding Medicine, 10*(1), 3–12.

ABM Clinical Protocol #14: Breastfeeding-Friendly Physician's Office: Optimizing Care for Infants and Children, Revised 2013. Grawey, A. E., Marinelli, K. A., Holmes, A. V. & the Academy of Breastfeeding Medicine, (2013). *Breastfeeding Medicine, 8*(2), 237–242.

ABM Clinical Protocol #15: Analgesia and Anesthesia for the Breastfeeding Mother, Revised 2012. Montgomery, A., Hale, T. W. & Academy of Breastfeeding Medicine (2012). *Breastfeeding Medicine, 7*(6), 547–553.

ABM Clinical Protocol #16: Breastfeeding the Hypotonic Infant. Academy of Breastfeeding Medicine (ABM). (2007). *Breastfeeding Medicine, 2*(2), 112–118.

ABM Clinical Protocol #17: Guidelines for Breastfeeding Infants with Cleft Lip, Cleft Palate, or Cleft Lip and Palate, Revised 2013. Reilly, S., Reid, J., Skeat, J., Cahir, P., Mei, C., Bunik, M. & the Academy of Breastfeeding Medicine. (2013). *Breastfeeding Medicine, 8*(4), 349–353.

ABM Clinical Protocol #18: Use of Antidepressants in Breastfeeding Mothers. Sriraman, N. K., Melvin, K., & Meltzer-Brody, S. (2015). *Breastfeeding Medicine, 10*(6), 290–299.

ABM Clinical Protocol #19: Breastfeeding Promotion in the Prenatal Setting. Academy of Breastfeeding Medicine (ABM) (2009). *Breastfeeding Medicine*, 4(1), 43–45.

ABM Clinical Protocol #20: Engorgement. Academy of Breastfeeding Medicine (ABM). (2009). *Breastfeeding Medicine, 4*(2), 111–113.

ABM Clinical Protocol #21: Guidelines for Breastfeeding and Substance Use or Substance Use Disorder, Revised 2015. Reece-Stremtan, S., & Marinelli, K. A. (2015). *Breastfeeding Medicine, 10*(3), 135–141.

ABM Clinical Protocol #22: Guidelines for Management of Jaundice in the Breastfeeding Infant Equal to or Greater than 35 Weeks' Gestation. Academy of Breastfeeding Medicine. (ABM). (2010). *Breastfeeding Medicine*, 5(2), 87–93.

ABM Clinical Protocol #23: Non-Pharmacologic Management of Procedure-Related Pain in the Breastfeeding Infant. Academy of Breastfeeding Medicine. (2010). *Breastfeeding Medicine, 5*, 315–319.

ABM Clinical Protocol #24: Allergic Proctocolitis in the Exclusively Breastfed Infant. Academy of Breastfeeding Medicine. (2011). *Breastfeeding Medicine, 6*(6), 435–440.

ABM Clinical Protocol #25: Recommendations for preprocedural fasting for the breastfed infant: "NPO" Guidelines. Academy of Breastfeeding Medicine. (2012). *Breastfeeding Medicine, 7*(3), 197–202.

Global Organizations and Documents

International Lactation Consultant Association (ILCA): www.ilca.org

International Board of Lactation Consultant Examiners (IBLCE): www.iblce.org

Academy of Breastfeeding Medicine: www.bfmed.org

Emergency Nutrition Network: www.ennonline.net

International Labor Organization. (2000). Maternity Protection Convention (Vol. C183). Geneva: International Labor Organization.

The Cochrane Collaboration: www.cochrane.org

United Nations Children's Fund. (1990). Innocenti Declaration on the Promotion, Protection, and Support of Breastfeeding. New York: UNICEF Nutrition Cluster.

United Nations Millennium Development Goals: http://www.unmillenniumproject.org/goals/

United Nations Sustainable Development Goals: http://www.undp.org/content/undp/en/home/mdgoverview/post-2015-development-agenda.html

World Alliance for Breastfeeding Action (WABA), World Breastfeeding Week: worldbreastfeedingweek.org

World Health Organisation. (2006). WHO Child Growth Standards based on length/height, weight and age. *Acta Paediatr. Suppl.*, 450, 76–85.

World Health Organisation. (2014). Every Newborn Action Plan. http://apps.who.int/iris/bitstream/10665/127938/1/9789241507448_eng.pdf?ua=1

World Health Organization (2005) Guiding Principles for Complementary Feeding of the Breastfed Child.

World Health Organization (WHO) & UNICEF. (1989). Protecting, Promoting and Supporting Breastfeeding: The Special Role of Maternity Services. Geneva, Switzerland: World Health Organization Nutrition Unit.

World Health Organization (WHO). (1978). Declaration of Alma-Ata: International Conference on Primary Health Care. Alma-Ata, USSR: Author.

World Health Organization (WHO). (1981). International Code of Marketing of Breastmilk Substitutes. Geneva, Switzerland: Author.

World Health Organization (WHO). (1985). Appropriate Technology for Birth (No. 0140-6736 (Print)). Geneva, Switzerland: Author.

World Health Organization (WHO). (1997). Care in Normal Birth: A Practical Guide. Geneva, Switzerland: Author.

World Health Organization (WHO). (1997). Hypoglycemia of the Newborn: Review of the Literature. Geneva, Switzerland: Author.

World Health Organization (WHO). (1998). Evidence for the Ten Steps to Successful Breastfeeding. (Vol. WHO/CHD/98.9). Geneva, Switzerland: Author.

WHO, UNICEF. (2014). Every Newborn: An Action Plan to End Preventable Deaths. Geneva: World Health Organization.

World Health Organization (WHO). (2003). *The Lancet* Child Survival Series. Geneva, Switzerland: Author.

World Health Organization (WHO). (2005). *The Lancet* Neonatal survival series. http://www.who.int/maternal_child_adolescent/documents/lancet_neonatal_survival/en/ Geneva, Switzerland: Author.

World Health Organization (WHO). (2004). Guiding Principles for Feeding Infants and Young Children During Emergencies. Geneva, Switzerland: Author.

World Health Organization (WHO). (2006). The WHO Child Growth Standards. Geneva, Switzerland: Author.

World Health Organization (WHO). (2007). Biomonitoring of Human Milk: A Protocol for Collection, Handling and Analysis of Samples at the Country Level. Geneva, Switzerland: Author.

World Health Organization (WHO). (2007). How to prepare formula for bottle-feeding at home. In Biomonitoring of Human Milk: A Protocol for Collection, Handling and Analysis of Samples at the Country Level. Geneva, Switzerland: Author.

World Health Organization (WHO). (2007). How to prepare formula for cup-feeding at home. In Biomonitoring of Human Milk: A Protocol for Collection, Handling and Analysis of Samples at the Country Level. Geneva, Switzerland: Author.

World Health Organization (WHO). (2007). Safe preparation, storage and handling of powdered infant formula. In Biomonitoring of Human Milk: A Protocol for Collection, Handling and Analysis of Samples at the Country Level. Geneva, Switzerland: Author.

World Health Organization (WHO). (2009). Acceptable Medical Reasons for Use of Breast-Milk Substitutes (Vol. WHO/NMH/NHD/09.01). Geneva, Switzerland: Author.

World Health Organization (WHO). (2009). Home Visits for the Newborn Child: A Strategy to Improve Survival (Vol. WHO/FCH/CAH/09.02). Geneva, Switzerland: Author.

World Health Organization (WHO). (2009). Infant and Young Child Feeding: Model Chapter for Textbooks for Medical Students and Allied Health Professionals. Geneva, Switzerland: Author.

World Health Organization (WHO) (2015). Monitoring & evaluation framework for antiretroviral treatment for pregnant and breast feeding women living with HIV and their infants. Geneva, Switzerland: Author. http://www.who.int/hiv/mtct/iatt-me-framework/en/

World Health Organization, & United Nations Children's Fund. (2003). Global Strategy for Infant and Young Child Feeding.

World Health Organization, & United Nations Children's Fund. (2009). Baby-Friendly Hospital Initiative: Revised, Updated and Expanded for Integrated Care. Geneva: World Health Organization.

World Health Organization. (1981). Resolution WHA 35.26 International Code of Marketing of Breast-milk Substitutes (Vol. WHA 35.26). Geneva: World Health Organization.

World Health Organization. (2004). Guiding Principles for Feeding Infants and Young Children During Emergencies. Geneva: World Health Organization.

World Health Organization. (2010). Guidelines on HIV and Infant Feeding 2010: Principles and Recommendations for Infant Feeding in the Context of HIV and a Summary of Evidence (pp. 58). Geneva: World Health Organization.

World Health Organization. (2014). Consolidated Guidelines on HIV Prevention, Diagnosis, Treatment and Care for Key Populations. Geneva: World Health Organization.

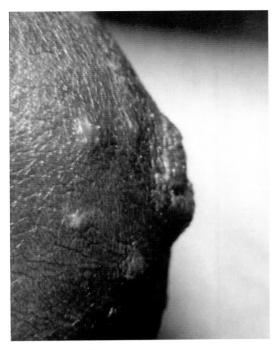

COLOR PLATE 1.
Courtesy of K. Jean Cotterman.

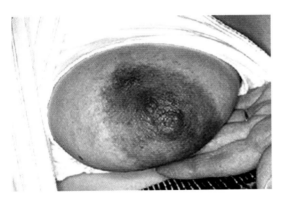

COLOR PLATE 2.

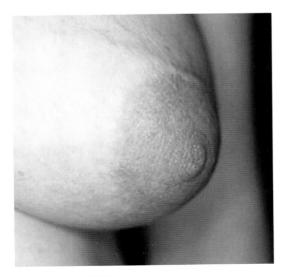

COLOR PLATE 3.

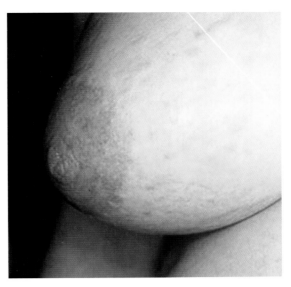

COLOR PLATE 4.

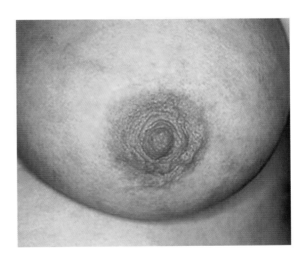

COLOR PLATE 5.

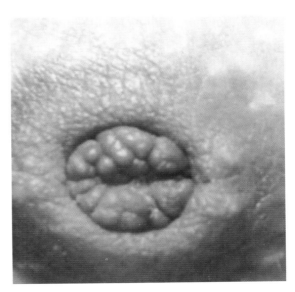

COLOR PLATE 6.
Courtesy of K. Jean Cotterman.

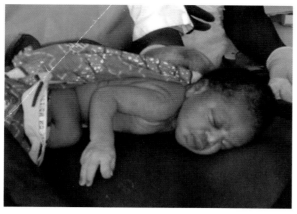

COLOR PLATE 7.

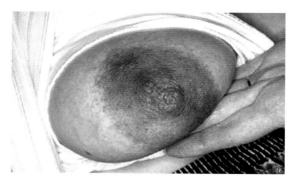

COLOR PLATE 10.

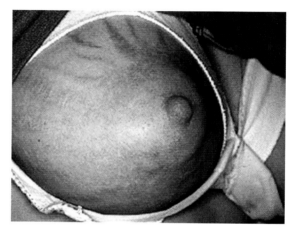

COLOR PLATE 11.

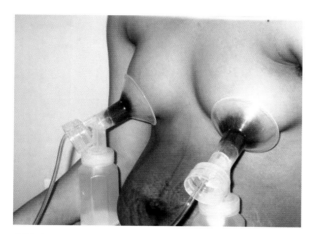

COLOR PLATE 8.
Courtesy of K. Jean Cotterman.

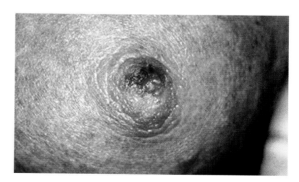

COLOR PLATE 12.
Courtesy of Greg Notestine.

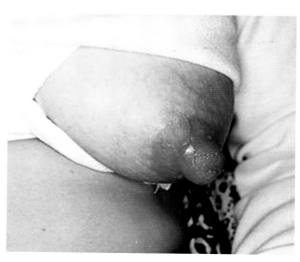

COLOR PLATE 9.

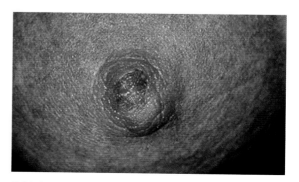

COLOR PLATE 13.
Courtesy of Greg Notestine.

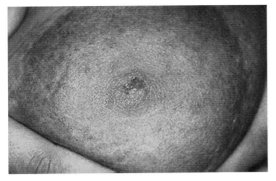

COLOR PLATE 14.
Courtesy of Greg Notestine.

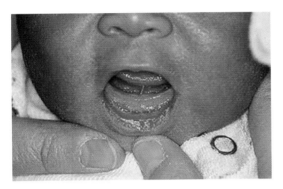

COLOR PLATE 15.
Courtesy of Greg Notestine.

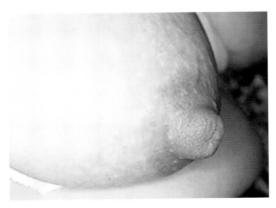

COLOR PLATE 16.

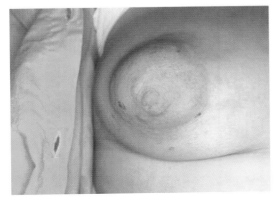

COLOR PLATE 17.

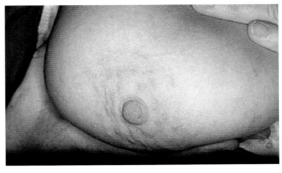

COLOR PLATE 18.

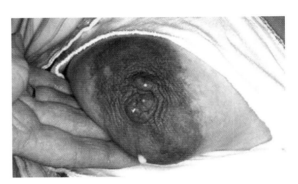

COLOR PLATE 19.

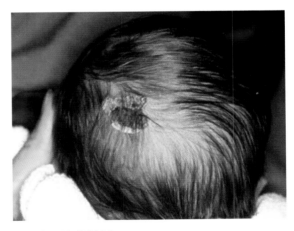

COLOR PLATE 20.

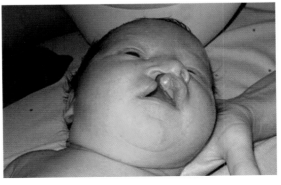

COLOR PLATE 21.
Courtesy of Catherine Watson Genna.

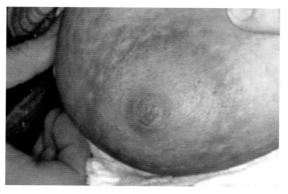

COLOR PLATE 22.

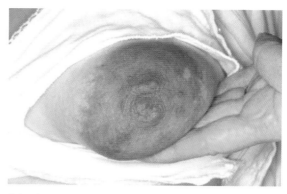

COLOR PLATE 26.

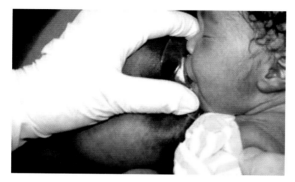

COLOR PLATE 23.
Courtesy of K. Jean Cotterman.

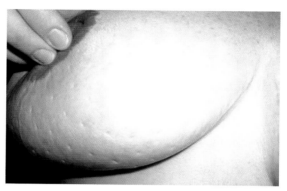

COLOR PLATE 27.
Courtesy of Catherine Watson Genna.

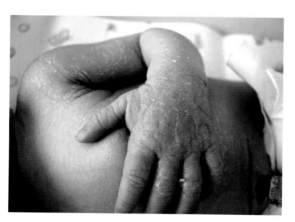

COLOR PLATE 24.
Courtesy of Catherine Watson Genna.

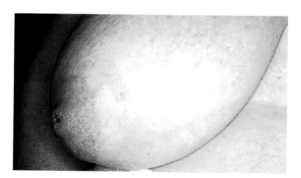

COLOR PLATE 28.

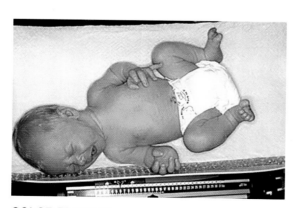

COLOR PLATE 25.

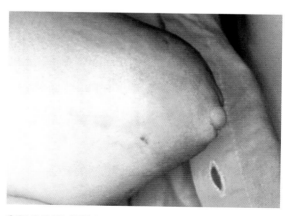

COLOR PLATE 29.

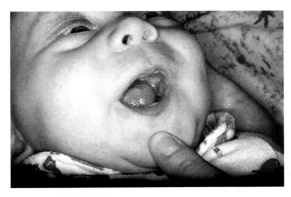

COLOR PLATE 30.

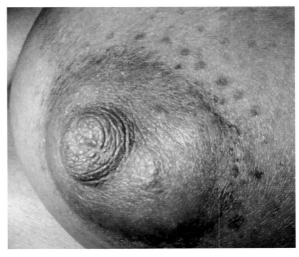

COLOR PLATE 33.
Courtesy of K. Jean Cotterman.

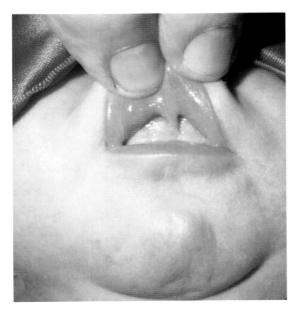

COLOR PLATE 31.
Courtesy of K. Jean Cotterman.

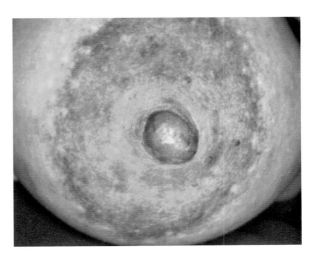

COLOR PLATE 34.

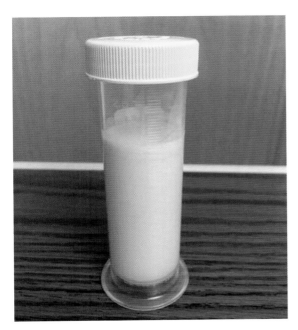

COLOR PLATE 32.
Courtesy of Laura Atkinson.

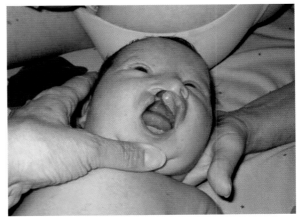

COLOR PLATE 35.
Courtesy of Catherine Watson Genna.

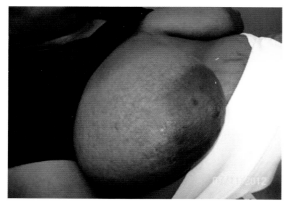

COLOR PLATE 36.
Courtesy of K. Jean Cotterman.

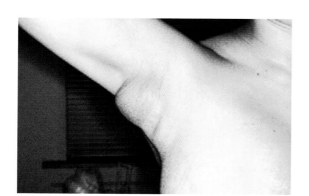

COLOR PLATE 37.

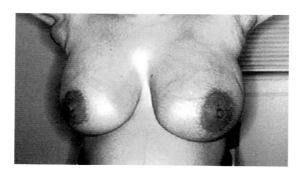

COLOR PLATE 38.

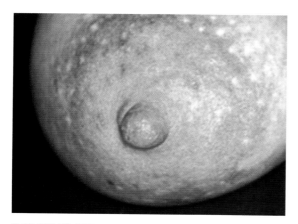

COLOR PLATE 39.

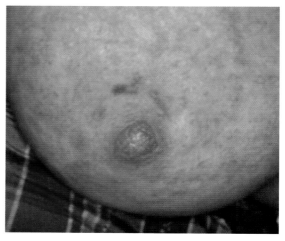

COLOR PLATE 40.

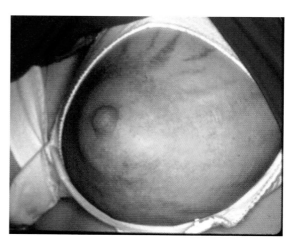

COLOR PLATE 41.

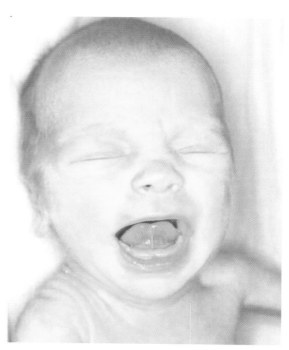

COLOR PLATE 42.

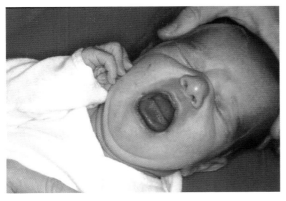

COLOR PLATE 43.

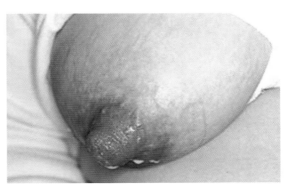

COLOR PLATE 46.

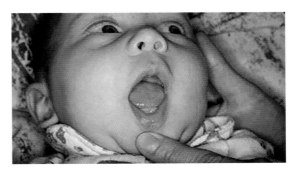

COLOR PLATE 47.

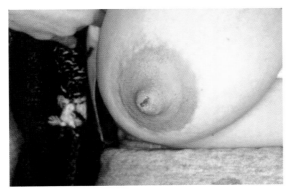

COLOR PLATE 44.

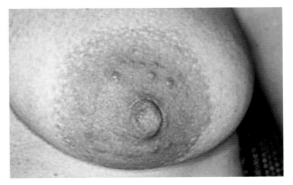

COLOR PLATE 48.

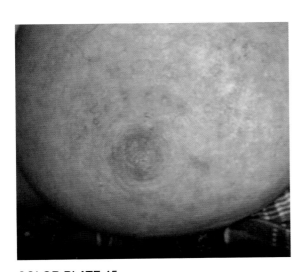

COLOR PLATE 45.

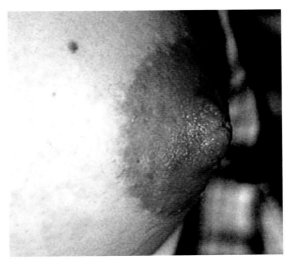

COLOR PLATE 49.
Courtesy of Greg Notestine.

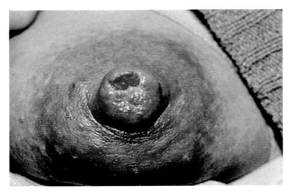

COLOR PLATE 50.
Courtesy of Greg Notestine.

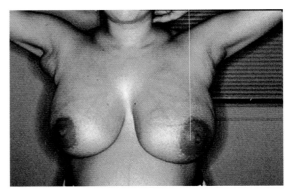

COLOR PLATE 53.

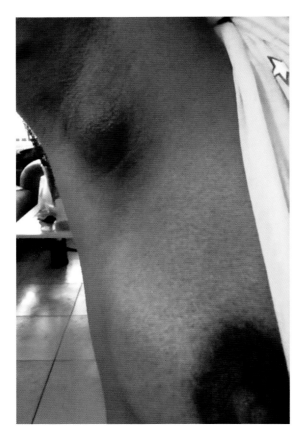

COLOR PLATE 51.
Courtesy of Jarene Fleming.

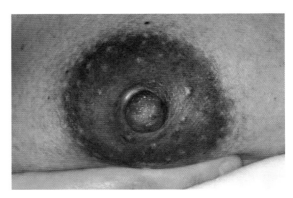

COLOR PLATE 54.

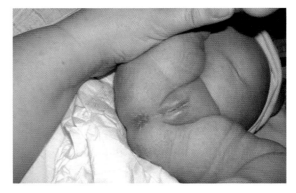

COLOR PLATE 55.
Courtesy of Erika Nehlsen.

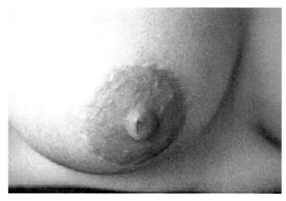

COLOR PLATE 52.

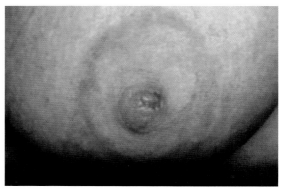

COLOR PLATE 56.

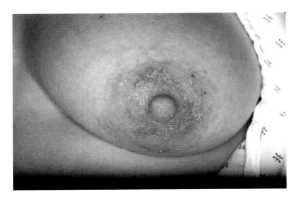

COLOR PLATE 57.

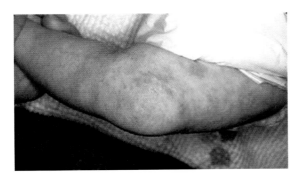

COLOR PLATE 58.

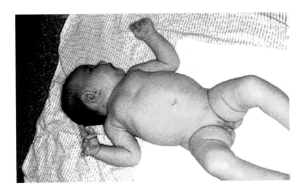

COLOR PLATE 59.

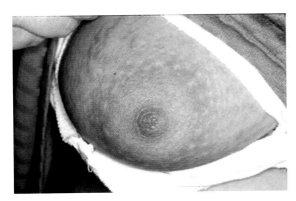

COLOR PLATE 60

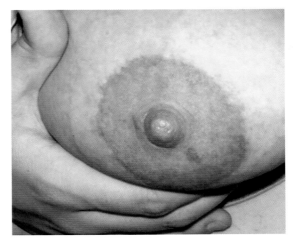

COLOR PLATE 61.
Courtesy of K. Jean Cotterman.

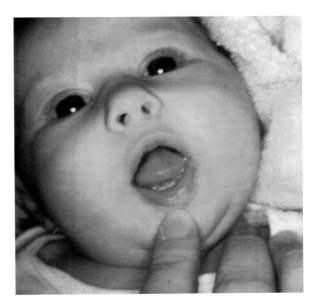

COLOR PLATE 62.

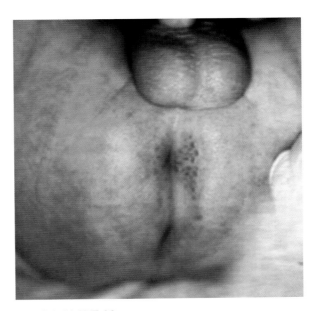

COLOR PLATE 63.

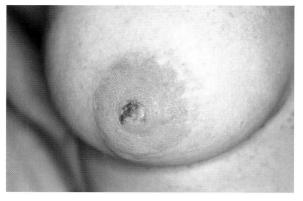

COLOR PLATE 64.

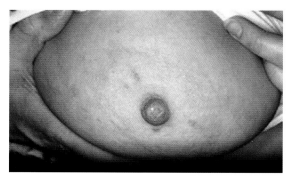

COLOR PLATE 68.

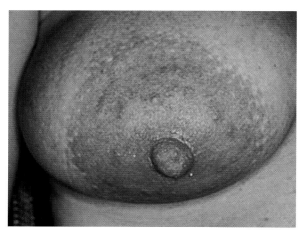

COLOR PLATE 65.

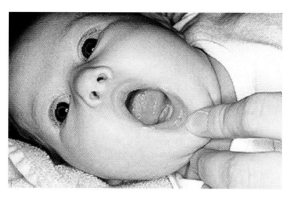

COLOR PLATE 69.

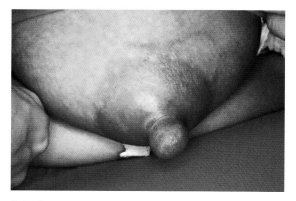

COLOR PLATE 66.

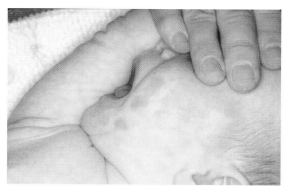

COLOR PLATE 70.

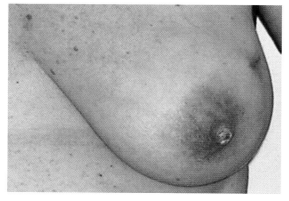

COLOR PLATE 67.
Courtesy of Catherine Watson Genna.

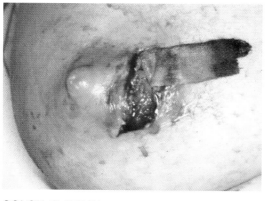

COLOR PLATE 71.

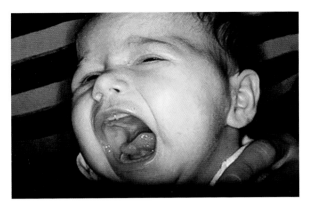

COLOR PLATE 72.

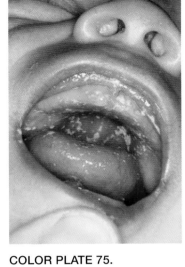

COLOR PLATE 75.

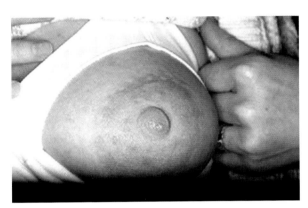

COLOR PLATE 73.

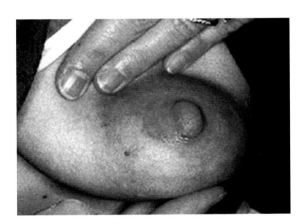

COLOR PLATE 76.

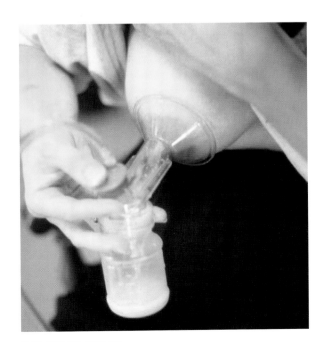

COLOR PLATE 74.

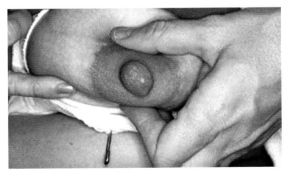

COLOR PLATE 77.

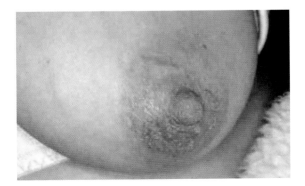

COLOR PLATE 78.

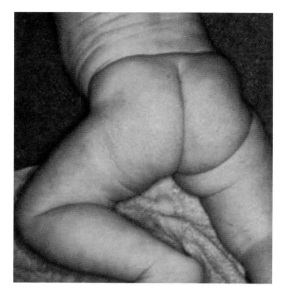

COLOR PLATE 79.

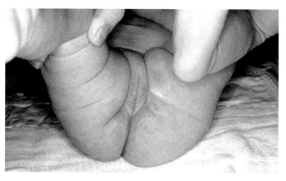

COLOR PLATE 83.

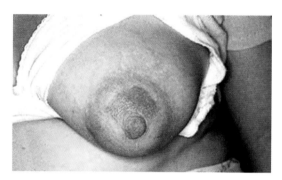

COLOR PLATE 80.

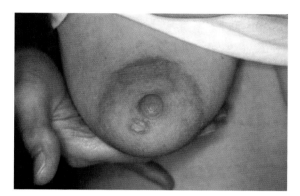

COLOR PLATE 84.

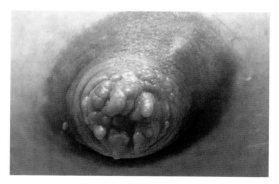

COLOR PLATE 81.
Courtesy of Carole Dobrich.

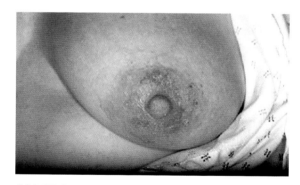

COLOR PLATE 85.

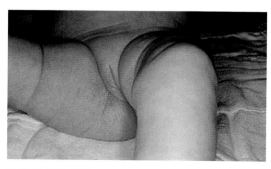

COLOR PLATE 82.

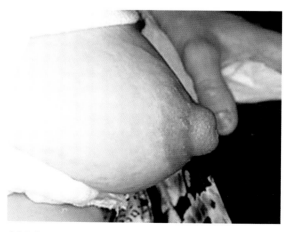

COLOR PLATE 86.

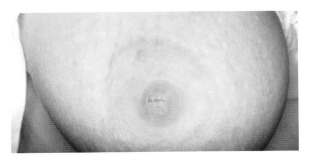

COLOR PLATE 87.

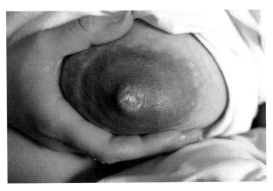

COLOR PLATE 91.
Courtesy of Catherine Watson Genna.

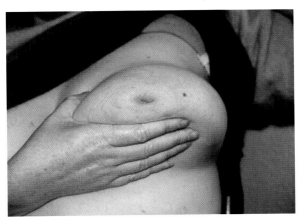

COLOR PLATE 88.
Courtesy of K. Jean Cotterman.

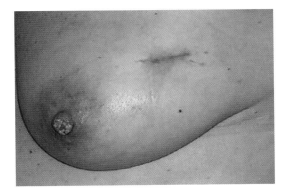

COLOR PLATE 92.
Courtesy of Catherine Watson Genna.

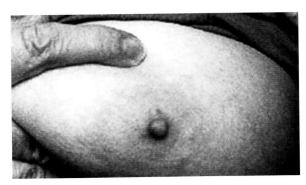

COLOR PLATE 89.

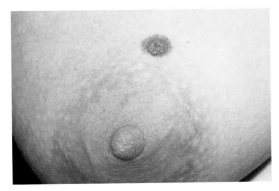

COLOR PLATE 93.
Courtesy of Carole Dobrich.

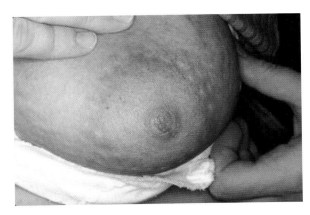

COLOR PLATE 90.
Courtesy of Catherine Watson Genna.

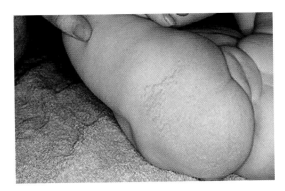

COLOR PLATE 94.

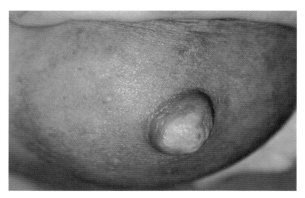

COLOR PLATE 95.
Courtesy of Catherine Watson Genna.

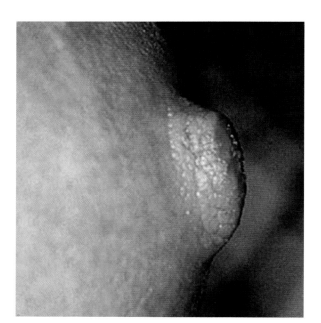

COLOR PLATE 96.
Courtesy of Greg Notestine.

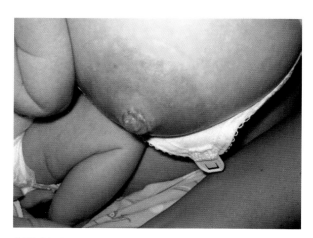

COLOR PLATE 97.
Courtesy of Catherine Watson Genna.

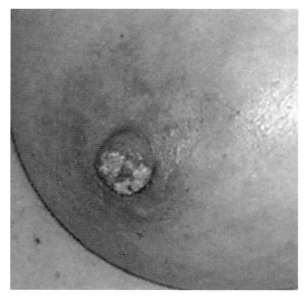

COLOR PLATE 98.
Courtesy of Catherine Watson Genna.

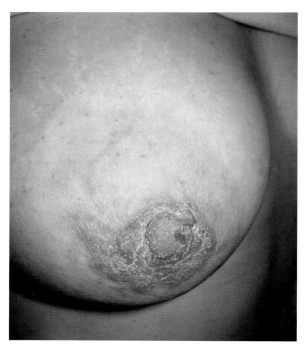

COLOR PLATE 99.
Courtesy of Catherine Watson Genna.

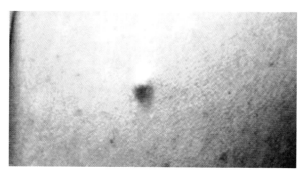

COLOR PLATE 100.

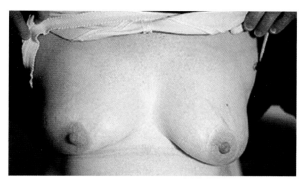

COLOR PLATE 101.

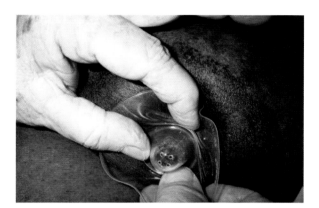

COLOR PLATE 102.

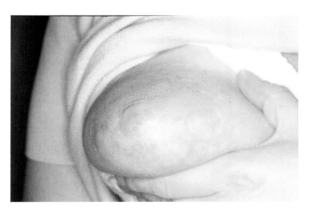

COLOR PLATE 103.

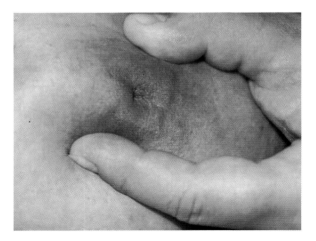

COLOR PLATE 104.
Courtesy of K. Jean Cotterman.

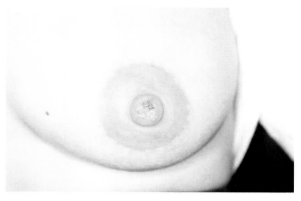

COLOR PLATE 105.

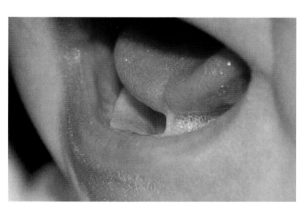

COLOR PLATE 106.
Courtesy of Greg Notestine.

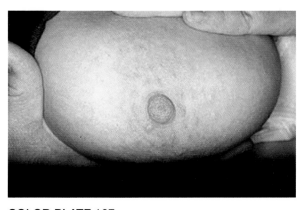

COLOR PLATE 107.

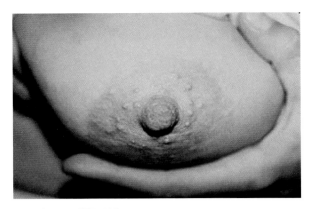

COLOR PLATE 108.
Courtesy of Greg Notestine.

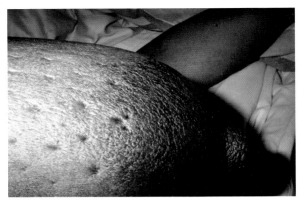

COLOR PLATE 109.
Courtesy of K. Jean Cotterman.